MEDICAL LIBRARY ASSOCIATION *Guides*

The Medical Library Association Guide *to* Finding Out About Complementary *and* Alternative Medicine

The Best Print and Electronic Resources

GREGORY A. CRAWFORD

Neal-Schuman Publishers, Inc.
New York London

The information in this book is intended to help the reader locate information about complementary and alternative medicine. It is not intended to replace the advice of a qualified health care professional. While every effort has been made to ensure accuracy and currency of the facts presented, this information should not be used to make decisions about medical care. Please consult with your physician before making any decisions regarding medical treatment.

Contact information and Web addresses listed in this book were accurate at the time the manuscript went to press.

Published by Neal-Schuman Publishers, Inc.
100 William St., Suite 2004
New York, NY 10038

Printed and bound in the United States of America.

The paper used in this publication meets the minimum requirements of American National Standard for Information Sciences—Permanence of Paper for Printed Library Materials, ANSI Z39.48-1992.

Library of Congress Cataloging-in-Publication Data

Crawford, Gregory A.
The Medical Library Association guide to finding out about complementary and alternative medicine : the best print and electronic resources / Gregory A. Crawford.
p. cm. — (Medical Library Association guides)
Includes bibliographical references and index.
ISBN 978-1-55570-727-9 (alk. paper)
1. Alternative medicine—Bibliography. 2. Alternative medicine—Computer network resources—Directories. I. Medical Library Association. II. Title.

Z6675.A42C73 2010
[R733]
016.6155—dc22

2010020401

Contents

Preface

The use of complementary and alternative medicine (CAM) has grown tremendously over the past few years. Medical schools now include information about CAM in their courses, doctors refer patients to practitioners of CAM, magazines often include articles on CAM, and television shows, including the news, frequently spotlight such therapies. Finding helpful information, however, can still be difficult. True, the Internet can be used, but judging the quality and accuracy of the information provided may be frustrating. Many magazine articles and books abound, but it can be hard to discern the ones that provide the best help. Library collections and reference librarians can be consulted, but their information is only as good as their sources.

The Medical Library Association Guide to Finding Out About Complementary and Alternative Medicine: The Best Print and Electronic Resources is a direct result of my own interest in CAM, both as a client and as a practitioner, and my work as a librarian. The impetus for writing this book was twofold. First, there did not seem to be a good current book aimed at reference librarians or collection development specialists that could assist them in their work. Second, I was eligible for a research sabbatical. As the director of the library at the Harrisburg campus of the Pennsylvania State University, I wanted to pursue research that would be both personally fulfilling and useful to the profession. The first topic that popped into my head was complementary and alternative medicine. After an examination of the available literature, the main source that I could identify was *Alternative Medicine Resource Guide* by Francine Feuerman and Marsha J. Handel, but this work has become dated [1]. Thus, I applied for and was granted the sabbatical to compile a book that I hope will be useful to librarians for answering basic reference questions on CAM, for building collections that will be helpful for patrons who seek additional information on these therapies, and for providing readers' advisory for materials on CAM.

Personally, I have been interested in alternative therapies for many years. Several years ago, my wife gave me a birthday present of learning Reiki and being attuned to Reiki I. Later, I was attuned to Reiki II, and then, after a decade of practicing Reiki, I became a Reiki master/teacher. During that same time span, I completed the Surya program taught by Dr. Michael Mamas. Surya healing is also known as transgradient touch and counseling since it combines hands-on energy work while providing spiritual counseling to our clients. Through the Surya program I also became a teacher of Surya meditation. Always curious, I completed the Doctor of Naturopathy degree through the Trinity College of Natural Health. Thus, complementary and alternative therapies have been of great importance to me and to my understanding of health, although I still have checkups with my regular physician and believe that traditional allopathic medicine should be incorporated, when necessary, into a healthy lifestyle. I regularly use a variety of alternative treatments, including chiropractic, acupuncture, Rolfing, massage, and hands-on healing. In addition, I take a variety of herbs, vitamins, and nutritional supplements to enhance my well-being. Even if the positive results that I have experienced arise merely from the placebo effect, I am grateful for the relief that they provide.

How to Use This Book

After an introduction that details the growth in the use of CAM within the United States, the first chapter provides an extensive listing of general works, covering many aspects of complementary and alternative approaches to health and healing. The remaining chapters follow a set structure that mirrors the overall goals of the work as a whole. First, each chapter presents general information on a specific type of complementary and alternative medicine, for example, ayurveda, chiropractic, Reiki, or yoga. This section of the chapter includes the history of the therapy, its use, and the training required for a practitioner and can be used to answer basic reference questions. Instead of using copious footnotes, I have listed the major sources of information I consulted under a general "Sources" heading. The second section of each chapter includes a selected listing of books, websites, and periodicals (journals and magazines) with an annotation detailing the coverage of each item. Thus, this section can be used for collection development and reader's advisory.

Due to the varying amount of materials available, some types of CAM receive their own chapters while others are combined with related therapies. For example, Reiki has its own chapter instead of being covered in the chapter on energy healing since a large number of books and websites are devoted to it. Similarly, the Alexander Technique, the Feldenkrais Method, and Rolfing all receive individual chapters rather than being included under "therapeutic massage and bodywork." In contrast, the Rosen Method and Hellerwork are included in the chapter on therapeutic massage and bodywork since fewer information resources are devoted to them.

Resource Selection

All the materials included in the chapter listings are in English. The majority of the books are published in the United States, although a significant number are published in foreign countries, predominantly in the United Kingdom and Canada. Due to cost, the ISBN is usually given for the paperback edition if both hardback and paperback editions are available. Most important, the materials are readily available through bookstores, book jobbers, Amazon, Barnes and Noble, Borders, or the publishers themselves. I have included only the most recent edition of each book, and all of the books were in print when they were examined for inclusion.

The materials listed are not intended to be completely comprehensive but comprise the best and most reliable representative selection of what is available. With that said, I tried to cast a wide net to capture as many good English language sources as possible on the topics discussed. After examination, many sources were excluded due to the nature and quality of their contents. Some are more controversial than others. Some are more technical than others and may only be of true interest to health care practitioners; those are included here if the more consumer-oriented publications were not comprehensive or reliable. Most of the books and magazines are relatively inexpensive, although a few are inordinately expensive. Due to the changing nature of the publishing industry and the discounts available through book jobbers and online retailers, book and magazine prices have not been included. Almost 1,000 items are included in the various chapters, representing 606 books, 160 websites, and 221 periodicals. All website URLs were reverified prior to publication.

Although I was already familiar with many of the therapies listed under the rubric of complementary and alternative medicine, I have learned a great deal during the writing of *The Medical Library Association Guide to Finding Out About Complementary and Alternative Medicine: The Best Print and Electronic Resources* about other modalities and have become even more fascinated with the many approaches that can be used to provide healing and support to those who are suffering. It is my hope that this Medical Library Association Guide will help my colleagues in other libraries and will, even in a small way, make other people healthier.

Reference

1. Francine Feuerman and Marsha J. Handel, *Alternative Medicine Resource Guide* (Lanham, MD: Medical Library Association & Scarecrow Press, 1997).

Acknowledgments

I would like to thank the Pennsylvania State University, the University Libraries, Penn State Harrisburg, and my coworkers at the Penn State Harrisburg Library, especially Ruth Runion-Slear, the interlibrary loan supervisor, for their support while I worked on this book. Also, my wife, Merle, and my son, Christopher, continue to be inspirations to me, and I appreciate their ongoing support of me, of my pursuits in alternative health, and of life in general. Special thanks go to Charles Harmon of Neal-Schuman Publishers and the various reviewers who provided excellent feedback throughout the preparation of the manuscript. I also appreciate the support of the Medical Library Association and their sponsorship of the book.

Introduction

When one thinks of complementary and alternative medicine, the first question is usually, "What is it?" Generally abbreviated CAM, complementary and alternative medicine can conjure up a variety of meanings. To some, anyone practicing CAM is a "quack." To others, allopathic (or Western) medicine itself is accused of being nothing but a system that pushes toxic drugs onto compliant, unquestioning patients. The truth, of course, lies somewhere in the middle. As Andrew Weil says,

> Alternative medicine is now the fastest-growing sector of American health care. Despite continuing objections from the rearguard of the scientific establishment, many forward-looking doctors have begun to recognize the virtues of complementary medicine. As for the American consumer, millions are voting with their feet and their pocketbooks for treatments other than those conventional physicians are trained to provide. Alternative medicine is clearly moving into the mainstream. [1]

In fact, Weil is the founder and director of the Arizona Center for Integrative Medicine at the College of Medicine, University of Arizona, where he is Clinical Professor of Medicine and Professor of Public Health. The Center for Integrative Medicine seeks to introduce allopathic physicians to the world of CAM so that they can incorporate it into their medical practices. Many additional hospitals and medical schools have established similar programs, and some CAM therapies are a regularly accepted part of medical care.

One great driving force behind this trend is the number of people using CAM, often as an adjunct to traditional medical care. According to a 1998 article in the *Journal of the American Medical Association* that examined the trends in the use of alternative medicine in the United States, 42.1 percent of the respondents to the survey indicated that they had used an alternative therapy during the previous year [2]. These therapies included, among others, herbal medicine, massage, megavitamins, energy healing, and homeopathy. In addition, most of these individuals paid the expenses out of their own pockets, although 36 percent had some of the expenses covered by insurance. The authors of the article estimated that there were 629 million visits to alternative medicine practitioners in 1997 versus 427 million in 1990. These are startling numbers when one considers that there were an estimated 386 million visits to all primary care physicians in 1997 and 388 million in 1990. They also conservatively estimated that $27 billion was spent on CAM services and products during 1997, a figure that rivals the estimated $29.3 billion spent in 1997 for out-of-pocket expenditures for all U.S. physician services, including out-of-pocket expenditures for hospitalizations. According to the National Center for Health Statistics, by 2007, this amount had grown to an estimated $33.9 billion [3]. The 2007 survey also indicated that 38.1 million adults in the United States made an estimated 354.2 million visits to practitioners of CAM. These figures are sure to continue to grow.

In 2002, the National Health Interview Survey found that 36 percent of American adults had used some form of CAM during the 12 months prior to the study, and if prayer is included, then 62 percent reported using CAM [4]. This study indicated that the most frequently used modalities were prayer, natural products, deep breathing exercises, meditation, chiropractic care, yoga, massage, and diet-based therapies. The most frequently cited reasons for using CAM were back pain and problems, head or chest colds, neck pain or problems, join pain or stiffness, and anxiety or depression. Women used CAM more frequently than men. In addition, with the exclusion of prayer, use of CAM increased as the level of education rose and as income grew. Those living in urban areas were more likely to use CAM than those who lived in rural areas.

In December 2008, the National Center for Complementary and Alternative Medicine (NCCAM) and the National Center for Health Statistics released the findings from the 2007 National Health Interview Survey [5]. This study discovered that the use of CAM during the 12 months prior to the survey increased to over 38 percent of American adults. The most frequently used therapies were nonvitamin, nonmineral natural products, followed by deep breathing exercises, meditation, chiropractic or osteopathic manipulation, massage, and yoga. Between 2002 and 2007 the use of acupuncture, massage therapy, and naturopathy increased. Similar to 2002, the conditions most frequently treated with CAM were musculoskeletal problems such as back pain, neck pain, joint pain, and arthritis. The next most frequently treated conditions were anxiety, high cholesterol levels, and head or chest colds. Mirroring the results from 2002, women used CAM more frequently than men, and those with greater levels of education, especially those with college and graduate education, used CAM more frequently. For the first time, the survey also examined the use of CAM by children and found that almost 12 percent of children had used CAM during the previous 12 months. The most commonly used therapies for children were natural products, chiropractic, deep breathing exercises, and yoga. The most frequently used natural products were echinacea and fish oil supplements. The conditions treated for children were similar to those of adults and included back and neck pain, head or chest cold, and anxiety and stress. In addition, 2.5 percent of children were treated for attention deficit/hyperactivity disorder or attention-deficit disorder using CAM therapies.

According to Blumenthal, in 1997 a total of over $441 million was spent solely on herbal supplements in food, drug, and mass market retail outlets in the United States [6]. The leading products sold were ginkgo (over $90 million in sales), ginseng ($86 million), and garlic ($71 million). Echinacea and St. John's wort each accounted for over $45 million in sales. These statistics, however, do not show the true scope of the market for herbs. It was estimated that the retail value of herbs sold in the United States for 1996 alone was approximately $3.24 billion, an average of $54 per person [7]. This amount does not include the money spent on vitamins and mineral supplements.

Thus, CAM represents a significant and growing presence in the medical landscape of the United States. Libraries must be cognizant of this trend so that they can supply materials that discuss these topics to their customers, yet deciding what to collect can be difficult. A recent search of the Amazon.com book database for the term "alternative health" yielded over 5,100 hits, while "alternative medicine" resulted in almost 21,000.

These searches, of course, did not find most of the books on topics related to CAM, especially those on specific therapies.

It is a difficult task to define the scope of complementary and alternative medical therapies. In its 2002 survey, NCCAM listed 27 different types of CAM therapies, including prayer, while the 2007 survey included 36 types of CAM and excluded prayer. The National Library of Medicine includes over 70 separate entries for therapies or approaches that could be labeled under the heading "complementary and alternative medicine." Thus, to compile a manageable listing of materials has been a formidable challenge and one that had to be focused on only the major forms of CAM that are most heavily used as determined by the NCCAM. For this work, I have attempted to cover primarily non-Western medical systems, natural healing techniques, manipulative techniques, and energetic healing therapies. Many of the books in the chapter on general works also discuss many of the lesser known and used therapies. As a result, there are many items that had to be left out, but I sincerely hope that this compilation will be useful to both librarians and to those who seek additional information on these therapies for their own health or for the health of their loved ones.

References

1. Andrew Weil, "Introduction," in *The Best Alternative Medicine: What Works? What Does Not?*, Kenneth R. Pelletier (New York: Simon & Schuster, 2000), 23.
2. David M. Eisenberg et al., "Trends in Alternative Medicine Use in the United States, 1990–1997," *Journal of the American Medical Association* 128, no. 18 (November 11, 1998): 1569–1575.
3. Richard L. Nahin, Patricia M. Barnes, Barbara J. Stussman, and Barbara Bloom, "Costs of Complementary and Alternative Medicine (CAM) and Frequency of Visits to CAM Practitioners: United States, 2007," in *National Health Statistics Reports*, no. 18 (Hyattsville, MD: National Center for Health Statistics, 2009).
4. Patricia M. Barnes, Eve Powell-Griner, Kim McFann, and Richard L. Nahin, "Complementary and Alternative Medicine Use among Adults: United States, 2002," in *Advance Data from Vital and Health Statistics*, no. 343 (Hyattsville, MD: National Center for Health Statistics, 2004).
5. Patricia M. Barnes, Barbara Bloom, and Richard L. Nahin, "Complementary and Alternative Medicine Use among Adults and Children: United States, 2007," in *National Health Statistics Reports*, no. 12 (Hyattsville, MD: National Center for Health Statistics, 2008).
6. Mark Blumenthal et al., ed., *The Complete German Commission E Monographs: Therapeutic Guide to Herbal Medicines* (Austin: American Botanical Council, 1998), 11.
7. Barbara Johnston, "One-Third of Nation's Adults Use Herbal Remedies: Market Estimated at $3.24 Billion," *HerbalGram* 40 (1997): 49.

Chapter 1

General Resources

This chapter covers a wide spectrum of materials, from highly technical overviews of complementary and alternative medicine to works of a general nature. Thus, some books will appeal more to health care professionals, while others will be of interest to those with a simple desire to learn more about these therapies or those who wish to use an alternative therapy for their own health. Books on specific types of therapy are included in the chapters on those therapies.

Annotated Bibliography

Print Resources

- Adams, Jon, ed. 2007. *Researching Complementary and Alternative Medicine*. New York: Routledge. 153 pp. ISBN: 0415367743; 9780415367745.
  The author's aim in compiling the articles in this book is to bring together the current state of thinking about the research enterprise related to complementary and alternative medicine (CAM) in order to advance our understanding of its efficacy and use. The book is divided into two parts. Part 1, "Methods in Practice," examines the methods used in researching CAM and the methodological challenges that face researchers. The second part, "Issues from the Field," addresses issues of evidence, the practitioner as researcher, public health, and the involvement of the consumer in CAM research. For those interested in the developing research on complementary and alternative therapies, this work will be of great interest.
- Al-Achi, Antoine. 2008. *An Introduction to Botanical Medicines: History, Science, Uses, and Dangers*. Westport, CT: Praeger Publishers. 188 pp. ISBN: 0313350094; 9780313350092.
  The author covers all aspects of the use of botanical medicines. The individual chapters address botanicals with anticancer activity, botanicals for cardiovascular and circulatory system, botanicals for skin disorders, botanicals for the endocrine system, gastrointestinal botanicals, botanicals for men's health, botanicals for women's health, botanicals for psychiatric disorders, and antimicrobial, antifungal, antiviral, and antiparasitic botanicals. The final chapter discusses natural remedies for pain control and herbal safety.
- Baer, Hans A. 2004. *Toward an Integrative Medicine: Merging Alternative Therapies with Biomedicine*. Walnut Creek, CA: AltaMira Press. 204 pp. ISBN: 0759103011; 9780759103016.
  In this book, the author presents his views on the transformation of the American health care system as alternative modes of therapy begin to gain acceptance by the practitioners of conventional medicine. He describes how those who practice alternative therapies have fought for legitimacy, especially chiropractors, naturopaths, acupuncturists, homeopaths, and bodyworkers. His observations are especially

useful for anyone interested in health care issues, including health care policy and economics.

- Barnes, Patricia M., Powell-Griner, Eve, McFann, Kim, and Nahin, Richard L. 2004. "Complementary and Alternative Medicine Use among Adults: United States, 2002." *Advance Data from Vital and Health Statistics*, no. 343. 20 pp. No ISBN. Hyattsville, MD: U.S. Department of Health and Human Services, Centers for Disease Control and Prevention, National Center for Health Statistics.
  Summarizing data from the 2002 National Health Interview Survey conducted by the Centers for Disease Control and Prevention's (CDC) National Center for Health Statistics, this report provides the results of interviews of 31,044 adults age 18 years, which indicate that 62 percent used some form of the 27 CAM therapies on the survey during the past 12 months when prayer for health reasons is included. Even when prayer is removed, 36 percent had used CAM within the past 12 months. The most commonly used CAM therapies were prayer for one's own health, prayer by others for one's health, natural products, deep breathing exercises, participation in a prayer group for one's own health, meditation, chiropractic care, yoga, massage, and diet-based therapies. The most common ailments treated by CAM were back pain or back problems, head or chest colds, neck pain or neck problems, joint pain or stiffness, and anxiety or depression. It is estimated that in 1997, the U.S. public spent between $36 billion and $47 billion on CAM therapies, with between $12.2 billion and $19.6 billion paid out of pocket to CAM providers such as chiropractors, acupuncturists, and massage therapists. This is more than the U.S. public paid out of pocket for all hospitalizations in 1997 and about half that paid for all out of pocket physician services. The majority of people use CAM as a complement to conventional medicine, not as an alternative. One of the major concerns is the interaction or interference that some herbal products can have on the pharmacology of some pharmaceutical drugs. CAM users often do not inform their conventional health care providers of their use of such products.
- Bausell, R. Barker. 2009. *Snake Oil Science: The Truth about Complementary and Alternative Medicine*. New York: Oxford University Press. 324 pp. ISBN: 0195383427; 9780195383423.
  Written by a biostatistician and research methodologist, this book emphasizes high-quality scientific evidence in its critique of alternative medicine. Throughout the book, the author explains how scientific research is conducted and provides a good description of the state of research on CAM. The author explores the placebo effect and how it is responsible for most of the positive results that have been reported for alternative therapies. This is a compelling book that will be of interest to both proponents and doubters in the efficacy of CAM therapies.
- Bivins, Roberta E. 2007. *Alternative Medicine? A History*. New York: Oxford University Press. 238 pp. ISBN: 0199218870; 9780199218875.
  Examining the past four centuries of medical history, this book focuses specifically on medical systems that are now considered alternative or complementary. The first chapter harkens back to the seventeenth century, a time when customers were often highly dissatisfied with the level of medical care they received. Chapter 2 examines the rise of medical systems, such as homeopathy and mesmerism, which challenged

the dominant medical practices of the eighteenth century. In Chapter 3, acupuncture during the nineteenth century is discussed, while the last chapter discusses multicultural medicine with the example of germ theory in India.

- Callahan, Daniel, ed. 2002. *The Role of Complementary and Alternative Medicine: Accommodating Pluralism. Hastings Center Studies in Ethics Series.* Washington, DC: Georgetown University Press. 214 pp. ISBN: 1589010167; 9781589010161.
  The essays included in this collection cover a broad territory related to complementary and alternative medicine. Chief among the topics are the efficacy of these therapies and the methodologies used to study them. Specifically, the essays address the assessment of efficacy in biomedicine, cultural diversity and ethics personal experience, spirituality in clinical care, interpreting the results of clinical trials, the nature of evidence, and the quest for holism in medicine. Although educated readers and health care providers will be able to understand the arguments presented, the main audience is researchers of health care.

- Cohen, Michael H. 2003. *Future Medicine: Ethical Dilemmas, Regulatory Challenges, and Therapeutic Pathways to Health Care and Healing in Human Transformation.* Ann Arbor: University of Michigan Press. 359 pp. ISBN: 0472112813; 9780472112814.
  Written for physicians and allied health care professionals, complementary and alternative medicine practitioners, mental health care professionals, attorneys, regulators, policymakers, and other interested people, this book seeks to examine the legal, ethical, and bioethical issues surrounding the movement of conventional medicine toward the inclusion of integrative and energy medicine. Topics covered include the ethics of referring patients to complementary and alternative practitioners, the implications of touch therapy in mental and spiritual health care and the changing definition of death. The author provides an interesting discussion of issues that will become increasingly important as more patients combine conventional and alternative therapies.

- Collinge, William. 1996. *The American Holistic Health Association Complete Guide to Alternative Medicine.* New York: Warner Books. 361 pp. ISBN: 0446672580; 9780446672580.
  Designed for the general reader who is seeking information on alternative treatments, this book presents basic information on traditional Chinese medicine, ayurveda, naturopathy, homeopathy, mind/body medicine, osteopathic medicine, chiropractic, and massage therapy and bodywork. For each, the author gives the key principles, variations within the tradition, procedures and techniques used, scientific support, strengths and limitations, practitioner–patient relationship, evaluation of personal results, relationship with other forms of medicine, costs, and choosing a practitioner.

- Committee on the Use of Complementary and Alternative Medicine by the American Public, Institute of Medicine. 2005. *Complementary and Alternative Medicine in the United States.* Washington, DC: National Academies Press. 337 pp. ISBN: 0309092701; 9780309092708.
  Commissioned in September 2002 by the National Institutes of Health, this report details the use of CAM within the United States. The Committee met between February 2003 and May 2004 and the report was generated from articles and other information on CAM therapies, evaluation of evidence, CAM-related decision making, and education on CAM. It is estimated that more than a third of American adults use some

form of CAM each year, with total number of visits to CAM providers exceeding those to primary-care physicians. In addition, an estimated 15 million adults take herbal remedies or high-dose vitamins in addition to their prescription drugs. Finally, the amount of annual out-of-pocket costs for CAM is estimated to exceed $27 billion. Very little research has been done on the cost-effectiveness of CAM, and more studies are needed both on CAM therapies themselves as well as on ways that they can be integrated into conventional medicine.

➤ Cuellar, Norma G. 2006. *Conversations in Complementary and Alternative Medicine.* Sudbury, MA: Jones and Bartlett. 282 pp. ISBN: 0763738883; 9780763738884.
This book will be of interest to anyone who wishes to learn more about complementary and alternative medicine. It consists of interviews with practitioners of a variety of therapies who were asked questions whose answers would be of interest to both health care providers and to patients. Modalities covered include traditional Chinese medicine, ayurveda, homeopathy, naturopathic medicine, biofeedback, hypnosis, music therapy, yoga, acupuncture, and Reiki, among others. The interviews personalize the discussion and make the approach taken by the author a refreshing alternative to learning about the modalities in other ways.

➤ Cutler, Ellen W. 2003. *The Food Allergy Cure: A New Solution to Food Cravings, Obesity, Depression, Headaches, Arthritis, and Fatigue.* 1st pbk. rev. ed. New York: Harmony Books. 333 pp. ISBN: 0609809008; 9780609809006.
The author provides a detailed discussion of the types of allergies that can be caused by food, of testing for sensitivities using applied kinesiology, and of treatment to overcome food-related allergies. Treatments described that assist the body's natural healing process include acupressure, energy medicine, immunology, enzyme therapy, and nutrition.

➤ Di Stefano, Vincent. 2006. *Holism and Complementary Medicine: Origins and Principles.* Crows Nest, NSW, Australia: Allen & Unwin. 205 pp. ISBN: 1741148464; 9781741148466.
In the first part of this book, the author places the modern practice of complementary medicine into its historical context, including its origin in antiquity and its development through the Middle Ages until modern times. The second part focuses on the principles of complementary medicine in comparison to allopathic medicine. Of special note are the discussion of holism, the healing relationship, and the therapeutic aims of holistic medicine. For those who seek to understand the history of alternative and complementary modalities and how they can fit with Western medicine, this is an important book.

➤ Erickson, Pamela I. 2008. *Ethnomedicine.* Long Grove, IL: Waveland Press. 123 pp. ISBN: 157766521X; 9781577665212.
In this short book, the author introduces the reader to ethnomedicine and examines the historical origins of medical systems, theories of disease causation that underlie the various medical traditions, and lessons that can be learned through the study of ethnomedicine.

➤ Ernst, Edzard. 2008. *Healing, Hype, or Harm? A Critical Analysis of Complementary or Alternative Medicine.* Charlottesville, VA: Societas. 178 pp. ISBN: 1845401182; 9781845401184.

In this work, the editor brings together chapters by a variety of experts to examine the world of complementary and alternative medicine. The authors address general issues such as the popularity of CAM therapies, the use of evidence in health care, the role of compassion, research on CAM, and legal issues. Other contributors focus on more specific issues such as CAM and politics, homeopathy, chiropractic, the placebo effect, and patient choice. Although most of the authors are from the UK, the book raises serious questions about CAM and its use. Thus, practitioners of both conventional medicine and alternative therapies will find much of interest in these pages.

➤ Ernst, Edzard. 2008. *Oxford Handbook of Complementary Medicine.* New York: Oxford University Press. 424 pp. ISBN: 0199206775; 9780199206773.
Using an evidence-based approach, this work provides information on complementary and alternative medicine in an easily accessible format, making it useful to doctors, nurses, medical students, and other health care professionals as well as patients. In addition, sections cover topics such as costs, safety, regulation, and legal and ethical issues for using CAM. The main part of the book provides helpful information on specific conditions such as the CAM treatments available, a ranking of the evidence for their effectiveness, an assessment of their risks and benefits, and a discussion of their effectiveness in relation to conventional treatment.

➤ Ernst, Edzard, Pittler, Max H., and Wider, Barbara, eds. 2006. *The Desktop Guide to Complementary and Alternative Medicine: An Evidence-Based Approach.* 2nd ed. Philadelphia: Mosby Elsevier. 556 pp. ISBN: 0723433836; 9780723433835.
The purpose of this book is to provide relevant, reliable, up-to-date information on the clinical evidence of complementary and alternative therapies. The book is divided into four main sections. The first section lists 46 conditions, from acne to upper respiratory tract infection, and gives clinical evidence for the effectiveness of CAM therapies and recommendations on their use. The second section focuses on 21 specific therapies, giving the background of the therapy, traditional concepts, scientific rationale, practitioners, conditions frequently treated, typical session, clinical evidence, and risks. The next session discusses herbal and nonherbal medicines, such as aloe, coenzyme Q10, and saw palmetto, with special attention given to the clinical evidence of their efficacy and the risks associated with using them. The final section discusses diagnostic methods, prevalence of CAM use, the reasons people use CAM, legal and ethical issues of using CAM, safety issues, and a cost evaluation of CAM.

➤ Ernst, Edzard, Pittler, Max H., and Wider, Barbara. 2007. *Complementary Therapies for Pain Management: An Evidence-Based Approach.* Edinburgh, NY: Elsevier Mosby. 349 pp. ISBN: 072343400X; 9780723434009.
The purpose of this book is to provide relevant information on the control of pain using complementary therapies based on clinical evidence. The authors first discuss concepts of pain as related to alternative therapies such as ayurveda, homeopathy, and traditional Chinese medicine. Then they provide very brief descriptions of 29 therapies, from acupuncture to yoga, from aromatherapy to massage and from chiropractic to spiritual healing. Various alternative remedies such as arnica, comfrey, feverfew, lavender, leeches, and willow are then presented with structured entries that include the source of the medicine, its main constituents, examples of traditional uses, conditions frequently treated, clinical evidence, dosage, risks, risk–benefit

assessment, and references. The next section gives different pain syndromes along with summaries of the clinical evidence for use of various CAM therapies. In summary, the book provides useful, albeit brief, information on different CAM therapies as well as their use in pain management.

- Fadlon, Judith. 2005. *Negotiating the Holistic Turn: The Domestication of Alternative Medicine.* Albany: State University of New York Press. 157 pp. ISBN: 079146315X; 9780791463154.
  Using ethnographic methods and quantitative data, the author examines the changing nature of alternative medicine and explains its growing popularity and use. Specifically, she studied the dissemination, practice, teaching, and consumption of a variety of alternative therapies in Israel. She concludes that alternative medicine has become "domesticated"; that is, it has become familiar to most people and an accepted complement to traditional medicine. Although the research focuses on Israel, many of her conclusions may well apply to the United States and will be of interest to health care practitioners as well as to policymakers.
- Feuerman, Francine, and Handel, Marsha J. 1997. *Alternative Medicine Resource Guide.* Lanham, MD: Medical Library Association; Scarecrow Press. 335 pp. ISBN: 0810832844; 9780810832848.
  Although now becoming somewhat dated as a result of new discoveries and the availability of new materials, this is still a useful guide to the resources of alternative medicine. The book is divided into two sections. The first is a resource guide to specific products and services such as organizations, schools, and treatment centers that specialize in alternative therapies. The second section provides a selective bibliography of books, journals, and newsletters on specific types of therapies such as ayurvedic medicine, homeopathy, reflexology, polarity therapy, yoga, meditation, and aromatherapy.
- Field, Tiffany. 2009. *Complementary and Alternative Therapies Research.* Washington, DC: American Psychological Association. 235 pp. ISBN: 1433804018; 9781433804014.
  Focusing primarily on psychotherapy, the author examines the efficacy of complementary and alternative therapies including massage therapy, acupressure, reflexology, acupuncture, tai chi and chi gong, yoga, aromatherapy, and meditation. A special chapter is devoted to complementary and alternative therapies in pediatric populations.
- Fontaine, Karen Lee. 2005. *Complementary & Alternative Therapies for Nursing Practice.* 2nd ed. Upper Saddle River, NJ: Pearson Prentice Hall. 510 pp. ISBN: 0131512544; 9780131512542.
  Written for nurses, this book serves as an introductory text to the principles, techniques, clinical research, healing practices, and health promotion methods related to complementary and alternative therapies. Over 20 different modalities are discussed. For each, the author covers the history and background, preparation to practice, major concepts, view of health and illness, diagnostic methods, treatment, and research. Of special interest to nurses are the uses of the therapy in integrated nursing practice, the "Using Research to Heal" sidebar that summarizes a research article and the "Try This" sidebar that gives a specific exercise to introduce the therapy to the reader.

- Freeman, Lynda W. 2009. *Mosby's Complementary & Alternative Medicine: A Research-Based Approach*. 3rd ed. St. Louis, MO: Mosby Elsevier. 608 pp. ISBN: 0323053467; 9780323053464.
  Designed not only for health care providers and students, this source gives any educated reader a comprehensive overview of the field of CAM based on current research on the efficacy of such therapies. Coverage includes a wide variety of alternative therapies as well as the personal experiences of researchers and practitioners of the different modalities. The appendixes provide additional information on CAM resources and contacts.
- Fundukian, Laurie J., ed. 2009. *The Gale Encyclopedia of Alternative Medicine*. 3rd ed. 4 vols. Detroit: Gale, Cengage Learning. 2688 pp. ISBN: 1414448724 (set); 9781414448725 (set).
  The four volumes in this encyclopedia provide over 800 articles on therapies, herbs and remedies, and diseases and conditions. Sidebars contain short biographies of important pioneers in the field of alternative medicine. The articles on therapies and herbs/remedies include information such as origins, benefits, preparations, precautions, side effects, research, and additional resources. For diseases and conditions the entries provide definitions, descriptions, causes and symptoms, diagnosis, treatment, allopathic treatment, expected results, prevention, and resources. Many entries include photographs, tables, or line drawings. This is a very useful reference resource that provides helpful information in an accessible format.
- Gevitz, Norman, ed. 1988. *Other Healers: Unorthodox Medicine in America*. Baltimore: Johns Hopkins University Press. 302 pp. ISBN: 0801837103; 9780801837104.
  This collection of writings explores the history of alternative medicine from the early nineteenth century to the late twentieth century in the United States. Individual chapters are devoted to the botanical movement, health reform movements, the water-cure movement, homeopathy, osteopathic medicine, chiropractic, Christian science healing, divine healing, and folk medicine. Taken together, these writings provide a good history of the influence of alternative medical practices on the American public and on the practice of orthodox medicine.
- Goldstein, Michael S. 1999. *Alternative Health Care: Medicine, Miracle, or Mirage?* Philadelphia: Temple University Press. 278 pp. ISBN: 1566396786; 9781566396783.
  Not a book about specific alternative therapies, this work examines the place of alternative medicine in American society. The author writes about the emergence and growth of alternative medicine, changing views of health and illness, the core beliefs espoused by practitioners of alternative therapies such as holism and vitalism, the role of the spirit in medicine, the politics of alternative medicine, and the marketing and business of alternative medicine. Based solidly on the research literature of many fields, this is an important and interesting analysis of the growing role that alternative health care is playing in American medicine.
- Harrington, Anne. 2008. *The Cure Within: A History of Mind–Body Medicine*. New York: W. W. Norton. 336 pp. ISBN: 0393065634; 9780393065633.
  The author, a historian of science, provides an examination of the history of mind–body medicine based on stories told by doctors and patients. She uses such stories to build the cultural history of mind–body medicine and is not as concerned

with the clinical research literature on its effectiveness. She starts with the premise that many of us, including physicians, think or believe that stress causes disease and that positive thinking can actually help us heal. Using six narratives, she takes the reader through much of the twentieth century and the conflicts surrounding the effects of the mind on the body and, in doing so, helps us make sense of these events in American medicine.

➤ Haugen, David M., ed. 2008. *Alternative Medicine. Opposing Viewpoints Series.* Detroit: Greenhaven Press. 222 pp. ISBN: 0737738200; 9780737738209.
A compilation of pro and con arguments for alternative medicine, this work is especially aimed at high school and college students. For example, the first argument is that homeopathic medicine is effective, while the second is that it is ineffective. The four chapters ask the following questions: Does alternative medicine work? Why is alternative medicine popular? Can alternative and conventional medicine work together? and What should government do to research and regulate alternative medicine? For students and other interested readers, this is a good source for brief, well-argued discussions on several of the major issues surrounding alternative medicine.

➤ Huebscher, Roxana, and Shuler, Pamela A. 2004. *Natural, Alternative, and Complementary Health Care Practices.* St. Louis, MO: Mosby. 912 pp. ISBN: 0323016766; 9780323016766.
Designed for health care professionals, this work is also useful for anyone interested in complementary and alternative therapies. The first section is arranged by systems of the body and gives suggestions for natural, alternative, and complementary remedies that can help with ailments in each body system. For example, in the chapter on gastrointestinal concerns, the authors discuss the use of ayurveda, traditional Chinese medicine, homeopathy, and even Amish folk medicine for treating constipation, diarrhea, and irritable bowel syndrome. The second section gives brief descriptions of different healing modalities divided into alternative health care systems, mind-body-spirit interventions, biologic-basic therapies, manipulative and body based methods, and energy therapies.

➤ Johnston, Robert D., ed. 2004. *The Politics of Healing: Histories of Alternative Medicine in Twentieth-Century North America.* New York: Routledge. 386 pp. ISBN: 0415933390; 9780415933391.
By taking a look at the history of alternative medicine, the editor has two main goals for the book. First, the collection of articles documents the ways practitioners and laypeople both conceptualized and practiced alternative therapies during the twentieth century and, second, the survival of alternative medicine as a matter of politics. The articles address topics as broad as the antivaccination movement, feminism, homeopathy, the health food movement, antifluoridation, women's health care, and CAM as a social movement. Thus, the book will be of interest to policymakers, historians of medicine, physicians, practitioners, and those who use alternative treatments.

➤ Jonas, Wayne B., ed. 2005. *Mosby's Dictionary of Complementary & Alternative Medicine.* St. Louis, MO: Elsevier Mosby. 519 pp. ISBN: 0323025161; 9780323025164.
This is a very useful dictionary that focuses on commonly used terms drawn primarily from CAM practices and CAM literature. Thus, the work does not attempt to be comprehensive but to provide resources to patients and others who seek simple

definitions of unfamiliar terms. The definitions themselves are very short, with pronunciations given for unfamiliar words. The illustrations are clear and helpful. There are minor problems with the work. For example, there is no entry for craniosacral therapy, and under the entry "triple burner" there is a see reference to "triple heater," but no such entry exists.

- Kayne, Steven B. 2009. *Complementary and Alternative Medicine*. 2nd ed. Chicago: Pharmaceutical Press. 619 pp. ISBN: 0853697639; 9780853697633.
  Although written primarily for pharmacists, this book can serve as both a practical introduction and as a reference source for the major types of complementary and alternative therapies. It is especially useful for information on the products that are most frequently requested in pharmacies and in hospitals by patients using complementary and alternative therapies. Topics covered in individual chapters include homeopathy, medical herbalism, aromatherapy, flower therapies, traditional Chinese medicine, ayurveda, and naturopathy.

- Kayne, Steven B. 2010. *Traditional Medicine: A Global Perspective*. London: Pharmaceutical Press. 331 pp. ISBN: 0853698333; 9780853698333.
  Since much of the world lacks access to medicines and to health care providers, traditional therapies are, by necessity, the primary method of healing available. In this book, the author discusses traditional medicines found throughout the world and argues that providing access to safe and effective traditional therapies could be a major, if not critical, way of increasing overall access to health care.

- Koopsen, Cyndie, and Young, Caroline. 2009. *Integrative Health: A Holistic Approach for Health Professionals*. Sudbury, MA: Jones and Bartlett Publishers. 359 pp. ISBN: 0763757616; 9780763757618.
  This is a general book on a variety of complementary and alternative medical therapies for health professionals, but it is accessible to anyone with an interest in this topic. Chapters examine topics such as holistic stress management, health and the human spirit, energy healing, meditation, traditional Chinese medicine, ayurveda, humor, nutrition, and therapeutic massage and bodywork

- Lake, James, and Spiegel, David, eds. 2007. *Complementary and Alternative Treatments in Mental Health Care*. Washington, DC: American Psychiatric Publishing. 478 pp. ISBN: 1585622028; 9781585622023.
  This work examines the use of complementary and alternative therapies in treating mental illnesses. The first section presents background issues such as trends in the use of CAM in mental health care, legal and ethical issues, patient safety, and integrative approaches. The second section is a review of the evidence for using a variety of therapies and gives clinical guidelines for their use. Among the therapies discussed are herbal medicines, nutritional supplements, traditional Chinese medicine, homeopathy, ayurveda, exercise, meditation, spirituality, yoga, and qigong. This work will be especially useful for mental health care professionals, although patients may also find much of interest.

- Langwith, Jacqueline. 2009. *Alternative Medicine*. Detroit: Greenhaven Press. 181 pp. ISBN: 0737743336; 9780737743333.
  Although primarily for students, this compilation strives to present both sides of this controversial issue. For each topic, a positive and a negative argument is given. For

example, the first chapter examines the effectiveness of acupuncture, homeopathy, and chiropractic, with one section arguing for its effectiveness and a second arguing that it is ineffective. Chapter 2 addresses the question of whether alternative medicine helps fight disease, while the third chapter asks what role alternative medicine should play in health care in the United States. Thus, this is a highly balanced work that can answer many questions about the efficacy of alternative medicine.

➤ Larson, Christine A. 2007. *Alternative Medicine. Health and Medical Issues Today.* Westport, CT: Greenwood Press. 215 pp. ISBN: 0313337187; 9780313337185.
The audience for this book is the health care consumer and its goal is to provide an overview of alternative therapies, the controversies that surround them, and the scientific evidence about them. The first four chapters examine the origins of alternative medicine, the underlying theories on which it is based, the business of providing alternative care, and the nature of the consumers who use such therapies. The next six chapters examine controversies such as the efficacy of alternative therapies, their regulation by the government, the provision of coverage for their use by managed care providers, and the future of health and health care. For those who seek to be deeply involved in their own health care, this is an important book to read.

➤ Lewith, G. T., and Jonas, Wayne B., eds. 2002. *Clinical Research in Complementary Therapies: Principles, Problems and Solutions.* New York: Churchill Livingstone. 376 pp. ISBN: 0443063672; 9780443063671.
With the growth of the availability and use of complementary and alternative therapies has also come a need for clinical research into the efficacy of these therapies. This book attempts to provide a framework for such research. The first section deals with methods and strategies and examines topics such as the role of outcomes research in evaluating CAM, the use of clinical audits, conducting multicenter and large trials, and the importance of patient selection. The second section examines clinical research as related to specific therapies including herbal medicine, homeopathy, naturopathic medicine, and acupuncture.

➤ Mackenzie, Elizabeth R., and Rakel, Birgit, eds. 2006. *Complementary and Alternative Medicine for Older Adults: Holistic Approaches to Healthy Aging.* New York: Springer. 324 pp. ISBN: 0826138055; 9780826138057.
With a focus on the older adult, the chapters in this book discuss a range a alternative approaches that may benefit many readers. Among the therapies presented are therapeutic diets, supplements and herbs, homeopathy, music therapy, art therapy, massage therapy, acupuncture, yoga, ayurveda, meditation, and spirituality. For each therapy, the authors give a brief description of the modality, anecdotal reports of its usefulness, a discussion of its efficacy as reported in the scientific literature, and resources for additional information.

➤ Mantle, Fiona, and Tiran, Denise. 2009. *A – Z of Complementary and Alternative Medicine: A Guide for Health Professionals.* New York: Churchill Livingstone. 254 pp. ISBN: 0443103291; 9780443103292.
This is a pocket-size quick reference to CAM for health care providers. Covering a variety of therapies including aromatherapy, ayurveda, Bach flower remedies, chiropractic, hypnosis, hydrotherapy, homeopathy, massage, medical herbalism, osteopathy, nutrition, reflexology, Reiki, traditional Chinese medicine, and yoga. It discusses

what the therapy is, what it does, and any contraindications, precautions and interactions associated with its use.

- Matthews, Dawn D., ed. 2002. *Alternative Medicine Sourcebook: Basic Consumer Health Information about Alternative and Complementary Medical Practices*. 2nd ed. Detroit, MI: Omnigraphics. 618 pp. ISBN: 0780806050; 9780780806054.
Designed for the general reader, this guide examines alternative medical systems and therapies, mind–body interventions, dietary supplements, alternative treatments for specific diseases, and controversial cancer treatments. Among the systems and therapies covered in short chapters are acupuncture, ayurveda, traditional Chinese medicine, chiropractic, homeopathy, naturopathic medicine, yoga, hypnosis, meditation, aromatherapy, massage therapy, and Reiki. For those seeking brief information on a wide array of topics, this is a helpful book.

- Micozzi, Marc S., ed. 2006. *Fundamentals of Complementary and Integrative Medicine*. 3rd ed. St. Louis, MO: Saunders Elsevier. 636 pp. ISBN: 1416025839; 9781416025832.
Written for both students and practitioners in health-related fields, this text covers the major complementary and alternative therapies used by the patients whom physicians and other health care providers will see in their practices. Of special note are the sections that discuss the foundations and the contexts of complementary and integrative medicine, which vary drastically from conventional medicine. The rest of the work is devoted to chapters on the wide variety of therapies available today such as homeopathy, chiropractic, aromatherapy, humor, and arts therapy as well as lesser know modalities such as Tibetan medicine, Native American healing, and Latin American Curanderismo.

- Micozzi, Marc S., ed. 2007. *Complementary and Integrative Medicine in Cancer Care and Prevention: Foundations and Evidence-Based Interventions*. New York: Springer. 478 pp. ISBN: 0826103057; 9780826103055.
Focusing specifically on cancer care and prevention, the chapters of this book examine a wide variety of complementary and alternative therapies. The first set of chapters discusses the biology and ecology of cancer while the second set presents mind/body approaches such as guided imagery, expressive therapies, and religion and spirituality. Part 3 covers diet, nutrition, and natural products as related to cancer. Alternative systems of medicine, including naturopathy, ayurveda, traditional Chinese medicine, and homeopathy, are presented in part 4. The last part discusses several controversial therapies such as antineoplastons and hydrazine sulfate as well as the legal and regulatory issues of alternative cancer treatments. The last chapter reports on an anonymous cancer patient's experiences and perspective on choosing between conventional and alternative treatments. Although designed for medical students and practitioners, this work will be of great interest to anyone who has had a cancer diagnosis.

- Miller, Debra A., ed. 2009. *Alternative Therapies*. Detroit: Greenhaven Press. 207 pp. ISBN: 0737741295; 9780737741292.
Although designed primarily for high school and lower division college students, this anthology is still an excellent introduction to the world of alternative therapies. Coverage includes chiropractic, acupuncture, dietary supplements, homeopathy,

naturopathy, and massage therapy. Other chapters discuss the effectiveness, health benefits, and safety of such therapies, and one chapter even examines the use of natural remedies with pets. The authors discuss both the pros and the cons of using alternative therapies.

- Murcott, Toby. 2005. *The Whole Story: Alternative Medicine on Trial?* New York: Macmillan. 173 pp. ISBN: 1403945004; 9781403945006.
  Although he admits he is not a medical expert, the author has undertaken an examination of the research on the efficacy of complementary and alternative therapies as related in the medical literature. He discusses topics such as research on the placebo effect, the randomized control trial, genetic medicine, acupuncture, homeopathy, and osteopathy but also brings in insights from conventional medicine. He concludes that the approach to patient care exhibited by alternative therapies and their emphasis on treating the whole body, not just the symptoms, may be a new paradigm for all medical care, especially for the treatment of chronic conditions and degenerative diseases that are difficult to treat using conventional medicine.
- Murray, Michael T. 2009. *What the Drug Companies Won't Tell You and Your Doctor Doesn't Know: The Alternative Treatments That May Change Your Life—And the Prescriptions That Could Harm You*. New York: Atria Books. 339 pp. ISBN: 1416549331; 9781416549338.
  In this work, the author stresses that there are many natural treatment alternatives that can help in the treatment of common health concerns. He examines topics such as removing obstacles to a cure, the power of a healthy lifestyle, bias in medical studies, and how to get well. The appendixes include discussions of osteoporosis, dietary supplements for diabetes and high blood pressure, and what to look for in vitamin and mineral supplements.
- Nahin, Richard L., Barnes, Patricia M., Stussman, Barbara J., and Bloom, Barbara. 2009. "Costs of Complementary and Alternative Medicine (CAM) and Frequency of Visits to CAM Practitioners: United States, 2007." *National Health Statistics Reports*, no. 18 (July 30, 2009). 16 pp. No ISBN. Hyattsville, MD: U.S. Department of Health and Human Services, Centers for Disease Control and Prevention, National Center for Health Statistics.
  This report summarizes data derived from the 2007 National Health Interview Survey conducted by the CDC's National Center for Health Statistics. The data indicate that in 2007, U.S. adults spent approximately $33.9 billion on visits to CAM practitioners and purchases of CAM products, classes, and materials. Over 38.1 million adults made an estimated 354.2 million visits to CAM practitioners, with most of these visits to practitioners associated with manipulative and body-based therapies. Approximately $14.8 billion was spent on the purchase of nonvitamin, nonmineral natural products.
- Navarra, Tova. 2004. *The Encyclopedia of Complementary and Alternative Medicine*. New York: Facts on File. 276 pp. ISBN: 0816049971; 9780816049974.
  A true reference book, this encyclopedia provides short entries of a vast number of topics, arranged in the typical A to Z format. Over 400 entries are included that cover complementary and alternative medical therapies, organizations, herbs, people, and terms drawn from the therapies. For those seeking short, useful information and definitions of terms, this will be a helpful resource.

- Portilla, Elizabeth de la. 2009. *They All Want Magic: Curanderas and Folk Healing*. College Station, TX: Texas A&M University Press. 147 pp. ISBN: 1603440992; 9781603440998.
  This work focuses on curanderas, the traditional healers in Mexican culture, and was written by a curandera in training. The author relates stories that healers have shared with her. In addition, she covers the herbs and recipes used in their healing.
- Rakel, David, and Faass, Nancy, eds. 2006. *Complementary Medicine in Clinical Practice: Integrative Practice in American Healthcare*. Sudbury, MA: Jones and Bartlett. 553 pp. ISBN: 0763730653; 9780763730659.
  Composed of 70 separately authored chapters, this work covers the gamut of topics related to the use of complementary and alternative therapies in the clinical setting. It covers the themes, trends, and current information available on CAM including the use of these therapies in integrative medicine, research on their effectiveness, and new models of integrative medicine. The therapies discussed include nutrition, exercise and fitness, mind–body medicine, self-care such as meditation and breathing exercises, therapeutic massage, acupuncture, chiropractic, and herbal therapy. In contrast to many other works, this provides much more depth on the therapies covered.
- Rosenfeld, Isadore. 1997, ©1996. *Dr. Rosenfeld's Guide to Alternative Medicine: What Works, What Doesn't and What's Right for You*. New York: Ballantine Books. 342 pp. ISBN: 0449000745; 9780449000748.
  Dr. Rosenberg wrote this book to help bridge the gap between conventional medical doctors and alternative practitioners. In it, he provides short chapters on a wide array of alternative therapies that serve to introduce the reader to the basics on these alternative therapies. In total, he covers 26 different therapies from acupuncture to reflexology, from bee venom therapy to neuro-linguistic programming, and from enzyme therapy to light therapy. After a brief discussion of the specific therapy, which often includes an examination of the major uses of the therapy, the author answers the question "What is the bottom line?" and provides his thoughts on the efficacy of the therapy.
- Ruggie, Mary. 2004. *Marginal to Mainstream: Alternative Medicine in America*. New York: Cambridge University Press. 232 pp. ISBN: 0521542227; 9780521542227.
  In this book, the author seeks to provide answers to many questions concerning complementary and alternative medical therapies. She discusses the modalities considered to be complementary or alternative, their safety, their effectiveness, insurance coverage for CAM, the response of the medical community to the increasing use of CAM, and the future integration of CAM into traditional medical practice. Using arguments based on the research literature, including surveys of the use of CAM and clinical research on its effectiveness, she concludes that some of the therapies are safe and effective and that many are being integrated into current medical practice.
- Sampson, Wallace, and Vaughn, Lewis, eds. 2000. *Science Meets Alternative Medicine: What the Evidence Says about Unconventional Treatments*. Amherst, NY: Prometheus Books. 246 pp. ISBN: 1573928038; 9781573928038.
  Written for health care providers, consumers, and anyone interested in alternative therapies, this book presents the scientific evidence of the effectiveness of alternative medical treatments. The work is divided into four sections. The first examines the origins of alternative medicine and recent trends in its use. The second section focuses on psychology and the influence of belief on the efficacy of alternative therapies.

Several therapies and theories are discussed in the third section, including naturopathy, the human energy field, and colloidal silver. The final section examines ethics and risks of promoting unproven treatments. In general, the authors of the chapters present a negative view of the value of alternative therapies and argue that additional controlled scientific experiments must be done to determine if, in fact, there is value to the use of these therapies.

- Schlitz, Marilyn, Amorok, Tina, and Micozzi, Marc S., eds. 2005. *Consciousness and Healing: Integral Approaches to Mind–Body Medicine.* Philadelphia, PA: Elsevier Churchill Livingstone. 585 pp. ISBN: 0443068003; 9780443068003.
  A compilation of essays by 67 authorities on health and healing, this work seeks to create a new perspective on integrating consciousness and healing within mind–body medicine. The editors seek to define integral medicine as an approach that integrates personal relationships, emotions, meanings, and belief systems with the body, mind, spirit, society, and nature. To do this requires expanding beyond the current biomedical model employed by traditional medical practice to embrace other avenues of healing. The book is divided into five parts, each addressing an important issue. The first part defines integral medicine. Part 2 maps the healing system and examines mind–body medicine and its research, new perspectives on the body, re-visioning illness, and honoring the spectrum of life, including death. Part 3 seeks to understand healing as a move toward wholeness and incorporates psychology and spirituality. In the fourth part, other ways of knowing and integrating the wisdom derived from the world's healing systems are presented. The last part looks at the transformation of medicine and envisions a new model for health and healing. Although much research is presented in the individual essays, this is a philosophical call to re-create medicine as we know it and will be of interest not only to physicians but also to patients and policymakers.
- Schneirov, Matthew, and Geczik, Jonathan David. 2003. *A Diagnosis for Our Times: Alternative Health, from Lifeworld to Politics.* Albany: State University Press of New York. 230 pp. ISBN: 079145732X; 9780791457320.
  Written by a sociologist and a political scientist, this work reports on an anthropological and ethnographic study of two alternative health networks, one based in "New Age" thought and the other in a conservative Christian ethos. The study examines the health regimes followed by the clients of alternative practitioners, the derivation of meaning from health traditions, and the relationship of the alternative health movement and other movements for social change. The authors conclude that alternative health movements are actually social movements that expose people to new values and new ways of living. Thus, these movements may have great implications for culture and for health care.
- Segala, Melanie, ed. 2003. *The Life Extension Foundation's Disease Prevention and Treatment: Scientific Protocols that Integrate Mainstream and Alternative Medicine.* Expanded 4th ed. Hollywood, FL: Life Extension Media. 1535 pp. ISBN: 0965877752; 9780965877756.
  Covering 130 ailments and conditions, this resource provides treatment protocols based on the scientific literature. The ailments and conditions range from the relatively mild and acute such as jet lag to the life-threatening and chronic such as breast cancer and HIV and AIDS. Each entry follows a similar format that can vary depending on

the ailment and condition but usually offers a discussion of the ailment, its causes and manifestations, treatments, and the use of vitamins, minerals, herbs, and other supplements and nutrients. A short section on prevention, a summary of suggestions for treatment, places to find additional information, and product availability are also given. All suggestions are based on clinical research and provide brief citations. A companion website includes the full citation information. This is a comprehensive resource that provides scientifically based suggestions for treating and preventing many diseases and illnesses that will be of use to many library patrons.

➤ Segen, Joseph C. 1998. *Dictionary of Alternative Medicine.* Stamford, CT: Appleton & Lange. 407 pp. ISBN: 0838516203; 9780838516201.
This dictionary provides short entries on over 5,000 terms related to alternative health therapies. Specific therapeutic modalities (such as acupuncture and homeopathy), herbs (such as goldenrod and red clover), people (such as Deepak Chopra and Andrew Weil), and technical terms from the various alternative health disciplines (such as colonic lavage and mechanotherapy) are included.

➤ Serlin, Ilene Ava, ed. 2007. *Whole Person Healthcare.* 3 vols.: vol. 1, *Humanizing Healthcare*; vol. 2, *Psychology, Spirituality, and Health*; vol. 3, *The Arts and Health.* Westport, CT: Praeger. 1,128 pp. ISBN: 0275992314 9780275992316.
With chapters written by experts in fields as diverse as medicine, psychology, public policy, religion, and the arts, this set of books seeks to provide a model for the practice of mind–body medicine with the goal of treating the whole person, not just the symptoms. The first volume addresses the concept of humanizing health care and provides the foundations for the practice of integrative health care, such as the development of treatment protocols, the assessment of the efficacy of alternative practices, the provision of health care to marginalized populations, and the creation of public policy. The second volume focuses on the role of psychology and spirituality in health care and on issues such as the meaning of illness, the role of spirituality, pastoral care, and research into therapies such as yoga and prayer. The final volume delves into the role of art in health and discusses the use of art, music, dance, drama, and poetry as therapy. Taken together, the three volumes help guide medical and other health care providers toward the integration of a variety of mind–body techniques into the practice of medicine.

➤ Shapiro, Rose. 2008. *Suckers: How Alternative Medicine Makes Fools of Us All.* London: Harvill Secker. 296 pp. ISBN: 1846550289; 9781846550287.
Often infused with humor, this book examines the world of alternative medicine and its efficacy. In addition to therapies such as homeopathy and acupuncture, which are labeled as reputable, the author also covers methods such as nutraceuticals, ear candling, and ergogenics, which she calls bizarre. The heart of the work is an examination of the research on alternative medicine that concludes that there is no hard evidence that they actually work as proponents claim.

➤ Shealy, C. Norman, and Church, Dawson. 2008. *Soul Medicine: Awakening Your Inner Blueprint for Abundant Health and Energy.* 2nd ed. Santa Rosa, CA: Energy Psychology Press. 295 pp. ISBN: 1604150106; 9781604150100.
Written by two well-known experts in the field of holistic medicine and vibrational healing, this book examines the role of the spirit in healing and the basics of energy

medicine, its use in treating common ailments, and recent scientific research on the therapeutic effects of prayer, energy healing, acupressure, and other similar techniques.

- Sherman, John. 2005. *Do-It-Yourself Natural Health: Natural Health Trio: Acupressure, Aromatherapy, & Herbal Therapy*. Monterey, CA: New Found Therapies. 228 pp. ISBN: 0970941129; 9780970941121.
  The goal of this book is to provide the reader with the knowledge to treat over 60 common ailments using acupressure, essential oils, and herbs. Thus, the author gives very basic instructions for performing acupressure on oneself, using aromatherapy oils, and taking herbs. He then describes 12 common herbs that can be used with many different ailments and discusses the 10 primary pressure points on the body. Next, he lists 47 common ailments along with the acupressure points, essential oils, and herbs to use in their treatment. The final section gives hints on topics such as enhancing the immune system and rejuvenating tired eyes and hands. This is a very practical manual that can be a good introduction to a variety of alternative therapies that can be tried in the privacy of one's own home.

- Singh, Simon, and Ernst, Edzard. 2008. *Trick or Treatment: The Undeniable Facts about Alternative Medicine*. New York: W. W. Norton. 342 pp. ISBN: 0393066614; 9780393066616.
  Using scientific evidence as their guide, the authors examine efficacy of many of the alternative treatment methods that are growing in popularity internationally. The authors build their argument carefully, first introducing the scientific method and how it can be used to examine CAM therapies. Then they examine acupuncture, homeopathy, chiropractic, and herbal medicine. They conclude that the results are mixed, with some positive results found for acupuncture, chiropractic, and herbal medicine, although their efficacy, according to the research literature, is limited in scope. They found no support for homeopathy. Although many may disagree with their conclusions, this is an interesting examination of complementary and alternative therapies that provides much food for thought as well as fodder for additional research.

- Spencer, John W., and Jacobs, Joseph J. 2003. *Complementary and Alternative Medicine: An Evidence-Based Approach*. 2nd ed. St. Louis, MO: Mosby. 632 pp. ISBN: 0323020283; 9780323020282.
  The purpose of this book is to examine the research evidence on the efficacy of complementary and alternative therapies and the claims made by proponents of these therapies. Unlike many other works that are arranged by specific types of modalities, the main section of this work is arranged by clinical disease or illness. Chapters examine the effectiveness of alternative therapies in treating asthma and allergies, cancer, atherosclerotic vascular disease, diabetes mellitus, neurologic disorders, psychiatric disorders, alcohol and chemical dependency, and pain. Then, the efficacy of the therapies in special populations of children, women, and elderly patients is addressed. The final section examines legal and ethical issues, medical training, and future trends in the use of complementary and alternative medicine. Since this is a technical work based on the scientific literature, the main audience consists of health care providers, researchers, and policymakers.

➤ Steinfeld, Alan. 2003. *Careers in Alternative Medicine*. Rev. ed. *The Career Resource Library*. New York: Rosen. 192 pp. ISBN: 0823937542; 9780823937547.
Although somewhat dated, this is still a good basic source for information on careers in alternative medicine. The author provides brief background on a variety of alternative and supplementary therapies yet shortchanges some modalities such as homeopathy, which is only mentioned in the text but receives no specific discussion. In general, for each therapy, a brief description and certification requirements, if any, are given. Sometimes a webpage for a certifying or professional organization is given. The section "For More Information" lists only schools of acupuncture and two organizations that focus on the Alexander Technique.

➤ Strozier, Anne L., and Carpenter, Joyce, eds. 2008. *Introduction to Alternative and Complementary Therapies*. Binghamton, NY: The Haworth Press. 297 pp. ISBN: 0789022052; 9780789022059.
Designed for psychotherapists and counselors, this book explores a variety of alternative and complementary approaches to psychotherapy that can work with standard therapeutic interventions. The topics covered include mindfulness and meditation, spirituality, poetry therapy, art therapy, psychodrama, dance/movement therapy, music therapy, animal-assisted therapy, and touch therapies. Although this is not a how-to book on using the therapies, the chapters do provide sufficient detail to give the therapist a basic understanding of the modalities and their use in therapy.

➤ Tierney, Gillian. 2007. *Opportunities in Holistic Health Care Careers*. Rev. ed. New York: McGraw Hill. 190 pp. ISBN: 007146767X; 9780071467674.
Although it does not cover all of the different modalities of complementary and alternative healing, this is one of the most current books on pursuing a career in these forms of health care. The author focuses on 11 specific forms of CAM: acupuncture and traditional Chinese medicine, chiropractic, holistic dentistry, energy healing (which includes Reiki, therapeutic touch, and polarity therapy), herbalism (which also includes aromatherapy and flower essences), massage therapy (including reflexology and craniosacral therapy), midwifery, holistic medicine, naturopathic medicine, osteopathic medicine, and yoga. A final chapter briefly presents ayurveda, biofeedback, feng shui, homeopathy, and iridology. For each modality covered, the author gives the philosophy of the modality, the types of patients and problems generally seen, the types of treatment offered, the employment setting and working conditions, the training and qualifications required, the salary and job outlook, professional organizations, licensing information, and programs or schools offering training in the modality.

➤ Tovey, Philip, Easthope, Gary, and Adams, Jon, eds. 2004. *The Mainstreaming of Complementary and Alternative Medicine: Studies in Social Context*. New York: Routledge. 180 pp. ISBN: 0415267005; 9780415267007.
This edited volume speaks to the sociology of complementary and alternative medicine. The essays raise issues related to the traditional medical profession and its patients, the claims of evidenced-based medicine, and how the demands of consumer expectations are met within the realm of health care. In addition, one of the major issues raised is the relationship between scientific knowledge and power and how that relationship is being challenged by alternate therapies. Thus, the work will be of interest to policymakers, health sociologists, and health care students and professionals.

- Trivieri, Larry. 2001. *The American Holistic Medical Association Guide to Holistic Health: Healing Therapies for Optimal Wellness.* New York: John Wiley. 438 pp. ISBN: 0471327433; 9780471327431.
  Written for anyone interested in understanding the concept of holistic medicine and alternative therapies, this book is aimed at giving information to those who wish to participate in their own healing. More limited than some other resources, the author focuses on nutritional medicine, environmental medicine, mind–body medicine, osteopathic medicine, chiropractic, botanical medicine, bodywork, naturopathic medicine, homeopathy, ayurveda, traditional Chinese medicine and acupuncture, and yoga. For each therapy, the entry includes fast facts, a brief history, how the therapy works, a case history that focuses on the therapy, selecting a practitioner, and other helpful resources.
- Trivieri, Larry, and Anderson, John W. 2002. *Alternative Medicine: The Definitive Guide.* 2nd ed. Berkeley, CA: Celestial Arts. 1233 pp. ISBN: 1587611414; 9781587611414.
  In this comprehensive work, the author covers 40 different alternative therapies and a vast array of health conditions. In addition to the well-known alternative therapies such as acupuncture, chiropractic, and homeopathy, lesser known therapies such as cell therapy, hyperthermia, NAET (Nambudripad's Allergy Elimination Techniques), and prolotherapy are included. Substantial information is given on over 30 different groups of health conditions, ranging from addictions to women's health. The final section is an A–Z listing of an additional 100 conditions for which briefer information is given. Due to its breadth of coverage, this is a worthwhile addition to most library collections.
- Trudeau, Kevin. 2006. *More Natural "Cures" Revealed: Previously Censored Brand Name Products that Cure Disease.* Elk Grove Village, IL: Alliance Publishing Group. 358 pp. ISBN: 0975599542; 9780975599549.
  In this book, the author provides useful information on how to avoid disease by avoiding illness-causing agents that surround us and by eating the right foods and taking the proper supplements. Although he spends too much time attacking the government, especially the FDA and the pharmaceutical industry, much of his information is helpful. Sometimes, though, the reader must dig to find the helpful nuggets.
- Trudeau, Kevin. 2007, ©2004. *Natural Cures "They" Don't Want You to Know About.* Elk Grove Village, IL: Alliance. 572 pp. ISBN: 0975599593; 9780975599594.
  Although written in a polemical style, this book does provide some good advice drawn from a variety of complementary and alternative sources. The author provides suggested cures for 50 common illnesses, but for many of the cures touted in the book, the reader needs to access the author's website which requires the payment of a monthly fee.
- Weil, Andrew. 2000, ©1995. *Spontaneous Healing: How to Discover and Enhance Your Body's Natural Ability to Maintain and Heal Itself.* New York: Alfred A. Knopf. 376 pp. ISBN: 0804117942; 9780804117944.
  Integrating a variety of approaches to health, the author seeks to provide readers with a means to increase their overall health and to promote healing. The first part of the book addresses healing itself and the systems that support it and reports on the author's own journey of discovery. The second section discusses ways of optimizing

the healing system, including diet, the use of tonics and supplements, exercise and rest, and protecting oneself from toxins. The final section focuses on what to do if you get sick. Overall, this is an excellent book that will introduce the reader to a variety of alternative health techniques that can be of assistance in increasing one's health and vitality and addressing illness.

- Weil, Andrew. 2004. *Natural Health, Natural Medicine: The Complete Guide to Wellness and Self-Care for Optimum Health*. Rev. ed. Boston: Houghton Mifflin. 432 pp. ISBN: 0618479031; 9780618479030.
  Written by one of the most well-known advocates of integrative medicine, this is an easy-to-read guide to preventing disease. Weil addresses questions about diet, air, exercise, relaxation, and social interactions. In addition, he provides suggestions on how to avoid heart attacks, strokes, and cancer by protecting the immune system. He also introduces natural treatments to common ailments using vitamins, supplements, and herbs.
- Weil, Andrew. 2006. *8 Weeks to Optimum Health: A Proven Program for Taking Full Advantage of Your Body's Natural Healing Power*. Rev. ed. New York: Knopf. 306 pp. ISBN: 0307264920; 9780307264923.
  Providing a week-by-week program for enhancing one's current condition and promoting lifelong health, this book combines ideas from a variety of sources such as ayurveda, nutritional herbology, and the use of vitamins and supplements. The chapter for each week provides projects to be accomplished during the week, dietary tips, suggestions for the use of supplements, and exercises, both physical and mental/spiritual. Recipes are included that can help meet the dietary changes suggested. Each chapter also has one or more healing stories that illustrate the principles being discussed. The last section of the book presents customized plans for specific populations such as those over 50, men or women, those who live in big cities, those who are overweight, and those who have a risk for cancer. This is a highly practical book that distills many of the theories available in other books into suggestions that can be immediately applied for better health.
- Wengell, Douglas A., and Gabriel, Nathen. 2008. *Educational Opportunities in Integrative Medicine: The A-to-Z Healing Arts Guide and Professional Resource Directory*. Atlanta, GA: Hunter Press. 291 pp. ISBN: 0977655245; 9780977655243.
  This is an excellent guide for those who have an interest in pursing training in any of the fields associated with integrative medicine. The first section examines those professions that require specific educational degrees followed by licensure such as chiropractic, acupuncture, and massage therapy. The second sections discusses 40 different non-degree programs that often have no licensure or certification programs such as aromatherapy, the Feldenkrais Method, herbal medicine, Pilates, and zero balancing. For each field, the entry provides a good description of the field, the training or education required, related organizations, periodicals, and selected online resources.
- Wiancek, Deborah A. 2000. *The Natural Healing Companion: Using Alternative Medicines: What to Buy, How to Take, and When to Combine for Best Results*. Emmaus, PA: Rodale. 531 pp. ISBN: 157954245X.
  This reference work provides basic information on a variety of topics. Remedies, including herbs, supplements, homeopathic remedies, and Chinese formulas, are

given for over 230 diseases and conditions. The section on herbs lists 128 different herbs, their use, dosage, characteristics, and cautions. Similarly, other sections list vitamins, minerals, and other supplements, homeopathic remedies, and Chinese medicines.

- Wisneski, Leonard A., and Anderson, Lucy. 2009. *The Scientific Basis of Integrative Medicine*. 2nd ed. Boca Raton, FL: CRC Press. 422 pp. ISBN: 1420082906; 9781420082906.
  Designed for physicians and other health practitioners, this resource provides a systems approach to integrative medicine. Specifically, the authors give an overview of the classic physiological system and then address psychoneuroimmunology, which they see as a way to integrate the physiological systems with other medical and healing techniques. Other chapters focus on the stress system, the relaxation system, energy medicine including nonthermal electromagnetic therapies and lasers, and the pineal gland. The final chapter examines the role of the spirit or soul in medicine.
- Yuan, Chun-Su, Bieber, Eric J., and Bauer, Brent A. 2006. *Textbook of Complementary and Alternative Medicine*. 2nd ed. Boca Raton, FL: Taylor & Francis. 794 pp. ISBN: 1842142976; 9781842142974.
  Originating in a CAM course for medical students, this book is designed for practicing physicians, medical students, and other health care professionals who have an interest in complementary and alternative therapies based on current scientific research. The first section examines commonly used CAM therapies such as herbalism, homeopathy, meditation, prayer, acupuncture, traditional Chinese medicine, and chiropractic. The second section presents CAM therapies for common medical conditions including cardiovascular disease, insomnia, diabetes, obesity, cancer, and premenstrual syndrome.

Internet Resources

- The Alternative Medicine Foundation, www.amfoundation.org/index.htm.
  The goal of the Alternative Medicine Foundation is to provide responsible and reliable information about alternative medicine to the public and health professionals. The site includes a wealth of information such as introductions to CAM for professionals and patients, a directory of useful databases, tips on choosing a practitioner, summaries of modalities such as energy work and naturopathy, and discussions of health issues such as autism spectrum disorders and managing pain.
- The Alternative Medicine Homepage, www.pitt.edu/~cbw/internet.html.
  Produced by the Falk Library of Health Sciences at the University of Pittsburgh, this webpage covers many aspects of alternative medicine, including associations and organizations, databases, diseases and conditions, fraud and quackery, government resources, mailing lists and newsgroups, and directories of practitioners.
- Alternative Medicine, Mayo Clinic, www.mayoclinic.com/health/consumer-health/MY00434/DSECTION=alternative-medicine.
  Produced by the Mayo Clinic as part of its consumer health information service, this webpage includes basic information on complementary and alternative medicine and therapies. It features articles on topics such as colon cleansing, probiotics, colloidal silver, acupuncture, and noni juice.

- Complementary and Alternative Medicine, Creighton University School of Medicine, altmed.creighton.edu.
  Designed to help answer the question "Do alternative therapies work?" this site provides resources for professionals, students, and the general public on complementary and alternative medicine. It includes original articles on various aspects of alternative medicine written by Creighton faculty and medical students as well as links to external sites that provide additional information on various aspects of alternative medicine.
- Complementary and Alternative Medicine, National Cancer Institute, www.cancer.gov/cancertopics/treatment/cam.
  Available in English and Spanish, these pages provided by the National Cancer Institute provide information on the use of complementary and alternative therapies in the treatment of cancer.
- The Continuum Center for Health and Healing, www.healthandhealingny.org.
  An initiative of Beth Israel Medical Center, the Continuum Center for Health and Healing is a resource for information on a wide variety of information on all aspects of health and healing including health conditions complementary and alternative therapies, and traditional and indigenous healing systems. The site includes detailed information on 30 different CAM therapies such as the history and philosophy of the modality, its treatment approaches, how it works and when to use it, what you need to know about treatment, and the training and licensing of practitioners.
- National Center for Complementary and Alternative Medicine, nccam.nih.gov.
  The NCCAM is a preeminent source of authoritative information on complementary and alternative health. As part of the National Institutes of Health, its mission is to explore complementary and alternative healing practices using rigorous scientific methods, train researchers in complementary and alternative medicine, and disseminate authoritative information to the public and professionals. The site provides a wealth of information from research-based discussions of treatments and conditions to details on the use of specific herbs.
- New York Online Access to Health, www.noah-health.org/en/alternative.
  NOAH seeks to provide online access to accurate, timely, relevant, and unbiased consumer health information in both English and Spanish. The page on alternative healing approaches includes articles on techniques such as acupuncture, aromatherapy, chiropractic, herbal medicine, homeopathy, meditation, Reiki, and vitamins, minerals, and supplements.
- The Rosenthal Center, www.rosenthal.hs.columbia.edu.
  Based in the Department of Rehabilitation Medicine of Columbia University's College of Physicians and Surgeons, the Rosenthal Center seeks to examine alternative therapies with academic focus and scientific rigor. The center conducts and facilitates research on the action, effectiveness, and safety of CAM therapies; educates medical professionals on the integration of CAM into conventional medicine; and acts as an information resource on CAM for the international medical community.
- Weil Lifestyle, LLC, www.drweil.com.
  Based on the work of Dr. Andrew Weil, this website covers all aspects of health and healing, including the use of vitamins and supplements, healthy aging, and creating

an optimum health plan. The heath centers tab covers topics such as bone and joint health, cancer, colds and flu, diabetes, heart health, and mental health. This is an excellent source for good information on all aspects of maintaining a healthy lifestyle.

Periodicals/Magazines/Journals

- *Alternative & Complementary Therapies*, published by Mary Ann Liebert Inc. Publishers, 1995– . Bimonthly. ISSN: 1076-2809. www.liebertpub.com/act.
  An academic journal, *Alternative & Complementary Therapies* seeks to provide the latest information available on alternative therapies and their integration into the clinical practice of medicine. Articles include profiles of innovative clinics and clinicians, integrative approaches for treating chronic illnesses, the use and biochemistry of herbal remedies, legal issues surrounding the use of CAM therapies, and mind–body approaches to the management of health and disease.
- *Alternative Medicine Alert*, published by A H C Media LLC, 1997– . Monthly. ISSN: 1096-942X. www.ahcpub.com/products_and_services/?prid=162&spcid=0,1& mtyid=5&cetid=0,1&pdr=1&clntr=0&clntru=/clinical_trials/?clu=162 &mtid=c.
  This monthly newsletter provides evidence-based, clinically proven information on complementary and alternative medicine that can be useful to medical professionals in their practices.
- *Alternative Medicine Review*, published by Thorne Research Inc., 1996– . Bimonthly. ISSN: 1089-5159. www.thorne.com/practitioners/alternative_ medicine_review.jsp.
  A peer-reviewed journal, *Alternative Medicine Review* publishes original articles, abstracts, and literature reviews that provide accurate and clinically relevant information on CAM to practicing medical professionals.
- *Alternative Therapies in Health and Medicine*, published by InnoVision Communications, 1995– . Bimonthly. ISSN: 1078-6791. www.alternative-therapies.com.
  Dedicated to exploring the integration of alternative therapies with conventional medical practices, this peer-reviewed journal examines the use of alternative therapies in the prevention and treatment of disease, healing illness, and promoting health.
- *Alternative Therapies in Women's Health*, published by A H C Media LLC, 1998– . Monthly. ISSN: 1522-3396. www.ahcpub.com/products_and_services/?prid=358&spcid=0,1,12&mtyid=5&cetid=0,1,2&pdr=0&clntr=0&clntru=/clinical_trials/?clu= 358&mtid=c.
  Focusing specifically on women's health, this newsletter provides access to clinically important information on herbs, dietary supplements, and alternative medical techniques. It includes summaries of the latest in scientific research, especially on botanical preparations and complementary and alternative therapies as used for the treatment of women and the promotion of women's health.
- *Awareness Magazine*, published by Awareness Publishing Group Inc., 1993– . Bimonthly. No ISSN. www.awarenessmag.com.
  A bimonthly consumer magazine, *Awareness Magazine* is devoted to the improvement of both the life of our planet and the lives of its readers. It includes articles on issues such as alternative and complementary treatments, natural health products, fitness, personal growth, spirituality, and the environment.

- *Be Well*, published by Alexandra Gayek, 2004– . Monthly. ISSN: 1549-0017. www.scienceofbeingwell.net/subscribe.html.
  Freely available online, *Be Well* provides inspiration and encouragement to those with an interest in alternative medicine. Articles and features include true healing stories, simple tips for living a healthier life, reports on medical and scientific research, and listings of useful resources.
- *BMC Complementary and Alternative Medicine*, published by BioMed Central Ltd., 2001– . Irregular. ISSN: 1472-6882. www.biomedcentral.com/bmccomplementalternmed.
  Published in an open-access, online format, this journal presents original research on all aspects of complementary and alternative medicine. It especially explores the biological mechanisms of the actions of CAM therapies, their efficacy, their safety, their costs, and the ways they are used in clinical settings.
- *CAM Lifestyle Magazine*, published by Target Publishing Ltd., 2007– . Bimonthly. No ISSN. www.camlifestyle.co.uk.
  Published in the United Kingdom, this magazine is designed for those who wish to learn more about complementary and alternative medicine. The magazine covers topics such as nutrition and diet, creating a healthy lifestyle, understanding the science behind CAM therapies, and working with one's medical practitioner to incorporate CAM into treatment.
- *Complementary and Alternative Medicine: Focus on Research and Care*, published by National Institutes of Health, National Center for Complementary and Alternative Medicine, 2009– . Three times per year. ISSN: 1556-388X. nccam.nih.gov/news/ newsletter/.
  Formerly titled *CAM at the NIH, Complementary and Alternative Medicine* is the newsletter of the National Center for Complementary and Alternative Medicine. As such it reports on the work of the NCCAM, summarizes current news and research about CAM, and gives useful hints on the use of CAM therapies, herbal remedies, and supplements.
- *Complementary Health Practice Review*, published by Sage Science Press, 1995– . Three times a year. ISSN: 1533-2101. chp.sagepub.com.
  This scholarly journal seeks to provide a forum for both alternative health care practitioners and traditional health care professionals who incorporate alternative methods into their practices. It covers all aspects of the use of complementary and alternative therapies, including the cultural, social, political, economic, and legal implications. In addition, the journal presents trends in CAM practice.
- *Complementary Therapies in Clinical Practice*, published by Churchill Livingstone, 1995– . Four times a year. ISSN: 1744-3881. www.elsevier.com/locate/ctcp.
  Previously devoted to complementary therapies in nursing and midwifery, this journal now includes articles on all aspects of complementary and alternative medicine. The major articles are peer reviewed and address issues such as implementing CAM in clinical settings, legal and ethical issues, social trends, best practices, policy development, and therapeutic information.
- *Complementary Therapies in Medicine*, published by Churchill Livingstone, 1993– . Four times a year. ISSN: 0965-2299. www.elsevier.com/locate/issn/09652299.
  Complementary Therapies in Medicine is an international, peer-reviewed journal of interest to all those who seek reliable information on complementary and

complementary therapies including health care practitioners, CAM therapists, nurses, academics, social scientists, researchers, health care managers, and patients.

- *Consumer Health Digest*, published by National Council Against Health Fraud Inc., 1977– . Weekly. ISSN: 0890-3417. www.ncahf.org/digest10/index.html.
  Published weekly as an electronic newsletter, *Consumer Health Digest* seeks to provide useful, trustworthy information on all aspects of health, including complementary and alternative medicine. The newsletter publishes summaries of research reports, current legislation, recent enforcement actions, and news items from around the world.
- *Dr. Robert Jay Rowen's Second Opinion*, published by Second Opinion Newsletter, 1991– . Monthly. ISSN: 1068-2953. www.secondopinionnewsletter.com.
  Dedicated to reporting on healing breakthroughs, especially within the realm of complementary and alternative health, this newsletter discusses topics as broad as heart disease, cancer, fatigue, diabetes, and autism.
- *Evidence-Based Complementary and Alternative Medicine*, published by Oxford University Press, 2004– . Quarterly. ISSN: 1741-427X. ecam.oxfordjournals.org.
  An international, peer-reviewed journal, *Evidence-Based Complementary and Alternative Medicine* publishes rigorous research on complementary and alternative medicine. Also included are articles on clinical studies, methodology, and theory.
- *Focus on Alternative and Complementary Therapies: An Evidence Based Approach*, published by Pharmaceutical Press, 1996– . Quarterly. ISSN: 1465-3753. www.pharmpress.com/fact.
  This scholarly journal examines the literature of both modern Western medicine and complementary and alternative medicine to present the results in an analytical and impartial manner that can be used by practicing health care providers as well as medical researchers.
- *Gerson Healing Newsletter*, published by Gerson Institute, 1984– . Bimonthly. No ISSN. www.gerson.org/membership/newsletters.htm.
  This is the official newsletter of the Gerson Institute, which is dedicated to treating disease using alternative, nontoxic methods including such techniques as organic foods, juicing, coffee enemas, detoxification, and natural supplements that help the body heal itself.
- *The Harvard Mental Health Letter*, published by Harvard Health Publications Group, 1984– . Monthly. ISSN: 1057-5022. www.health.harvard.edu/newsletters/Harvard_Health_Letter.
  Designed for both health care professionals and general readers, this newsletter focuses on news and research related to mental health. Topics include nutrition, food therapy, herbal supplements, and other alternative treatments, in addition to research drawn from the medical literature.
- *Healing Garden Journal*, published by Healing Garden Journal, 2000– . Bimonthly. ISSN: 1942-2768. healinggardenjournal.com.
  The purpose of *Healing Garden Journal* is to be a resource for those seeking total well-being in their bodies, minds, and spirits. The journal promotes environmental

and social awareness and advocates wellness through the use of natural foods, fitness, and alternative and complementary health care.

- *Heart & Soul*, published by Heart and Soul Enterprises, 1993–2003 (ceased), resumed 2004– . Quarterly. ISSN: 1092-1974. www.heartandsoul.com.
  Aimed at African-American women, this magazine covers issues such as health, fitness, and living an environmentally friendly life.
- *Holistic Life: Take Control of Your Own Health/Ponga el Control de su Salud en Usted Mismo*, published by New York Institute for Holistic Life, 1991– . Three times per year. ISSN: 1060-2615. www.vidaholistica.com/holistic_life_journal.htm.
  A bilingual newsletter including both Spanish and English, *Holistic Life* strives to provide knowledge related to complementary and alternative medical modalities and how they can affect one's health.
- *Integrative Medicine: A Clinician's Journal*, published by InnoVision Communications, 1999– . Bimonthly. ISSN: 1546-993X. www.imjournal.com.
  With a focus on integrating conventional and natural medicine, this journal provides both research-based and practical information to health care professionals. Articles include methods of preventing and treating illness with the goal of providing optimal patient care.
- *International Journal of Applied Research in Natural Products*, published by Healthy Synergies Publications, 2008– . Quarterly. ISSN: 1940-6223; healthy-synergies.com/default.aspx.
  An international open access journal, this publication provides peer-reviewed articles that report on the latest in applied research in natural products. Coverage includes functional foods, dietary supplements, nutraceuticals, and other natural health-related natural products. The goal of the journal is to help practitioners in preventing and managing chronic and infectious diseases.
- *The Internet Journal of Alternative Medicine*, published by Internet Scientific Publications LLC, 2002– . Semi-annual. ISSN: 1540-2584. www.ispub.com/ostia/index.php?xmlFilePath=journals/ijam/front.xml.
  A free, full-text, online academic journal, *The Internet Journal of Alternative Medicine* covers all aspects of complementary and alternative health. Each issue includes original research articles as well as reviews of other research.
- *Journal of Accord Integrative Medicine*, published by Accord Complementary Institute, 2005– . Bimonthly. ISSN: 1932-4642. accordinstitute.org.
  Integrating acupuncture, Chinese medicine, qigong, parapsychology, and somatic science with Western medicine, this journal publishes articles on current scientific research, theories, technologies, and methods. It also includes historical reviews, book reviews, and clinical observations.
- *Journal of Alternative and Complementary Medicine: Research on Paradigm, Practice, and Policy*, published by Mary Ann Liebert Inc. Publishers, 1993– . Ten times a year. ISSN: 1075-5535. www.liebertpub.com/products/product.aspx?pid=3.
  This is an interdisciplinary journal for research in alternative and complementary medical therapies. The goal of the journal is to publish articles that use rigorous research methodologies and articles on clinical care, case studies, and health policy.

- *Journal of Alternative Medicine Research*, published by Nova Science Publishers Inc., 2009– . Quarterly. ISSN: 1939-5868. www.novapublishers.com/catalog/product_info.php?products_id=6404.
  The peer-reviewed *Journal of Alternative Medicine Research* is an international, multidisciplinary forum for research that examines a holistic approach to alternative and conventional medicine, health and social issues and policy, epidemiology, rehabilitation, quality of life, and other aspects of human development over the lifespan.
- *Journal of Complementary & Integrative Medicine*, published by Berkeley Electronic Press, 2004– . Three times a year. ISSN: 1553-3840. www.bepress.com/jcim.
  This online journal publishes research articles, review articles, and discussion papers on all aspects of complementary and alternative medicine, including the efficacy and safety of the various therapies represented. It includes controlled clinical trials and observational studies, case reports, historical studies of CAM, biological and pharmacological activity, and the quality of CAM products.
- *Life Extension Magazine*, published by Life Extension Foundation, 1994– . Monthly. ISSN: 1524-198X. www.lef.org/magazine/mag_all.html.
  Published by the Life Extension Foundation, a major provider of information on anti-aging supplements and therapies, this magazine summarizes the latest research findings from the medical, health, and nutritional fields.
- *Lilipoh: A Quarterly Guide to Health, Nutrition and the Environment*, published by Lilipoh Publishing Inc., 1996– . Quarterly. No ISSN. www.lilipoh.com.
  Through its articles, *Lilipoh* examines illness as a phenomenon that is reflective of both the spirit and the body. It covers topics as varied as holistic health, well-being, creativity, spirituality, gardening, education, art, and social health.
- *Mayo Clinic Health Letter*, published by Mayo Clinic, 1983– . Monthly. ISSN: 0741-6245; bookstore.mayoclinic.com/products/newsletterDetails.cfm?mpid=22.
  Produced by the world-renowned Mayo Clinic, the *Mayo Clinic Health Letter* is filled with accurate and practical news and information on topics such as arthritis, high blood pressure, heart disease, nutrition, exercise, new medical treatments, and more. Each monthly issue includes health tips, answers to medical questions, and full color medical illustration to help the reader understand the medical topics covered.
- *Mayo Clinic Women's HealthSource*, published by Mayo Clinic, 1997– . Monthly. ISSN: 1091-0220. bookstore.mayoclinic.com/products/newsletterDetails.cfm?mpid=23.
  Dedicated to the health of women, this newsletter seeks to provide medical and lifestyle information that can help women lead healthier lives.
- *Natural Glow*, Glow Publications Inc., 2002– . Monthly. ISSN: 1538-8468; stretched-pixel.com/portfolio/web/samples/natural_glow/home.html.
  Aimed primarily at younger women, this magazine publishes articles on health issues, beauty and skin care, nutrition and vegetarianism, spa and aromatherapy, fitness and yoga, and other related topics.
- *Natural Lifestyle: Love Life, Live Well—Naturally*, published by Target Publishing Ltd., 2002– . Monthly. No ISSN. www.nat-lifestyle.com.
  A British magazine, *Natural Lifestyle* provides articles and information designed to help its readers and their families lead healthier and more natural lifestyles. It

includes features and departments on natural products, remedies, diet, nutrition, and research in health and alternative therapies.

- *Natural Living Magazine*, published by Natural Living Lifestyles Inc., 2007– . Quarterly. ISSN: 1939-6562. naturalla.com/index.html.
  This California based magazine examines green trends, environmentally friendly lifestyles, and natural living. It provides tips and information to make living a greener and healthier lifestyle easier.
- *Natural Solutions: Vibrant Health, Balanced Living*, published by InnoVision Health Media, 1994– . 10 times a year. ISSN: 1940-8153. www.naturalsolutionsmag.com.
  Focusing on all types of alternative medicine, this magazine includes feature articles as well as summaries of research from medical journals, conferences, and newsletters.
- *New Frontier: Magazine of Transformation*, published by New Frontier Education Society, 1981– . Monthly. ISSN: 0886-4616. newfrontier.com/2.
  New Frontier publishes articles and interviews on topics as varied as holistic health and medicine, metaphysics, yoga, natural foods, astrology and important world news.
- *New Visions Magazine*, published by New Visions Magazine Inc., 1988– . Bimonthly. No ISSN. www.newvisionsmagazine.com.
  Covering healthy living, wellness, spirituality, astrology, and alternative therapies, this magazine is designed for general readers who have an interest in improving their lives.
- *NewLife: America's Guide to a Healthy Life, Body, and Spirit*, published by Serenity Health Organization Inc., 1986– . Bimonthly. ISSN: 1088-1441. www.newlifemag.com.
  Focusing on holistic health, the environment, and on New Age ideologies, this magazine strives to promote the full potential of all individuals. It publishes articles on living a healthy and spiritual lifestyle.
- *Nutritional Wellness*, published by M P A Media, 2006– . Quarterly. ISSN: 1559-8705. www.nutritionalwellness.com.
  Devoted to providing reliable information on nutrition, this newsletter is designed for doctors. The goal is to provide information on topics such as whole foods, herbs, homeopathy, and other natural nutritional products that doctors may use in the treatment of their patients.
- *The Open Complementary Medicine Journal*, published by Bentham Open, 2008– . Irregular. ISSN: 1876-391X. www.bentham.org/open/toaltmedj/index.htm.
  An online, open access journal, this publication features both full length and shorter research articles and literature reviews in complementary and alternative medicine. As a peer-reviewed journal, its goal is to be a trusted source of information of current developments in CAM.
- *The Original Internist*, published by Clint Publications, 1994– . Quarterly. ISSN: 1529-4722. www.clintpublications.com.
  This magazine covers all aspects of natural health care, including methods such as chiropractic, homeopathy, osteopathy, and naturopathy.
- *Positive Health: Integrated Medicine for the 21st Century*, published by Positive Health Publications Ltd., 1994– . Monthly. ISSN: 1356-3963. www.positivehealth .com.
  Published in the United Kingdom, *Positive Health* is aimed at consumers who seek to live healthier lives. The magazine includes feature article, summaries of research,

case studies, and book reviews on healing modalities as diverse as nutrition, massage, acupressure techniques, and aromatherapy.

- *Prevention: Smart Ways to Live Well*, published by Rodale Inc., 1950– . Monthly. ISSN: 0032-8006. www.prevention.com/health.
  A monthly magazine, *Prevention* publishes articles on nutrition, preventive medicine, fitness, natural living, and drugless therapies such as the use of herbs. The emphasis of the magazine is on a healthy lifestyle and self-improvement.
- *Total Health for Longevity*, published by Total Health Holdings LLC, 1979– . Bimonthly. ISSN: 0274-6743. www.totalhealthmagazine.com.
  A magazine with an emphasis on anti-aging, this publication presents strategies to live a long, healthy life. Articles cover topics such as nutrition, diet, fitness, travel, spirituality, and mind–body interactions.
- *Tufts University Health & Nutrition Letter*, published by Tufts University, 1983– . Monthly. ISSN: 1526-0143. www.healthletter.tufts.edu.
  The goal of this publication is to provide consumers with information that can directly affect their health. Topics include health and nutrition advice in addition to information drawn from fields as diverse as public policy, biomedicine, epidemiology, and psychology.
- *University of California, Berkeley, Wellness Letter: The Newsletter of Nutrition, Fitness, and Self-Care*, published by Health Letter Associates, 1984– . Monthly. ISSN: 0748-9234. www.wellnessletter.com.
  Designed for physicians, nutritionists, and other health care professionals as well as the general reader, this newsletter seeks to translate major medical research into practical advice that can be applied in our daily lives. It includes coverage of both traditional medicine as well as topics such as nutrition, diet, exercise, self-care, and preventive medicine.
- *Well Being Journal: Heralding the Integration of Medicine with Physical, Mental, Emotional, Spiritual & Social Aspects of Healing*, published by Well Being Inc., 1991– . Bimonthly. ISSN: 1559-4955. www.wellbeingjournal.com.
  Well Being Journal publishes articles on natural healing, complementary and alternative medicine, energy healing, nutrition, herbs, and the relationship of spirituality to health. The magazine also includes personal stories of hope and healing written by individuals who have experienced the restoration of health by using various healing methods.

Chapter 2

The Alexander Technique

Background and History

The Alexander Technique is named after Frederick Matthias Alexander, a Tasmanian actor born in 1869 who was famous for his recitations of Shakespearean speeches. After regularly performing these speeches, he lost his voice. During this time, Alexander noticed that he lost his voice only when he was reciting, not during regular conversation. This caused him to look for the reason that he would lose his voice only during his recitations. He examined himself in a mirror to see if he could spot the difference between his normal speaking patterns and his recitation patterns. He determined that prior to reciting he was tensing his neck muscles, causing his head to move back, tightening his throat muscles and forcing a short deep breath. Thus, he concluded, if he did not do these things, his voice would return. Although it was more difficult than he thought it would be to correct these problems, he succeeded in not tensing his neck muscles, which caused the other two problems to disappear and his voice to return. He then experimented with the way he held his head to see if that could help him project his voice, but he found that other muscles tensed and he was less able to recite properly. Thus, he determined that his voice was not the problem, but the mechanics of the body. He discovered that the position of his head influenced his whole body. Alexander continued to monitor his body, especially his head position, while walking, standing, talking, and gesturing.

For over 50 years, Alexander refined his techniques. He also began to treat patients referred to him by physicians, especially for speech problems and other physical ailments such as back pain. In 1904, Alexander moved to London where he established a school for young children in 1924. In 1914 with the beginning of World War I, he split his time between London and the United States for over a decade. His first school for teachers of his technique opened in London in 1930. He lived in the United States during much of World War II.

Alexander died in 1955. Since his death, the Alexander Technique has continued to be taught, especially in colleges, universities, and acting schools.

Primary Uses and Actions

Many common ailments and physical complaints are the result of incorrect posture or incorrect use of the body. The Alexander Technique can help alleviate these problems by teaching proper body mechanics. Among the ailments that can be ameliorated by learning the Alexander Technique are depression, muscle fatigue, migraine headaches, sciatica, hypertension, stress-related disorders, backaches, circulatory problems, respiratory problems, and speech problems. Actors, dancers, singers, and musicians have been especially drawn to the Alexander Technique due to its ability to help them prevent muscle injuries due to misuse or overuse.

Training

Certification for Alexander Technique teachers is available from Alexander Technique International. Candidates for certification must have completed Alexander Technique training, a process that can take up to three years. In addition, they must demonstrate their knowledge of the concepts and principles of the technique and their ability to teach these skills to others. There are no licensing requirements in any state to teach the Alexander Technique.

Sources

Bloch, Michael. 2004. *F. M., The Life of Frederick Matthias Alexander: Founder of the Alexander Technique*. London: Little, Brown.

Gelb, Michael J. 1995. *Body Learning: An Introduction to the Alexander Technique*. New York: Henry Holt and Company.

See also FELDENKRAIS METHOD; THERAPEUTIC MASSAGE AND BODYWORK

Annotated Bibliography

Print Resources

- Alcantara, Pedro de. 1999. *The Alexander Technique: A Skill for Life*. Marlborough, UK: Crowood Press. 128 pp. ISBN: 1861262868; 9781861262868.
  Written in an easy-to-read style, this book presents the principles of the Alexander Technique in an understandable and straightforward manner. The author gives examples of what to expect in an Alexander lesson and discusses how the technique can affect both emotions and health and well-being. Separate chapters focus on sports and exercise and on the performing arts.
- Bloch, Michael. 2004. *F. M., The Life of Frederick Matthias Alexander: Founder of the Alexander Technique*. London: Little, Brown. 276 pp. ISBN: 0316728640; 9780316860482.
  This is a good biography of the founder of the Alexander Technique. Although it does not address the principles and practices of the Alexander Technique directly, the book does give background that makes a study of the technique more interesting.
- Brennan, Richard. 2004. *The Alexander Technique Manual: Take Control of Your Posture and Your Life*. London: Connections Book Publishing. 144 pp. ISBN: 185906163X; 9781859061633.
  Based on the practice of the Alexander Technique, the goal of this book is to help us understand ourselves and how we work so that we can lead more rewarding lives. To achieve this goal, the author presents the basic principles of the technique and demonstrates how they can be applied. Wonderfully illustrated with color photographs, the chapters provide easy exercises that reinforce the principles being presented. Special chapters on applying the Alexander Technique to sports and to pregnancy and childbirth are also included.
- Conable, Barbara, and Conable, William. 1995. *How to Learn the Alexander Technique: A Manual for Students*. 3rd ed., rev. and enlarged. Columbus, OH: Andover Press. 154 pp. ISBN: 0962259543; 9780962259548.

This book is designed to aid in the study of the Alexander Technique, especially for those who are currently taking a course in the technique. All the major concepts of the technique are presented in an understandable manner, and good illustrations provide visual context to these concepts. The author also includes a chapter on body mapping that can assist in learning the Alexander Technique.

- Craze, Richard. 2003. *Teach Yourself Alexander Technique*. Chicago: McGraw-Hill. 149 pp. ISBN: 0071429727; 9780071429726.
  Introducing the major tenets of the Alexander Technique, this is a wonderful, small book. Through the use of simple line drawings, the major concepts are well illustrated and the reader can begin to apply these concepts immediately. The strength of the book lies in its showing how the technique can be used in everyday situations, whether working at a computer or changing a baby's diapers.
- Dimon, Theodore. 1999. *The Undivided Self: Alexander Technique and the Control of Stress*. Berkeley, CA: North Atlantic Books. 234 pp. ISBN: 1556432941; 9781556432941.
  Building on the theories of F. M. Alexander, the author broadens his vision to that of the mind and body functioning as a unified system. Understanding this mind/body system is necessary before one can become conscious of action and behavior. Of specific concern is tracing symptoms to the incorrect working of the system, thereby providing a way to understand the origin of the symptoms and suggesting ways to change the mind/body system in order to alleviate them.
- Gelb, Michael J. 1995. *Body Learning: An Introduction to the Alexander Technique*. New York: Henry Holt and Company. 180 pp. ISBN: 0805042067; 9780805042061.
  This is a good, practical introduction to the Alexander Technique. Divided into four parts, it presents a history of Alexander and the discovery of his technique, the major operational ideas of the technique, learning how to learn, and the questing spirit, which delves into using the Alexander Technique for organizational change. The author answers many questions on the technique and presents the balanced resetting state procedure. This is a good first book for those interested in the Alexander Technique.
- Gray, John. 1991. *The Alexander Technique: A Complete Course in How to Hold and Use Your Body for Maximum Energy*. New York: St. Martin's Press. 176 pp. ISBN: 0312064942; 9780312064945.
  The author presents easy-to-follow directions for incorporating the principles of the Alexander Technique into daily life. Throughout, the theories of F. M. Alexander are explained and then put into practice through various exercises. One of the strengths of this book are the sections titled "Working on Oneself," which seek to instill the principles when no teacher is available. Once these basic principles are mastered, the intermediate and later lessons presented in parts 2 and 3 can be attempted with better understanding.
- Harer, John B., and Munden, Sharon. 2009. *The Alexander Technique Resource Book: A Reference Guide*. Lanham, MD: Scarecrow Press. 161 pp. ISBN: 0810854317; 9780810854314.
  The goal of this book is to provide access to the wealth of information on the Alexander Technique, including general texts and articles; resources related to the performing arts, especially dance, music, and theater; resources on sport, fitness, and recreation; resources for health and medicine; electronic resources; and journals and

audiovisual materials. The last chapter is a directory of worldwide Alexander Technique associations.

- MacDonald, Robert, and Ness, Caro. 2000. *Secrets of Alexander Technique.* New York: DK Publishing. 224 pp. ISBN: 0789467720; 9783822856475.
  This little book provides a good introduction to F. M. Alexander, his technique, and his basic principles. The bulk of the book presents specific exercises that may be used in an Alexander Technique class such as sitting down, reading without strain, writing freely, working efficiently at the keyboard, conscious driving, constructive rest, squatting, walking, and proper breathing. The last section puts the Alexander Technique into the context of daily life and activities including exercising, swimming, horseback riding, pregnancy and childbirth, injury and pain, and digestion.

- McEvenue, Kelly. 2002. *The Actor and the Alexander Technique.* New York: Palgrave Macmillan. 148 pp. ISBN: 0312295154; 9780312295158.
  The author has written a good introduction to the Alexander Technique as seen through the lens of the actor.

- Nicholls, Carolyn. 2008. *Body, Breath & Being: A New Guide to the Alexander Technique.* Hove, UK: D & B. 159 pp. ISBN: 190446842X; 9781904468424.
  Using the experiences of individuals who have studied and benefited from the Alexander Technique, this guide provides practical information and exercises so readers can actually see how the technique may benefit them. Over 100 color photographs and diagrams enhance the text.

- Potter, Nicole, ed. 2002. *Movement for Actors.* New York: Allworth Press. 277 pp. ISBN: 1581152337; 9781581152333.
  Based on teachings derived from the Alexander Technique, the Feldenkrais Method, and a variety of other teachings, this book discusses movement that can be used to enhance an actor's presence on the stage or screen.

- Taylor, Anthony James. 2004. *Whatever You're Doing Now You Can Do It Better! Your Guide to the Alexander Technique.* San Luis Obispo, CA: Gil Books. 247 pp. ISBN: 0952632047; 9780952632047.
  This is a book about changing and improving your life based on the ideas and methods taught in classes on the Alexander Technique. After a brief biographical sketch of Alexander, each of the next chapters presents a core principle derived from the Alexander Technique. In addition to changing your posture and body mechanics, the goal of the book, and the Alexander Technique, is to give you the tools necessary to change your life, whether it is to be a better actor or musician, to become happier, to change careers, or to improve the quality of your life.

- Vineyard, Missy. 2007. *How You Stand, How You Move, How You Live: Learning the Alexander Technique to Explore Your Mind–Body Connection and Achieve Self-Mastery.* New York: Marlowe & Company. 322 pp. ISBN: 1600940064; 9781600940064.
  This is one of the best books available for the reader who wants a general introduction to the Alexander Technique. Written in a highly readable style, the book uses self-experiments to reinforce the concepts presented in the text. The goal of the book, which is the same as the goal of the Alexander Technique, is to improve movement through improved balance and coordination and reduced tension in the body. Such

improvement will help with maintaining health, recovering from injuries, improving posture, learning new skills, and being more graceful. Many case studies are presented to clarify the teachings.

- Weiss, Maria. 2009. *The Alexander Technique and the Art of Teaching Voice: Singing and Speaking with an Energetic, Free, and Beautiful Voice*. Saarbrücken, Germany: VDM Verlag Dr. Müller. 175 pp. ISBN: 3639122933; 9783639122930.
  This book focuses specifically on the principles and applications of the Alexander Technique to the teaching of voice. After giving background information on the technique, the author presents how the technique can assist in developing proper posture, breathing, and practice and performance techniques for vocal teachers and singers.

Internet Resources

- The Alexander Technique Center, www.alexandercenter.com.
  The Alexander Technique Center of Washington, DC, offers instruction in the Alexander Technique, private lessons, workshops, lectures, and a teacher-training program. The website has information for those interested in learning about the technique and special sections on using the technique for musicians, on ergonomics, and on the relationship between the American philosopher John Dewey and F. M. Alexander.
- Alexander Technique International, www.ati-net.com.
  Alexander Technique International is a worldwide organization of Alexander Technique teachers, students, and supporters of the Alexander Technique. Their website includes useful information about the organization itself and the technique, provides a directory of teachers, and lists workshops, articles, and other resources.
- The American Society for the Alexander Technique, www.alexandertech.org.
  The American Society for the Alexander Technique, the largest professional association of certified Alexander Technique teachers in the United States, maintains this website, which gives information on the Alexander Technique, lists classes and events, and provides bibliographies of books, videos, and teaching aids.
- The Complete Guide to the Alexander Technique, www.alexandertechnique.com.
  This website provides a good introduction to Alexander Technique with a multitude of links to articles, videos, and other resources. It also includes a listing of teachers of the technique.
- The Society of Teachers of the Alexander Technique, www.stat.org.uk.
  Maintained by the Society of Teachers of the Alexander Technique, this website abounds with useful information about the technique. Of special note are the pages on improved breathing, sport and fitness, self-development, and the use of the technique in the workplace.

Periodicals/Magazines/Journals

- *Exchange: Journal of the Alexander Technique International*, published by Alexander Technique International, 1992– . Three times per year. No ISSN. www.ati-net.com/exchange.php.

The official publication of the Alexander Technique International, this journal contains articles of interest to practitioners of the Alexander Technique and to their clients. It also includes articles on using the Alexander Technique to promote proper body awareness and health.

Chapter 3

Alternative Diagnosis Techniques

Background and History

Muscle Response Testing

The terms *muscle response testing*, *applied kinesiology*, *biokinesiology*, and *clinical kinesiology* all refer to a method of diagnosis using a client's body as a tool to determine allergies to specific triggers or nutritional deficiencies and to suggest appropriate remedies. The techniques vary, but the general idea is that the body itself will tell the diagnostician what is wrong when it is asked properly. For example, the body can be asked what it is allergic or sensitive to and what remedies will be beneficial through a protocol that tests the muscle strength of the patient. At its simplest, muscle response testing involves having the patient extend his or her arm while possible allergic triggers are held, one at a time, in his or her other hand over the solar plexus. The practitioner will then try to push down on the patient's arm, and if the arm is weak and is easy to push down, then that particular allergic trigger is responsible for the symptoms being experienced. Then, potential remedies are held, one at a time, and when the appropriate remedy is found, the arm will be difficult to push down. Other types of testing also employ the use of acupuncture/acupressure points. The point is pressed and then the arm is tested to determine the problem—whether allergic triggers or nutritional deficiencies—and the solutions. In clinical kinesiology, the patient is often lying down, and the muscle testing is done with the right arm held up perpendicular to the body while the practitioner tries to push the arm back down to the patient's side. Often a patient will be asked to place his or her left hand on the place that hurts and the testing is begun. The patient may be instructed to place his or her hand on other places and the test repeated to determine the source of the problem, which may be different from the place that the pain is manifested.

Applied kinesiology incorporates these ideas of muscle response testing and expands them into a variety of tests using various muscles and muscle groups of the body. Applied kinesiology is usually performed by chiropractors or other medical practitioners since it involves specific techniques designed for individual muscles and muscle groups. It also combines the use of the meridians and acupuncture points, lymphatic drainage techniques, and nutrition to treat identified problems.

Reams Testing

Reams testing is also known as RTBI—Reams Theory of Biological Ionization, biological ionization, or health by the numbers. The test is named after Dr. Cary Reams who sought to determine the perfect pH numbers for the human body. Reams testing analyzes the saliva and urine to help discover imbalances in the body's chemistry, especially the levels of sugar, urine, and saliva pH; urine salt; urine albumen; and urea. By maintaining the target numbers in each of these levels, the body will be able to maintain health. If the levels are not within the established range, it is thought that the individual may be at a greater risk for developing disease. To help obtain the optimal body chemistry, Dr. Reams developed the "Dr. Reams Process," which consists of body detoxification and purification; biochemical balancing through the use of herbs, minerals, and supplements; simple exercises for lymphatic function; and special foods that assist in cellular regeneration and maintenance.

Dried Blood Cell Analysis

Dried blood cell analysis studies the drying patterns of human blood to seek evidence of nutritional or organ weakness. Using a small sample of blood that is viewed under a high-powered microscope, dried blood cell analysis can help a practitioner screen for a variety of conditions including parasites, yeast, bacteria, nutritional deficiencies, and viruses. The analysis can supply information that helps in either referring the patient to the proper health care provider or prescribing appropriate herbs, supplements, and nutritional interventions.

Saliva Hormone Test

Generally used for women, the saliva hormone test is a simple test that can determine the levels of steroid hormones, especially estradiol, progesterone, and testosterone. The test is especially useful in identifying conditions such as depression, headaches, sleep disorders, mood swings, premenstrual syndrome, hot flashes, and diminished sex drive.

Primary Uses

These alternative diagnosis techniques assist the practitioner in determining the proper treatment. Reams testing and dried blood cell analysis are used primarily to determine nutritional deficiencies that can be corrected through supplements, herbal remedies, and changes in the diet. Muscle testing is used for two distinct purposes. For physicians and physical therapists, the testing of muscles may be simply to determine factors such as strength, injury, or neurological functioning. For alternative health practitioners, muscle testing is a way to diagnose allergies, food and chemical sensitivities, emotional problems, and nutritional deficiencies. The testing of the muscles is a way to have the body "speak" so that it can tell its own story. Muscle testing can also be used to determine appropriate remedies for treating the problem, rather than a trial and error method of suggesting remedies.

Training

There are no standards for training in the use of these diagnostic techniques. Some weekend classes are available, but many practitioners have learned them simply by reading a book or using the directions that come with the testing kits. In many cases, patients themselves are using home testing kits or mailing body samples to labs to obtain results. Classes on using these tools are now being offered at a variety of schools, especially those focusing on massage or natural health.

Sources

Lepore, Donald. 1985. *The Ultimate Healing System: Breakthrough in Nutrition, Kinesiology and Holistic Healing Techniques*. Pleasant Grove, Utah: Woodland Publishing.

Navarra, Tova. 2004. *The Encyclopedia of Complementary and Alternative Medicine.* New York: Facts on File.

See also IRIDOLOGY AND SCLEROLOGY

Annotated Bibliography

Print Resources

- Diamond, John. 1979. *Your Body Doesn't Lie: How to Increase Your Life Energy through Behavioral Kinesiology.* New York: Warner Books. 208 pp. ISBN: 0446358479; 9780446358477.
  In this book, the author explains the use of applied kinesiology to help determine various environmental and lifestyle factors that affect your body's energy. He also provides suggestions for activities that enrich energy and shows how to mitigate the effects of activities and situations that deplete energy The author calls his technique *behavioral kinesiology* since it is aimed more at the behavior and psychology of the individual rather than testing for specific remedies.
- Frost, Robert. 2002. *Applied Kinesiology: A Training Manual and Reference Book of Basic Principles and Practices.* Berkeley, CA: North Atlantic Books. 372 pp. ISBN: 1556433743; 9781556433740.
  This is an in-depth introduction to applied kinesiology for chiropractors and other health care professionals. It presents the basic principles of applied kinesiology, fundamental procedures of the technique, and more advanced techniques. The author details 33 specific muscle tests and gives suggested techniques for correcting the problems identified. Throughout the text, case histories are presented to increase the reader's understanding of the principles being discussed.
- Lepore, Donald. 1985. *The Ultimate Healing System: Breakthrough in Nutrition, Kinesiology and Holistic Healing Techniques.* Pleasant Grove, UT: Woodland Publishing. 402 pp. ISBN: 1885670087; 9781885670083.
  This is a well-illustrated manual on how to use muscle testing to determine allergens or sensitivities and the nutrients that can neutralize these allergens or sensitivities. The author provides a good introduction to the muscle testing technique that he uses and then discusses the role of allergies and their antidotes in the lives of patients. He continues by discussing methods of determining the appropriate nutrients to use to treat the problems of patients, including vitamins, minerals, amino acids, herbs, flower remedies, cell salts, and glandular extracts. Other chapters include discussions of specific diseases, addictions, pollution, drinking water, miracle foods (such as alfalfa and bee pollen), juice therapy, and a variety of other therapeutic techniques (such as color therapy, music therapy, and gem therapy).
- Levy, Susan L., and Lehr, Carol. 1996. *Your Body Can Talk: How to Use Simple Muscle Testing to Learn What Your Body Knows and Needs: The Art and Application of Clinical Kinesiology.* Prescott, AZ: Hohm Press. 367 pp. ISBN: 0934252688; 9780934252683.
  This book focuses on clinical kinesiology, which integrates the philosophies of anatomy, physiology, and acupuncture. Thus, the authors combine the application of acupuncture and the meridian system with muscle testing to help determine the causes of illness or health problems as well as their remedies. The book includes a

good discussion of acupuncture, energy and emotions, the chakras, energizing the immune system, curing candida, dealing with electromagnetic pollution, healing premenstrual syndrome, natural menopause, and the male energetic system.

- Valentine, Tom, and Valentine, Carole. 1985. *Applied Kinesiology: Muscle Response in Diagnosis, Therapy and Preventive Medicine.* New York: Thorsons Publishing Group. 144 pp. ISBN: 072251123X; 9780892813285.
  The goal of this book is to provide the information that a patient needs to know about applied kinesiology. It does not teach one to do such testing, but provides a good introduction to the theory and use of manual muscle testing in a clinical setting.

- Weinstock, David. 2010. *NeuroKinetic Therapy: An Innovative Approach to Manual Muscle Testing.* Berkeley, CA: North Atlantic Books. 131 pp. ISBN: 155643877X; 9781556438776.
  Based on the idea that after an injury, specific muscles cease working properly, thereby forcing other muscles to become overworked, NeuroKinetic Therapy permits the practitioner to evaluate clients and help restore function. The practitioner uses light pressure that the client resists to determine the strength or weakness of each muscle, revealing the sources of the injury while also retraining the client's body to be reprogrammed at the neural level by removing the compensation patterns that resulted from the injury. The book is organized anatomically, with each section giving clear photographs that demonstrate the correct positioning of the muscle accompanied by concise explanations and instructions.

Internet Resources

- Applied Kinesiology.com, www.appliedkinesiology.com.
  This site provides a good discussion of the basics of applied kinesiology and includes conditions that can be understood more fully using applied kinesiology and a directory of doctors who use the technique in their practices.

- Kinesiology Network, www.kinesiology.net.
  The Kinesiology Network provides access to kinesiology websites, schools and colleges, associations, information on applied kinesiology, kinesiology research, and one of the web's most complete databases of human muscles.

- Professional Applied Kinesiology, The International College of Applied Kinesiology, www.icakusa.com.
  The International College of Applied Kinesiology provides excellent information on applied kinesiology, its use in determining the cause of many medical conditions, scientific research on applied kinesiology, and a directory of doctors who use applied kinesiology.

- SalivaTesting.com, salivatesting.com.
  Although this is a commercial site, it does provide good general information on testing the saliva for the presence of hormones, especially estradiol (estrogen), progesterone, testosterone, and dehydroepiandrosterone (DHEA).

- Synergistic Kinesiology, www.synergistickinesiology.com.
  Featuring a different type of applied kinesiology called synergistic kinesiology, this website offers information on the use of kinesiology and muscle testing, the history

of kinesiology, and a comparison of approaching health from a holistic perspective and from the perspective of modern Western medicine.

Periodicals/Magazines/Journals

- *AK, The International Journal of Applied Kinesiology and Kinesiologic Medicine*, published by Castello Publishing, 1998– . Two to three times a year. ISSN: 1126-3970. www.kinmed.com.
  Worldwide in scope, this journal seeks to share the latest information on kinesiology with health care practitioners such as chiropractors, osteopaths, dentists, neurologists, cardiologists, and others in Europe, Australia, and North America.

Chapter 4

Aromatherapy and Essential Oils

Background and History

Smell has been important to the maintenance of health since the dawn of humanity. Some smells, such as rotting flesh, warned people that a carcass they found was not good to eat. Other smells, such as incense and flowers, were so pleasant that they were thought to be worthy of the gods. Ointment jars that contained scented oils from ancient sites such as the tombs of Egypt show that perfumes and aromatics have been used for millennia. Smells or aromas have also been used in healing for thousands of years and played important roles in many ancient medical practices and rituals. Herbs could be burned to release healing smoke, others would have their oils expressed through pressure or cooking and used either externally or internally, and still others would have been used as teas or foods. Thus, the use of aromatherapy and essential oils has a long history in the annals of the healing arts.

Today, aromatherapy generally refers to the use of essential oils, derived from the bark, leaves, petals, resins, roots, stalks, seeds, or stems of plants. Although essential oils have been used for centuries, modern aromatherapy is most often traced to René-Maurice Gattefossé, a French chemist who studied the cosmetic uses of essences. One day, while performing an experiment, he badly burned his hand. To help reduce the pain, he plunged his hand into a container of lavender essential oil that was sitting nearby. To his amazement, the burn healed completely without scarring. This led to additional research on essential oils and their therapeutic properties, especially their role as disinfectants and antiseptics. Gattefossé published his book *Aromathérapie* in 1928, thereby establishing the name of the field. Other researchers, such as Jean Valnet, built on Gattefossé's work, using essential oils for treating wounds during World War II. His 1964 book, *Aromathérapie, Traitement des Maladies par les Essences des Plants* [*Aromatherapy: Treatment of Illness by the Essences of Plants*], sought to teach other physicians the use of essential oils in medical treatments. In Italy, beginning in the 1920s, Dr. Renato Cayola, Dr. Giovanni Garri, and Professor Paolo Rovesti studied the psychological effects of essential oils, with special attention given to the treatment of anxious or depressed individuals.

Research continues on essential oils, and new ones are still being created, as are new mixtures of oils. Gary Young is one of the leading researchers and proponents for the use of essential oils to treat illnesses, whether physical, psychological, or spiritual. Along with others, he has helped expand the scope of essential oils and their uses by including essential oils in a variety of products including supplements, cosmetics, skin care products, massage oils, and soaps.

Primary Uses

Aromatherapy and essential oils can be used to treat many ailments, whether physical, psychological, or spiritual. Most resources on aromatherapy will list specific essential oils and the illnesses that they can correct. For example, lemon can be used to treat anxiety, digestive problems, and sore throats, but it can also help expel parasites. Frankincense is often used to treat allergies, headaches, and inflammation while also increasing spiritual awareness. Clove is indicated for use in infectious diseases, respiratory infections, and pain, and it can be used to treat arthritis, acne, and even warts.

As with any medicinal product, the production of an essential oil can radically affect its healing abilities. Thus, only therapeutic grade oils that are produced from organically grown plants that are properly distilled should be used on the human body or taken internally. Such oils are usually expensive and have not been diluted with a carrier oil.

The methods of applying essential oils are varied, and only a small amount is needed. Essential oils can be inhaled, either directly from the bottle, from a few drops on the hand, from drops in a bowl of hot water, or from drops on a cotton ball or tissue. They may also be diffused into the air using a cold-air diffuser. In some cases, direct application to the skin is warranted, especially in the case of many oils that act as antiseptics. In such cases, a carrier oil, such as almond oil, may need to be used to reduce the chance of skin irritation. In massage therapy, the oils are often combined with a neutral massage oil and applied directly to the skin. Essential oils that are labeled as Generally Regarded as Safe (GRAS) or certified as Food Additives (FA) by the U.S. Food and Drug Administration can be taken internally, either orally, rectally, or vaginally. Some oils, such as lemon, orange, peppermint, or those made from spices, can even be used in cooking. Their strength, however, is much greater than the spice itself, so care must be exercised to monitor the amount used.

Although many essential oils have proven antiseptic properties, they are believed to work on the subtle energetic level of the body. They promote healing by helping to relieve stress and soothing the emotions. Some researchers point to the chemical composition of various oils as part of their healing properties. Many oils can fight infections due to their antibacterial, antifungal, and antiviral properties. Other oils contain hormonelike molecules that help to balance the physiological systems of the body and can help stimulate the secretion of antibodies, hormones, and enzymes. Since the chemical structure of essential oils is similar to the structure of human cells and tissues, the oils are easily absorbed and accepted by the cells of the body and can diffuse quickly throughout the body. When diffused in the air, the oils provide negative ions that inhibit bacterial growth.

Training

Most aromatherapists are self-taught or have taken workshops or correspondence courses in aromatherapy, although many schools of alternative medicine and therapeutic massage now offer courses in aromatherapy. In the United States, there is no official agency or association that regulates aromatherapy, and no standards exist for its practice. The National Association for Holistic Aromatherapy, an organization founded in 1990 by six women who were studying aromatherapy, seeks to promote and elevate academic standards in aromatherapy education yet has no authority to certify or accredit aromatherapy programs. Similarly, the Aromatherapy Registration Council offers a voluntary examination that tests a student's knowledge of aromatherapy and those who pass can list "RA" (Registered Aromatherapist) as one of their qualifications to practice.

Sources

Buckle, Jane. 2003. *Clinical Aromatherapy: Essential Oils in Practice*. 2nd ed. Philadelphia: Churchill Livingstone.

Essential Oils: Desk Reference 2007. 4th ed. Orem, Utah: Essential Science Publishing.

Valnet, Jean. 1990. *The Practice of Aromatherapy: A Classic Compendium of Plant Medicines & Their Healing Properties*. Rochester, VT: Healing Arts Press.

See also FLOWER THERAPIES

Annotated Bibliography

Print Resources

➤ Baser, K. Hüsnü Can, and Buchbauer, Gerhard. 2010. *Handbook of Essential Oils: Science, Technology, and Applications*. Boca Raton, FL: CRC Press/Taylor & Francis. 975 pp. ISBN: 1420063154; 9781420063158.
Since more individuals are using essential oils, there is a growing need for production standards, more quality control parameters, and well-defined good manufacturing practices. To help fill this need, the authors have compiled this comprehensive handbook of the chemistry, pharmacology, and biological activity of essential oils as well as their production, uses, and regulation. They also cover sources, methods of production, analysis, storage, and transport of essential oils in addition to providing information on their use in aromatherapy.

➤ Buckle, Jane. 2003. *Clinical Aromatherapy: Essential Oils in Practice*. 2nd ed. Philadelphia: Churchill Livingstone. 416 pp. ISBN: 0443072361; 9780443072369.
The author, a registered nurse who integrates aromatherapy with her work, has written this book for health care professionals who seek to integrate aromatherapy into their clinical practices. The work is divided into two broad sections. The first section offers an overview of aromatherapy and essential oils. The second section focuses on the clinical use of aromatherapy and includes topics such as infection, insomnia, pain and inflammation, stress management, dermatology, immunology, oncology, and psychiatric care.

➤ Clark, Marge. 2008. *Essential Oils and Aromatics: A Step-by-Step Guide for Use in Massage and Aromatherapy*. Sandy, UT: Silverleaf Press. 95 pp. ISBN: 1933317736; 9781933317731.
Focusing on almost 50 of the most useful essential oils, this resource discusses the physical and emotional benefits of their use in aromatherapy and massage. The author discusses using the oils through diffusion, in bathing, for skin care, and in massage.

➤ Cooksley, Valerie Gennari. 2002. *Aromatherapy: Soothing Remedies to Restore, Rejuvenate and Heal*. Paramus, NJ: Prentice Hall Press. 400 pp. ISBN: 073520361X; 9780735203617.
This is a good, basic, yet complete introduction to the use of aromatherapy and essential oils. After a very short introductory section, the author provides a guide to the use of essential oils for over 100 common health challenges. She also gives useful, succinct descriptions of 30 essential oils that are frequently used by aromatherapists, including such information as the botanical name, the origin of the oil, extraction method, medicinal properties, safety precautions, and physical and psychoemotional benefits of using the oil.

- Davis, Patricia. 2005. *Aromatherapy, An A–Z: The Most Comprehensive Guide to Aromatherapy Ever Published.* Rev. and enlarged ed. London: Vermillion. 335 pp. ISBN: 009190661X; 9780091906610.
  Providing over 400 entries, this work covers 82 essential oils and more than 200 specific conditions. Although the guide is not the most comprehensive as indicated by its subtitle, it is a useful work that provides useful information in an easy-to-read format. The entries on specific conditions are the most helpful aspect of the work.
- *Essential Oils: Desk Reference.* 2007. 4th ed. Orem, UT: Essential Science Publishing. 558 pp. ISBN: 0943685494; 9780943685496.
  Providing the most up-to-date information on essential oils, this resource includes a wealth of information. After background discussions of the history of essential oils, how they work, their chemistry, their safety, and their production, the work gives detailed information on each oil such as the botanical family, the extraction method, its chemical constituents, its action, its traditional uses, and its indications for use in treating diseases and illnesses. Other sections include oil blends, hormonal therapy, massage techniques using essential oils, and a guide to using essential oils to treat specific illnesses, disorders, and diseases. The appendixes offer even more information, especially research on the use of essential oils.
- Keim, Joni, and Bull, Ruah. 2008. *Daily Aromatherapy: Transforming the Seasons of Your Life with Essential Oils.* Berkeley, CA: North Atlantic Books. 371 pp. ISBN: 1556436939; 9781556436932.
  Organized by season, this book presents 365 daily intention exercises that use essential oils to help transform one's life. The authors present one oil for each week of the month (covering 48 different oils) and discuss its effects on the reader's mind and spirit. Each intention exercise includes an affirmation, emotional self-discovery questions, a ceremony, a blessing, an activity, a visualization, and a prayer.
- Keville, Kathi. 2009. *The Little Book of Aromatherapy.* Rev. 1st ed. New York: Crossing Press. 167 pp. ISBN: 1580911951; 9781580911955.
  The purpose of this guide is to give readers basic information on using essential oil formulas for enhancing beauty, health, and overall well-being. The author presents the most common oils and their use for improving one's complexion, boosting emotions, and even healing specific disorders.
- Keville, Kathi, and Green, Mindy. 2009. *Aromatherapy: A Complete Guide to the Healing Art.* 2nd ed. Berkeley, CA: Crossing Press. 246 pp. ISBN: 1580911897; 9781580911894.
  This is a comprehensive guide to the art and science of aromatherapy, including the creation of therapeutic essential oils and herbal preparations for balancing body, mind, and spirit. The authors present more than 90 formulas for using essential oils in health and first aid, skin and hair care, massage, and relaxation.
- Lawless, Julia. 2002, ©1992. *The Encyclopedia of Essential Oils: The Complete Guide to the Use of Aromatic Oils in Aromatherapy, Herbalism, Health & Well-Being.* London: Thorsons. 226 pp. ISBN: 0007145187; 9780007145188.
  Divided into two parts, this book provides an introduction to aromatics and a survey of over 160 essential oils. The introductory section delves into the historical roots of

aromatherapy and herbalism, their actions on the body, how to use essential oils at home, and the blending of oils. The essential oils survey lists the family of the plant, synonyms, a general description, geographic distribution of the plant, other related species, use in herbal and folk tradition, action, extraction method, characteristics such as color and smell, principal chemical constituents, safety data, aromatherapy and home use, and other uses.

- Lis-Balchin, Maria. 2006. *Aromatherapy Science: A Guide for Healthcare Professionals.* Chicago: Pharmaceutical Press. 462 pp. ISBN: 0853695784; 9780853695783.
  Using an analytical and scientific approach, this book introduces the practices and principles of aromatherapy to health care professionals. The eight chapters provide information on the historical background and practice of aromatherapy, the chemistry and bioactivity of essential oils, the science of smell and its psychological effects, safety issues of aromatherapy, and clinical studies. The book also includes "monographs" on 68 essential oils that provide the related CAS numbers, species/botanical name, synonyms, other species, safety, including GRAS status, extraction and source, appearance and odor, aromatherapy uses, herbal uses, food and perfumery uses, chemistry, toxicity, bioactivities, antimicrobial (including antibacterial and antifungal) activities, antioxidant activity, clinical studies, use in pregnancy and lactation, pharmaceutical guidance, and use in babies and young children. The various appendixes present useful information, generally in chart format.
- Martin, Ingrid. 2007. *Aromatherapy for Massage Practitioners.* Philadelphia: Lippincott Williams & Wilkins. 320 pp. ISBN: 0781753457; 9780781753456.
  Divided into five parts, this work is designed as a textbook that introduces massage therapists to aromatherapy and instructs them on how to integrate it into their massage practices. The first part discusses essential oils and their effects on the body while also providing useful information on 50 common essential oils, focusing on their use in massage. Part 2 delves into practical matters such as the use of carrier oils, safety issues, and blending oils. Incorporating aromatherapy into a massage treatment is the core of Part 3. Specific client issues related to different body systems is discussed in Part 4, while care of the elderly and end-of-life care is considered in Part 5.
- Mojay, Gabriel. 1999. *Aromatherapy for Healing the Spirit: Restoring Emotional and Mental Balance with Essential Oils.* Rochester, VT: Healing Arts Press. 191 pp. ISBN: 0892818875; 9780892818877.
  The author blends concepts from Oriental medicine with the use of essential oils, especially in massage. He discusses the uses and benefits of 40 essential oils.
- Price, Shirley, and Price, Len, eds. 2007. *Aromatherapy for Health Professionals.* Philadelphia: Churchill Livingstone Elsevier. 576 pp. ISBN: 0443101345; 9780443101342.
  Aimed at health care professionals such as nurses, occupational therapists, and physiotherapists, this book is accessible to the motivated lay reader. Divided into four sections, all aspects of aromatherapy are covered. Section 1 covers the science of essential oils such as their chemistry, quality and safety, power and hazards, traditional uses, and modern research. The second section focuses on the practice of aromatherapy such as how essential oils enter the body, touch and massage, and aromatic medicine. The use of aromatherapy in various health care settings comprises section 3. Topics covered include primary health care, critical care, pregnancy and childbirth, learning

disabilities and autism, geriatric care, and palliative and supportive care. The final section delves into policy issues, with a major focus on the United Kingdom. The appendixes provide information on specific essential oils and on the uses of the oils with various diseases and symptoms.

- Rose, Jeanne. 1999. *375 Essential Oils and Hydrosols.* Berkeley, CA: Frog, Ltd. 251 pp. ISBN: 1883319897; 9781883319892.
  The author explores the science of aromatherapy, especially its botanical basis. Thus, she provides an excellent introduction to the scientific names and botanical classification of plants used for making essential oils, although no illustrations of the plants are given. The bulk of the book is devoted to the guide to essential oils. Each entry gives the family of the plant, its habitat and growth extent, its scent, its chemical components, and its medicinal properties, indications, and uses. This is one of the few books that discuss hydrosols, the pure water produced during the distillation process.

- Schiller, Carol, and Schiller, David. 2008. *The Aromatherapy Encyclopedia: A Concise Guide to Over 385 Plant Oils.* Laguna Beach, CA: Basic Health. 234 pp. ISBN: 1591202280; 9781591202288.
  Covering a multitude of different essential oils, this book includes chapters on topics such as the safety, handling, and selection of oils; vegetal oils, butters, and waxes; essential oils; infused oils; methods of application, dispersion, and inhalation of essential oils; the properties of oils; cross-references from botanical names to common names; and plant family name classification.

- Schnaubelt, Kurt. 1998. *Advanced Aromatherapy: The Science of Essential Oil Therapy.* Rochester, VT: Healing Arts Press. 138 pp. ISBN: 0892817437; 9780892817436.
  Although the title includes the word "advanced," this is a good introduction to the science of aromatherapy. The chapters include the history and rise of aromatherapy, the distillation and composition of essential oils, the effects of essential oils, self-treatment using the oils, choosing the appropriate oils, and application of essential oils for specific conditions. The author pays special attention to the chemical components of the oils and uses their chemical signatures to assist in determining the appropriate use of each of the oils he profiles.

- Shutes, Jade, and Weaver, Christina. 2008. *Aromatherapy for Bodyworkers.* Upper Saddle River, NJ: Pearson Prentice Hall. 374 pp. ISBN: 0131737376; 9780131737372.
  Aimed primarily at bodyworkers such as massage therapists and aromatherapists, this book covers the basics of aromatherapy and essential oils. The authors discuss essential oils chemistry, methods of blending oils, the use of oils on the skin, the physiology of olfaction, and applications and techniques of aromatherapy. They also cover the use of aromatherapy in massage and the use of aromatherapy with special populations and in special settings. The work concludes by discussing the business of aromatherapy and provides specific information on 48 commonly used essential oils.

- Tisserand, Robert B. 1985, ©1977. *The Art of Aromatherapy: The Healing and Beautifying Properties of the Essential Oils of Flowers and Herbs.* New rev. ed. Rochester, VT: Healing Arts Press. 321 pp. ISBN: 0892810017; 9780892810017.

Although somewhat dated, this work is still useful. Tisserand covers the history and basic principles of aromatherapy and essential oils. He includes discussions of aromatic baths, massage, and skin care while also giving practical hints and recipes for oil blends and oil infused waters, mouthwash, and cologne. He specifically discusses 28 essential oils.

➤ Tisserand, Robert, and Balacs, Tony. 1998. *Essential Oil Safety: A Guide for Health Care Professionals*. New York: Churchill Livingstone. 279 pp. ISBN: 0443052603; 9780443052606.
Although most books on aromatherapy may include a short section on the safety and the possible adverse effects of essential oils, this book focuses on these topics exclusively. The authors' goal in writing this book is to provide information to ensure the safe and effective use of essential oils while alerting aromatherapists and health care professionals to the potential hazards of using the oils. Of special interest are the chemical profiles of 95 essential oils that emphasize toxicological information. For each oil, the profile gives the botanical name, its family, the part of the plant from which the oil is derived, notable chemical constituents, standardized testing of toxicity, hazards, contraindications, cautions, maximum use levels, toxicity data and recommendations, comments, and other oils that have similar chemistry and/or hazards. The safety index provides charts of oral toxicity, skin irritation, sensitization, and phototoxicity of 177 essential oils. Although technical in nature, this is an essential book for collections on aromatherapy.

➤ Valnet, Jean. 1990. *The Practice of Aromatherapy: A Classic Compendium of Plant Medicines & Their Healing Properties*. Rochester, VT: Healing Arts Press. 279 pp. ISBN: 0892813989; 9780892813988.
Written by one of the "fathers" of aromatherapy, this is an excellent introduction to the practice of aromatherapy and the use of flower essences as agents of healing. Imbued with a scientific basis, the author discusses the healing power of plants, facts about essential oils, and the medicinal uses of the oils. He then provides detailed information on 40 common essential oils. For each oil, he provides the botanic name and genus, the principal known constituents, its healing properties, its indication for use, the methods of use, and additional helpful notes. No illustrations of the source plants are given. Other chapters include a therapeutic index of ailments and the essences used to treat them, case histories, formulae for medicinal wines and vinegars, elixirs, compound preparations, and how to gather and preserve aromatic plants.

➤ Wilson, Roberta. 2002. *Aromatherapy: Essential Oils for Vibrant Health and Beauty*. New York: Avery. 340 pp. ISBN: 1583331301; 9781583331309.
Divided into four parts, this work provides a good introduction to aromatherapy and the use of essential oils. Part 1 discusses the basic principles and history of aromatherapy, including the production of essential oils and hydrosols and the use of carrier oils. Part 2 covers 44 commonly used essential oils, from basil to ylang ylang. The third part focuses on the different ways aromatherapy can be used including air fresheners, baths, diffusers, inhalants, massage, and skin brushing. The last section lists 61 common conditions that can generally be treated with aromatherapy, from acne to a weakened immune system.

Internet Resources

- Aromatherapy Registration Council, www.aromatherapycouncil.org.
  The Aromatherapy Registration Council was formed as an independent organization to provide a public register of aromatherapists who have voluntarily demonstrated their knowledge of the core concepts of aromatherapy through successfully passing a registration examination. The examination is available to those who are self-taught as well as those who have completed aromatherapy coursework.
- AromatherapyPoint, www.aromatherapypoint.com.
  AromatherapyPoint seeks to provide reliable information on aromatherapy and essential oils as well as aromatherapy recipes and using aromatherapy for healing the body, spirit, and mind.
- AromaWeb, www.aromaweb.com.
  Providing over 300 pages about aromatherapy and essential oils, AromaWeb includes articles, profiles of essential oils and carrier oils, recipes, an aromatherapy business directory, and book descriptions.
- The International Federation of Aromatherapists, www.ifaroma.org.
  The International Federation of Aromatherapists promotes excellence within the aromatherapy profession, encourages the use of aromatherapy for health and well-being, supports ethical scientific research of essential oils, and advances professional standards of education and training. In addition to pages on aromatherapy and essential oils, the site also includes directories of aromatherapists and aromatherapy courses.
- National Association for Holistic Aromatherapy, www.naha.org.
  The goal of the National Association for Holistic Aromatherapy is to enhance public awareness of the benefits of aromatherapy. Their website provides helpful information about aromatherapy and its uses.
- A World of Aromatherapy, www.aworldofaromatherapy.com.
  This website includes many pages on the history of aromatherapy, the basics of using aromatherapy for healing, and the uses and properties of a variety of essential oils.

Periodicals/Magazines/Journals

- *AQ*, published by Aromatherapy Quarterly Inc., 1983– . Quarterly. ISSN: 0966-7164. No web address available.
  Aromatherapy is the skillful use of essential plant oils for medical, psychological, and spiritual applications. This journal explores the chemistry, therapeutic uses of aromatic plants, essential oils, and ancient perfumes, with related articles on travel and archeology.
- *Aromatherapy Journal*, published by the National Association for Holistic Aromatherapy, 2000– . Quarterly. ISSN: 1559-4084. www.naha.org/journal.htm.
  E-mailed to members of the NAHA in pdf format, *Aromatherapy Journal* covers issues, stories, and papers related to aromatherapy and its use as a healing technique. It also includes stories on other natural health modalities such as massage and acupuncture and issues such as the environment that may be of interest to aromatherapists.

- *Aromatherapy Thymes*, published by Aromatherapy Thymes Inc., 2006– . Quarterly. ISSN: 1533-7111. www.aromatherapythymes.com.
This magazine discusses the art and science of aromatherapy, including the practical use of essential oils for physical and emotional healing. Each issue includes an in-depth profile on a selected essential oil, information on essential oil safety, regulatory updates, and a calendar of events.
- *The Aromatherapy Times*, published by the International Federation of Aromatherapists, 1990s– . Quarterly. ISSN: 1748-1686. www.ifaroma.org/index.php?page=IFA_Journal&ID=71.
This informative publication covers developments in aromatherapy from around the world, including research, legislation, workshops, and lectures.
- *Aromatherapy Today*, published by Aromatherapy Today Publications, 1995– . Three times a year. ISSN: 1832-9829. aromatherapytoday.com.
An Australian publication, each issue includes an extensive profile on a specific essential oil in addition to features such as calendars of aromatherapy conferences, research reports, and other items.
- *Aromatic News*, published by Aromatic Plant Project, 2000– . Quarterly. No ISSN. www.aromaticplantproject.com/articles_news.html.
This newsletter provides a wealth of articles on the use of the essential oils of aromatic plants. The articles include information on the plants themselves, specific essential oils, carrier oils, producing oils, cooking, and specific conditions that can be treated using essential oils.
- *International Journal of Clinical Aromatherapy*, published by Essential Oil Resource Consultants, 2004– . Semi-annual. No ISSN. www.ijca.net.
An academic journal focusing on the clinical aspect of aromatherapy, this publication seeks to provide scholarly information on the use of essential oils in health care and related professions. Each issue focuses on a specific theme and includes peer-reviewed articles on the topic.
- *The International Journal of Essential Oil Therapeutics: Exploring the Bioactivity of Aromatic Plants*, published by Essential Oil Resource Consultants, 2007– . Quarterly. No ISSN. www.ijeot.com.
Covering the use of aromatherapy treatment in improving the mental, emotional, and physical health and well-being of clients, this journal provides a scholarly examination of essential oils and their application. The journal was previously titled *The International Journal of Aromatherapy*. Of special interest is the pharmacology, toxicology, drug interactions, safety, and clinical application of essential oils.
- *Journal of Essential Oil Research*, published by Allured Publishing Corp., 1989– . Bimonthly. ISSN: 1041-2905. www.jeoronline.com.
Focusing specifically on essential oil research and analysis, *JEOR* publishes studies on the chemical composition of aromatic plants and their use in flavorings and fragrances. Written by experts from around the world, the articles are peer-reviewed and scholarly in nature.

Chapter 5

Ayurveda

Background and History

Tracing its roots back for over 5,000 years, ayurveda is the traditional medicine of India. In Sanskrit, the word *ayurveda* is usually defined as the science of life, longevity, or daily living. "Ayu" means life or daily living, while "veda" means knowledge, knowing, or science. Thus, ayurveda is concerned with everything pertaining to human life, from birth to death, from health to disease, from depression to spiritual fulfillment. The practice of ayurveda seeks to create balance and health in one's life since illness is viewed as the manifestation of an imbalance in the body, mind, or soul. Treatment of illness is generally accomplished through the use of natural remedies such as herbs, food, surgery, yoga, meditation, and lifestyle changes.

Ayurveda was probably codified in the sixth century BCE, although its true origins are even older, dating back to the Indian sacred writings known as the Vedas (Rik, Sama, Yajur, and Atharva), which were brought to India by the Aryans, a people who invaded India from the northwest around 1500 BCE. The science of ayurveda is primarily based on a variety of ancient Sanskrit texts with two—corresponding to the two major schools of ayurveda—having preeminence. Probably the oldest extant work is the *Samhita* (collection or compendium) by Charaka, which was probably compiled in Kashmir and focuses primarily on internal medicine. The Charaka *Samhita* represents the work of the Atreya school of ayurvedic physicians. The *Samhita* of Sushruta, while also discussing internal medicine, emphasized surgery and is the basis of the Dhanvantari school of ayurvedic surgeons. The oldest extant texts probably date to between 100 BCE and 100 CE.

According to ayurveda, the universe is composed of five fundamental elements: ether, air, fire, water, and earth. These five elements manifest in the human body as the three doshas: vata (or vayu), pitta, and kapha. The three doshas, in turn, govern all physiological and psychological functions of the human body. Illness or disease results from an imbalance in the doshas due to a buildup of waste products (mala) in the body. Diagnosis of diseases can be made through a variety of techniques, including examination of the various pulses, the tongue, the face, the lips, the fingernails, and the eyes, and the taking of a detailed medical history.

Primary Uses

Ayurveda is a complete, holistic system of health and is more comprehensive than simply a medical system. It examines the individual in all aspects of his or her life, including not only the physical realm but also psychological and spiritual aspects. Similar in some respects to modern allopathic medicine, ayurveda is divided into several specialties including pediatrics, gynecology, obstetrics, ophthalmology, otolaryngology, general or internal medicine, geriatrics, surgery, and psychiatry, but it also includes toxicology, fertility and virility, and rejuvenation. Thus, all aspects of the human condition are addressed by ayurveda, whether body, mind, or spirit.

Since one of the major goals of ayurveda is increasing longevity, ayurvedic practitioners emphasize detoxification and rejuvenation to eliminate the potential for diseases in addition to treating specific illnesses and diseases. Therefore, there is often a dual nature to treatment: one part will treat an illness while another part will build the body up to resist disease. There is also an emphasis on maintaining a proper lifestyle that may include meditation, oil massages, and moderate exercise. Since herbs, foods, and spices are the primary healing agents, great attention is paid to proper nutrition and the preparation and consumption of food and drink. As a result, "prescriptions" may actually be specific recipes for preparing meals and beverages that can be consumed not just by the patient but by the whole family. In addition to the physical body, ayurveda is based ultimately in the realm of spirit. Thus, the spiritual development of the patient is extremely important. The ayurvedic practitioner may provide spiritual counseling and instruction in exercises such as meditation and pranayama (breathing exercises). The practitioner may also discuss the use of aromatherapy, yoga, sound therapy (such as the use of mantras and special music), and lifestyle changes.

Training

Ayurvedic physicians or practitioners, also known as vaidyas, receive extensive training. In India, there has been a resurgence in ayurvedic training since the founding of an independent India in 1947. For several centuries, especially under Muslim and British rulers, ayurveda was suppressed. Currently, there are 240 ayurvedic universities and colleges in India that flourish alongside allopathic medical schools. Under rules established by the Central Council of Indian Medicine, ayurvedic practitioners receive 5.5 years of training, which include a 1 year internship. At the end of their training, students receive the degree of Bachelor of Ayurvedic Medicine and Surgery. The Central Council of Indian Medicine (CCIM) was established in 1971, with the goal of regulating and standardizing ayurvedic education.

Outside of India, ayurvedic education is not well controlled. In the United States, ayurvedic education is a combination of resident-based and distance education. Since there is no American equivalent to the CCIM, the various programs stress different aspects of ayurveda and grant certifications and degrees that vary greatly in quality and educational depth. Schools such as the Ayurvedic Institute (www.ayurveda.com), the Mount Madonna Institute (www.mountmadonnainstitute.org), American University of Complementary Medicine (www.aucm.org), and the Ayurveda Academy (www.ayurvedaacademy.com) offer either full-time or part-time residential programs that include student clinics. Many others offer self-study programs.

Sources

Lad, Vasant. 1985. *Ayurveda: The Science of Self-Healing: A Practical Guide*. 2nd ed. Wilmot, WI: Lotus Press.

Svoboda, Robert E. 2004. *Ayurveda: Life, Health and Longevity*. Albuquerque, NM: The Ayurvedic Press.

Tirtha, Swami Sada Shiva. 2007. *The Ayurveda Encyclopedia: Natural Secrets to Healing, Prevention, & Longevity*. 2nd ed. Bayville, NY: Ayurveda Holistic Center Press.

See also YOGA; MEDITATION

Annotated Bibliography

Print Resources

➤ Chopra, Deepak. 2000. *Perfect Health: The Complete Mind Body Guide*. Rev. ed. New York: Three Rivers Press. 390 pp. ISBN: 0609806947; 9780609806944.
The founder of the Chopra Center for Well Being Dr. Chopra was trained in allopathic medicine and is board certified in internal medicine and endocrinology. After meeting Maharishi Mahesh Yogi in 1985, Chopra began to study ayurveda. Based on the principles of ayurveda, this book provides laypersons with a way to apply ayurvedic thought to their own lives in order to improve their health. Only the basics of ayurveda, such as the doshas, are presented. The bulk of the book focuses on how to use the ideas of ayurveda, such as herbs, proper diet, and proper daily routine and exercise to enhance one's health and life, with the result being a longer, healthier life.

➤ Godagama, Shantha, and Hodgkinson, Liz. 2004. *The Handbook of Ayurveda: India's Medical Wisdom Explained*. Berkeley, CA: North Atlantic Books. 128 pp. ISBN: 1556435010; 9781556435010.
Written by the founding president of the Ayurvedic Medical Association, UK, this short book provides an accessible introduction to the world of ayurveda, including the basic principles and the doshas. The author gives advice on proper nutrition and exercise, provides a plan for health and longevity, and discusses issues related to couples and mothers and babies. He also gives a short listing of ayurvedic products that can be useful for treating common ailments.

➤ Inglis, Kim, and Invernizzi, Luca. 2009. *Ayurveda: Asian Secrets of Wellness, Beauty and Balance*. Clarendon, VT: Tuttle. 144 pp. ISBN: 0804840873; 9780804840873.
The authors examine not only ayurveda but also Unani, Siddha, and Tibetan traditional medicine. The three sections of the book cover wellness, beauty, and balance. Thus, it includes topics such as massage, herbal healing, hair care, body wraps, water therapies, yoga, and meditation.

➤ Khalsa, Karta Purkh Singh. 2009. *The Way of Ayurvedic Herbs: A Contemporary Introduction and Useful Manual for the World's Oldest Healing System*. Twin Lakes, WI: Lotus Press. 400 pp. ISBN: 0940985985; 9780940985988.
Designed for the layperson interested in ayurveda, the author discusses the five elements, the basics of ayurveda, the doshas, ayurvedic diagnosis, and ayurvedic treatment. The chapter on food and diet in ayurveda includes sections on fasting and detoxification, milk products, ghee and butter, honey, lemon, salt, mung beans and kicharee, kanji, and more. A materia medica provides detailed information on almost 100 herbs, minerals, and formulas. In addition, treatments for a variety of specific diseases and ailments are detailed.

➤ Lad, Vasant. 1985. *Ayurveda: The Science of Self-Healing: A Practical Guide*. 2nd ed. Wilmot, WI: Lotus Press. 175 pp. ISBN: 0914955012; 9780914955009.

Written by Dr. Vasant Lad, the director of the Ayurvedic Institute in Albuquerque, New Mexico, this work provides an excellent introduction to ayurveda. The goal of the book is to help readers apply the principles of ayurveda to their lives so that they may live a healthier, happier, more fulfilling life. Thus, although the basic principles of ayurveda are discussed, they are presented in a brief format so that they are understandable to the informed layman. The chapters are divided into bite-sized chunks such as the human constitution, disease process, diagnosis, treatment, diet, and lifestyle and routine. There are useful tables, charts, and diagrams interspersed throughout the text. This is one of the best lay introductions to ayurveda.

➤ Lad, Vasant Dattatray. 2002. *Textbook of Ayurveda.* 2 vols.: vol. 1, *Fundamental Principles of Ayurveda*; vol. 2, *A Complete Guide to Clinical Assessment.* Albuquerque, NM: The Ayurvedic Press. ISBN: 1883725070; 9781883725075 (vol. 1); 1883725119; 9781883725112 (vol. 2).
Designed for serious students of ayurveda, this set can serve as a textbook for the professional study of ayurveda. Dr. Lad has compiled in English the most comprehensive discussion available on the science and practice of ayurveda. In the first volume, he presents the underlying principles of the ayurveda. In the second, he discusses ayurvedic clinical assessment. Finally, in the forthcoming third volume, he will provide detailed information on the management of diseases.

➤ Morningstar, Sally. 2008. *Ayurveda Made Simple: An Easy-to-Follow Guide to the Ancient Indian System of Health and Diet by Body Type, with Over 150 Color Photographs.* London: Southwater. 64 pp. ISBN: 1844765792; 9781844765799.
This little book gives a basic explanation of ayurveda, especially body types and the five elements. It then covers diet, massage techniques, and oils, herbs, colors, crystals, gems, exercise and tonics that can assist in maintaining the equilibrium of each body type.

➤ Morrison, Judith H. 1995. *The Book of Ayurveda: A Holistic Approach to Health and Longevity.* New York: Fireside. 192 pp. ISBN: 0684800179; 9780684800172.
Nicely illustrated, this book gives the reader a good introduction to ayurveda with the goal of helping the reader develop a lifestyle aimed at maximizing health, longevity, and enjoyment of life. After providing a simplified history of ayurveda, Morrison delves quickly into the three vital energies, the disease process, and maintaining wellness in today's fast-paced environment. She also includes charts to guide the reader through the process of assessing his or her constitutional type (vata, pitta, or kapha), ailments, and daily and morning routines. A lengthy food chart provides insight into the use of foods with particular constitutional types.

➤ Ninivaggi, Frank John. 2001. *An Elementary Textbook of Ayurveda: Medicine with a Six Thousand Year Old Tradition.* Madison, CT: Psychosocial Press. 286 pp. ISBN: 1887841334; 9781887841337.
This book does an excellent job in providing the basics of ayurveda in an understandable manner. The author, a psychiatrist at Yale School of Medicine, presents the history and development of ayurveda, its theoretical foundations, its concepts of human anatomy and physiology, health and disease processes, nutrition and diet, lifestyle and behavioral regimens, and ayurvedic therapies and medicines. The glossary is extremely helpful since it translates many of the Sanskrit terms used in the text.

- Ninivaggi, Frank John. 2008. *Ayurveda: A Comprehensive Guide to Traditional Indian Medicine for the West.* Westport, CT: Praeger. 349 pp. ISBN: 0313348375; 9780313348372.
  This is a good introduction to ayurveda. The author discusses its history and development, theoretical foundations, anatomy, physiology and digestion, prakruti and vikruti, the disease process, nutrition and diet, and lifestyle and behavioral regimens. He then presents ayurvedic therapies, panchakarma, and a materia medica. The book closes with a discussion of the cultivation of consciousness and the biopsychospiritual perspective in contemporary clinical psychiatry.

- Premila, M. S. 2006. *Ayurvedic Herbs: A Clinical Guide to the Healing Plants of Traditional Indian Medicine.* Binghamton, NY: The Haworth Press. 368 pp. ISBN: 0789017679; 9780789017673.
  With the growth of interest in ayurveda in the United States and Europe, this book is a welcome addition to the medical and herbal literature. The author seeks to bring together traditional information on ayurvedic herbs with the scientific research on these herbs. The results are presented in 12 chapters arranged by how the herbs affect the body, such as gastrointestinal agents, urinary tract drugs, antidiabetic agents, and dental and ophthalmological agents. For each herb, the Sanskrit, English, Hindi, and Tamil names are given. In addition, the entry includes a short introduction, a description of the plant, traditional uses, parts used, chemical constituents, pharmacology, clinical studies, and safety information.

- Ranade, Subhash, and Rawat, Rajan. 2008. *Ayurvedic Massage Therapy: Therapeutic Massage Techniques Based on the Ancient Healing Science of Ayurveda.* Twin Lakes, WI: Lotus Press. 133 pp. ISBN: 0940985993; 9780940985995.
  After introductory chapters on the history of massage, the basic principles of ayurveda, and ayurvedic anatomy and physiology the rest of book is devoted to ayurvedic massage techniques such as kerala massage and marma massage.

- Sharma, Hari M., and Clark, Christopher. 1998. *Contemporary Ayurveda: Medicine and Research in Maharishi Ayur-Veda.* New York: Churchill Livingston. 163 pp. ISBN: 0443055947; 9780443055942.
  Aimed at health care professionals and students, this book seeks to introduce ayurveda to a group grounded in allopathic or Western medicine. The authors argue that medicine needs a new model of treating patients that permits new approaches, such as those offered by ayurveda. They stress that the "consciousness model" of medicine is appropriate for treating patients, and they stress the model emphasis that the whole patient is treated, not just their symptoms. To familiarize physicians and others with ayurveda, the book includes chapters on the foundations of ayurveda, pathogenesis and diagnosis, diet and digestion, the herbal pharmacopeia, the rhythms of nature, purification therapies, exercise, and gynecology, obstetrics, and pediatrics.

- Svoboda, Robert E. 2004. *Ayurveda: Life, Health and Longevity.* Albuquerque, NM: The Ayurvedic Press. 258 pp. ISBN: 1883725097; 9781883725099.
  Svoboda, the first Westerner to graduate from an ayurvedic college and be licensed to practice ayurveda in India, has written an excellent, easily understood introduction to ayurveda. He provides good explanations of ayurveda's history, basic principles, and methods. Chapters such as those on anatomy, routines, food, pathology, diagnosis, and treatment give the reader sufficient insight into ayurveda that many of the principles

can be directly applied to one's own life. In addition, the concepts discussed in the chapters on medicinal substances, pharmacology, disease, and rejuvenation and virilization can provide guidance in the personal use of ayurveda.

- Tirtha, Swami Sada Shiva. 2007. *The Ayurveda Encyclopedia: Natural Secrets to Healing, Prevention, & Longevity*. 2nd ed. Bayville, NY: Ayurveda Holistic Center Press. 669 pp. ISBN: 0965804259; 9780965804257.
  This encyclopedia provides a comprehensive introduction to ayurveda. In addition to providing an excellent discussion of the fundamentals of ayurveda, the author presents easy to understand discussions of ayurvedic analysis, therapeutics, and the treatment of specific illnesses and diseases. One chapter, aptly named "Miscellaneous," discusses topics as broad as headaches, arthritis, dangerous spiritual practices, the use of herbs, recipes, and mutually incompatible foods. If a library could purchase only one book on ayurveda, this would be the best purchase.

Internet Resources

- AllAyurveda.com, www.allayurveda.com.
  Although not well designed, this site provides a wealth of information on ayurveda and its underlying principles. Of special note are the sections on applying the principles to one's own life and diet planning. The site also provides information on meditation, spiritual remedies, and the astrology of India.
- Ayurveda, Holistic Online.com, holisticonline.com/ayurveda/ayv_home.htm.
  This website provides a good introduction to ayurveda, its history, its basic concepts, and balancing the doshas.
- Ayurvedhealthcare.com, www.ayurvedhealthcare.com.
  A good source for general information on ayurveda, this site also has good information on a number of ailments, including remedies and recipes to treat them.
- The Ayurvedic Institute, www.ayurveda.com.
  Produced by the Ayurvedic Institute, one of the leading ayurvedic schools and ayurveda health spas outside of India, this website includes excellent information on the basic concepts and principles of ayurveda, food and nutrition, and ayurvedic cleansing methods.
- Ayurvedic Medicine, nccam.nih.gov/health/ayurveda.
  Provided by the National Center for Complementary and Alternative Medicine, this site provides a very basic introduction to ayurveda and its underlying basis of beliefs. Although the site lacks depth, it gives authoritative information from a well-trusted source.
- Ayurvedic Medicine, Taking Charge of Your Health, University of Minnesota, taking charge.csh.umn.edu/therapies/ayurveda/what.
  Provides an overview of ayurveda and includes sections on the safety of ayurveda and finding an ayurvedic practitioner.

Periodicals and Journals

- *Ancient Science of Life*, published by the International Institute of Ayurveda, 1981– . Quarterly. ISSN: 0257-7941. www.ayurvedajournals.org/index.php/asl.

Published in India, this is a scholarly journal devoted to publishing research papers on ayurveda and its related disciplines. It also covers other aspects of health care.

- *Ayurveda Today*, published by the Ayurvedic Institute. 1988– . Quarterly. No ISSN. www.ayurveda.com/online_resource/ayurveda_today_index.pdf.
  Ayurveda Today is the newsletter of the Ayurvedic Institute and is a benefit of membership in the Institute. It contains in-depth articles on a variety of aspects of ayurveda, recipes, information on herbs, and guidelines on living according to ayurvedic principles.
- *Elements: Ayurveda Health & Nutrition*, published by the International Society for Ayurveda and Health, 2003– . Three times a year. ISSN: 1557-0592. www.ayurvedahealth.org/elements.htm.
  The journal of the International Society for Ayurveda and Health, this publication provides articles on all aspects of ayurveda.
- *Light on Ayurveda: Journal of Health*, published by Light on Ayurveda Educational Foundation, 2002– . Quarterly. No ISSN. www.loaj.com.
  Written for all levels of interest, from students to experienced practitioners, this publication includes articles and case studies on many aspects of ayurveda and yoga. Recent issues have focused on the respiratory system, jyotish, yoga, stress, beauty, and fertility and sterility.

Chapter 6

Chiropractic

Background and History

Chiropractic is generally considered to be the second largest primary health care profession in the United States, with an estimated 53,000 chiropractors currently practicing. Chiropractic can trace its roots back to the ancient Chinese, Greeks, Indians, and Egyptians, among others, who practiced different forms of manipulation to help treat illness and physical ailments, especially lower back pain. Modern chiropractic history is usually traced to Daniel David Palmer, who lived in Davenport, Iowa, in the 1890s. Palmer, after pursuing a variety of careers, became a magnetic healer and used a form of hypnosis and "laying on of hands" for healing. In September of 1895, Palmer treated Harvey Lillard, a building maintenance man who 17 years earlier had become deaf after straining his back while working. Palmer first used his regular healing method, but was not successful. He then examined Lillard's spine and found that one vertebra was painful and out of place. Lillard confirmed that this was indeed the place in his spine that was hurt when he lost his hearing. Palmer repositioned the bone. Soon, Lillard confirmed that he could now hear better than before. Palmer then used this technique of spinal manipulation on other patients who showed improvement after their treatments. After these successes, Palmer sought a name for his technique. A patient of his, Rev. Samuel Weed, knew Greek and when asked for a Greek word for "done by hand," suggested the words *cheiero practikos*, which Palmer shortened to chiropractic.

In 1897 Palmer began to teach his technique in the Palmer School and Cure, which in 1907 became the Palmer School of Chiropractic. Among his first students were several medical doctors, osteopaths, and his son Bartlett Joshua Palmer, who lead the school until his death in 1961. Palmer and his students continued to experiment and to extend chiropractic techniques. Over time, two forms of chiropractic developed, straight and mixed. Straight chiropractic is the more traditional and conservative approach. It focuses on the correction of vertebral subluxations, or spinal misalignments, that affect nerve function. Since such an interruption in the proper functioning of the nerves results in interference with the functioning of the tissues, organs, and cells of the body, correcting subluxations can return the body to a state of health. Mixed chiropractic, in contrast, focuses on a greater analysis of the body and performing spinal and other adjustments that seek to reduce or eliminate disease or symptoms. Additional therapeutic techniques, such as ultrasound, laser acupuncture, nutritional counseling, and orthotics, may be used in addition to spinal manipulation.

Primary Uses and Actions

Chiropractic focuses on disorders of the musculoskeletal system and of the nervous system. It can be used to treat a variety of ailments but is most frequently used in the treatment of pain. Lower back pain has been the subject of several studies that show the efficacy of spinal manipulation. There is also some scholarly evidence that chiropractic treatment is effective in the reduction in pain associated with whiplash, neck pain, migraine headaches, and sciatica. Chiropractors practice a drug-free, hands-on approach to health care that includes patient examination, diagnosis and treatment in the form of spinal and joint manipulation. Often, chiropractors will recommend therapeutic and rehabilitative exercises, nutritional supplementation, and dietary and lifestyle changes.

Training

In general, chiropractic colleges require that their incoming students have completed a minimum of 90 semester hours of undergraduate education in a premedical program, although many students, if not most, will have graduated with a bachelor's degree prior to admission. Course work must include biology, organic and inorganic chemistry, physics, psychology, social sciences, English, and humanities. Once enrolled in a chiropractic college, the student must complete a minimum of 4,200 hours of classroom, laboratory, and clinical experience over four to five years. The first two years of chiropractic training include courses and laboratory work in anatomy, physiology, neuroanatomy, biomechanics, pathology, nutrition, and biochemistry. The final years include courses in manipulation and spinal adjustment and stress clinical experience in physical and laboratory diagnosis, neurology, orthopedics, geriatrics, pediatrics, and radiological technique. Once all requirements are completed, the student is awarded the degree of Doctor of Chiropractic.

Currently, there are 18 Doctor of Chiropractic programs in the United States accredited by the Council on Chiropractic Education. In addition, there are 2 Doctor of Chiropractic programs accredited in Canada, 6 in Australasia, and 4 in Europe. The Council on Chiropractic Education–International establishes accreditation standards so that chiropractic credentials are internationally portable. After graduation, doctors of chiropractic are required to pass the examinations offered by the National Board of Chiropractic Examiners, after which they may be licensed to practice in all 50 states, the District of Columbia, and in many nations around the world. Some states also require that state examinations that supplement the National Board tests be passed before a state license is granted.

Many chiropractic colleges also offer specialized postdoctoral training in fields such as orthopedics, neurology, sports injuries, nutrition, rehabilitation, radiology, industrial consulting, family practice, pediatrics, and applied chiropractic sciences. Once the chiropractor has completed such training, he or she may take specialty exams that permit the use of the title of "diplomate" status in the specialty.

Sources

Green, Bart N., Johnson, Claire, and Sportelli, Louis. 2004. *Opportunities in Chiropractic Careers*. Rev. ed. Chicago: VGM Career Books.

Palmer, D. D. 1997. *The Chiropractor*. Kila, MT: Kessinger.

Peterson, Dennis, and Wiese, Glenda. 1995. *Chiropractic: An Illustrated History*. St. Louis, MO: Mosby.

See also THE ALEXANDER TECHNIQUE; FELDENKRAIS METHOD; THERAPEUTIC MASSAGE AND BODYWORK

Annotated Bibliography

Print Resources

- Benedetti, Paul, and MacPhail, Wayne. 2002. *Spin Doctors: The Chiropractic Industry under Examination*. Tonawanda, NY: Dundurn Press. 296 pp. ISBN: 155002406X; 9781550024067.
  Although based largely on incidents and statistics from Canada, this book is an examination of the chiropractic profession and the theory of subluxations. The authors provide many examples of complications arising from incorrect chiropractic adjustments, including strokes, which are suffered by up to 200 Canadians each year. Decidedly antichiropractic, this is an interesting book that discusses many of the basic tenets of the profession of chiropractic and its practitioners.

- Coulter, Ian D. 1999. *Chiropractic: A Philosophy for Alternative Health Care*. Boston: Butterworth Heinemann. 117 pp. ISBN: 0750640065; 9780750640060.
  The author offers an exploration of the philosophy of chiropractic health care as an exemplar for other alternative health modalities, especially the role of lifestyle in the creation of disease. Although the book will be of greatest interest to chiropractic practitioners and students, it is also of interest to chiropractic patients, to allopathic physicians, and to those interested in alternative medical treatment. In addition, the author provides one way to understand the increasing popularity of complementary and alternative medicine.

- Green, Bart N., Johnson, Claire, and Sportelli, Louis. 2004. *Opportunities in Chiropractic Careers*. Rev. ed. Chicago: VGM Career Books. 140 pp. ISBN: 007141164X; 9780071411646.
  Providing a detailed look at the profession of chiropractic and its educational requirements, this is a highly useful book for anyone interested in pursuing a career in chiropractic. Its chapters give an overview of the profession, the history of chiropractic, the typical day of a chiropractor, education preparation and requirements, and financing a chiropractic education.

- Homola, Samuel. 1999. *Inside Chiropractic*. New York: Prometheus Books. 270 pp. ISBN: 1573926981; 9781573926980.
  Written by a chiropractor, this book takes issue with some of the treatment claims of chiropractic. The author states that he believes chiropractic is useful for back pain, neck pain, and musculoskeletal problems but not useful for the treating of illnesses. Chapters include discussions of subluxation, the causes of and remedies for back pain, chiropractic education, and the gadgets used by chiropractors. For those considering undergoing chiropractic treatment, this is a book that will surely pique their interest.

- Homola, Samuel. 2002. *The Chiropractor's Self-Help Back and Body Book: Your Complete Guide to Relieving Aches and Pains at Home and on the Job*. Alameda, CA: Hunter House. 296 pp. ISBN: 089793377X; 9780897933773.

Back pain is one of the most common ailments for which people seek treatment. This book gives advice on how to treat not only back pain but also head, neck, arm, wrist, hip, leg, and shoulder pain with easy to do home exercise and stretches. Other chapters discuss self-help programs for spinal arthritis, for preventing and easing back pain during pregnancy, and for protecting a painful back during sex. The author also provides information on choosing the appropriate specialist or chiropractor to treat pain, especially back pain.

➤ Lenarz, Michael, and St. George, Victoria. 2003. *The Chiropractic Way: How Chiropractic Care Can Stop Your Pain and Help You Regain Your Health without Drugs or Surgery*. New York: Bantam Books. 357 pp. ISBN: 0553381598; 9780553381597.
Written for those who are considering chiropractic treatment or for patients who wish to understand more about their treatment, this book provides a good introduction to the practice of chiropractic. In the first part, the authors discuss the fundamentals of chiropractic philosophy and practice, how it works, and how its philosophy promotes health and well-being. Part 2 focuses on choosing a chiropractor and gives hints on what to expect during a visit to a chiropractor. It also adds chapters on exercise, proper eating, and relaxation and meditation. The third part broadens the scope of the book to discuss health care in general. Overall, this is an excellent introduction not only to chiropractic but also to choosing a healthy lifestyle.

➤ McDonald, William P., Clum, Gerald W., Cleveland, Ashley E., and Phillips, Reed B. 2009. *Chiropractic Peace*. Norwalk, IA: Foundation for Chiropractic Education and Research. 192 pp. ISBN: 0615279597; 9780615279596.
Written primarily for chiropractic leaders, students, faculty, and practitioners, this book examines the political, sociological, philosophical, and historical issues of the chiropractic profession. The goal is to end the infighting between chiropractors classed as mixers and those classed as straights and to provide a concept of chiropractic care that will accommodate all chiropractors who practice according to basic chiropractic principles.

➤ Norton, Matthew K. 2008. *Where Does It Hurt? Surprising Stories and Insights for Releasing Pain and Restoring Whole Body Health*. New York: Body Mind Press. 253 pp. ISBN: 097997870X; 9780979978708.
The author, a chiropractor with 25 years of experience, shares his ideas and strategies for assisting in the healing of his clients. Using real-life stories, the book presents the author's approach, which is based on using the nervous system to restore health and well-being.

➤ Palmer, D. D. 1997. *The Chiropractor*. Kila, MT: Kessinger. 115 pp. ISBN: 156459775X; 9781564597755.
A reprint of the 1914 edition by the founder of chiropractic, this book takes the reader back to the early days of chiropractic treatment. Important both for its historical significance and for its influence on the practice of chiropractic, the book still has relevance and is an important source of information on the function of the chiropractor and the theoretical basis for much of the treatment used even today in chiropractic therapy.

- Paton, Scott. 2009. *Health beyond Medicine: A Chiropractic Miracle*. Ramsey, NJ: Healthcare Unity Press. 335 pp. ISBN: 0981808301; 9780981808307.
Written by a chiropractor whose gentle chiropractic technique restored his baby's health after doctors could not help, this book addresses what the author calls a broken health care system. After chapters on the insurance industry, vaccines, and antibiotics, the author discusses how chiropractic care can enhance health. He then discusses exercise, nutrition, sleep, and positive living.
- Peterson, Dennis, and Wiese, Glenda. 1995. *Chiropractic: An Illustrated History*. St. Louis, MO: Mosby. 509 pp. ISBN: 0801677351; 9780801677359.
With over 900 illustrations, this work is a fascinating look at the history of chiropractic. The authors trace the history of the profession around the world beginning in ancient times. Individual chapters focus on American medicine in the nineteenth century, Daniel David Palmer, the early twentieth century, the Great Depression and World War II, the postwar years, and the period from the 1960s through the early 1990s. Among the more interesting chapters are the ones on chiropractic adjusting techniques and equipment.
- Reizer, John L. 2002. *Chiropractic Made Simple: Working with the Controlling Laws of Nature*. Otsego, MI: PageFree Publishing. 107 pp. ISBN: 1589610393; 9781589610392.
The purpose of this book is to educate the general public about chiropractic, how it works, and how it can be beneficial to one's health. The author tackles such topics as the inherent intelligence of the body, the concept of subluxation and its effects on health, the safety of chiropractic care, choosing a chiropractor, and the education and licensure of chiropractors. For anyone interested in receiving chiropractic care, this is a good introduction to the profession and its techniques.

Internet Resources

- American Chiropractic Association, www.acatoday.org.
The website of the American Chiropractic Association provides information on chiropractic both for patients such as health tips and a locator service for doctors of chiropractic and for chiropractors such as lobbying information, insurance, and educational opportunities. It also gives access to articles from the *ACA News* and the *Journal of the American Chiropractic Association*.
- Chirobase, www.chirobase.org.
As the subtitle to Chirobase states, this site is "Your skeptical guide to chiropractic history, theories, and practices." Created by Quackwatch, it seeks to provide scientific and accurate information about chiropractic that can help the consumer understand chiropractic care and the often dubious practices of some chiropractors.
- The Chiropractic Resource Organization, www.chiro.org/wordpress.
Designed as a blog, this site features a variety of resources not only about the practice and history of chiropractic but also nutrition, case reports, pediatrics, radiology, and clinical documentation.
- ChiroWeb.com, www.chiroweb.com.
A site for both chiropractors and patients, ChiroWeb.com offers discussion forums, news, webcasts, and classified advertising related to chiropractic.

- Federation of Chiropractic Licensing Boards, www.fclb.org.
  Founded in 1926, the FCLB consists of governmental regulatory boards that regulate chiropractic licensure. The website features links to the chiropractic regulatory boards from Australia, Canada, Mexico, and each of the states of the United States in addition to resources for consumers and those interested in chiropractic education.
- International Chiropractors Association, www.chiropractic.org.
  This website is aimed primarily at chiropractors from around the world and provides information on chiropractic positions, news, legislation, and education.
- PlanetChiropractic.com, www.planetc1.com.
  Begun as online community for chiropractors who wished to share information with one another, the site lists seminars and schools, provides access to news articles and a blog, and acts as a directory of chiropractors in many U.S. cities.
- The World Chiropractic Alliance, www.worldchiropracticalliance.org.
  Founded in 1989 as an advocacy organization, the World Chiropractic Alliance seek to provide both educational opportunities and political action for the practice of chiropractic. In addition, the site features news articles, position papers, press releases, and links to chiropractic resources.
- YourSpine.com, www.yourspine.com.
  YourSpine.com provides consumer information based on chiropractic on pain, women's health, men's health, children's health, and chronic conditions. It also has a search feature that helps the user find chiropractors by zip code, although the listings are incomplete. The site is produced and maintained by Chiropractic America, LLC.

Periodicals/Magazines/Journals

- *ACA News*, published by American Chiropractic Association, 2005– . Monthly. ISSN: 0744-9984. www.acatoday.org/level2_css.cfm?T1ID=34&T2ID=218.
  The professional monthly magazine of the American Chiropractic Association, *ACA News* provides timely and relevant information about legislative, insurance and media-related issues potentially affecting doctors of chiropractic.
- *The American Chiropractor*, published by The American Chiropractor, 1979– . Bimonthly. ISSN: 0194-6536. www.theamericanchiropractor.com.
  This professional trade journal seeks to cover the field of chiropractic and other related health care modalities.
- *Chiropractic and Osteopathy*, published by BioMed Central Ltd., 1996– . Irregular. ISSN: 1746-1340. www.chiroandosteo.com/home.
  Covering all aspects of evidence-based information, this journal reports on clinical research of interest to chiropractors, osteopaths, and related health care professionals.
- *Chiropractic Economics*, published by Doyle Group, 1954– . Eight times a year. ISSN: 1087-1985. www.chiroeco.com.
  Chiropractic Economics is designed to help chiropractors who wish to build and operate their practices more efficiently by offering practical, step-by-step business-management information.

- *Chiropractic History*, published by Association for the History of Chiropractic, 1981– . Semi-annual. ISSN: 0736-4377. www.historyofchiropractic.org/mc/page.do?sitePageId=53364&orgId=ahc.
  This journal publishes papers, book reviews, and short articles on the history of chiropractic and other alternative health practices.
- *The Chiropractic Journal*, published by the World Chiropractic Alliance, 1986– . Monthly. ISSN: 1542-3190. www.worldchiropracticalliance.org/tcj.
  For over 20 years, *The Chiropractic Journal* has published information on the enhancement of chiropractic practice, legislative developments, insurance regulations, and products of interest to chiropractors.
- *The Chiropractic Report: An International Review of Professional and Research Issues*, published by Chiropractic Report, 1987– . Bimonthly. ISSN: 0836-1444; chiropracticreport.com/portal.
  A scholarly journal, *The Chiropractic Report* publishes articles on professional, clinical, and research developments of interest to professional chiropractors.
- *Chiropractic Wellness and Fitness Magazine*, published by Chiropractic Wellness and Fitness Magazine, 2000– . Monthly. ISSN: 1559-4092 www.cwfmonline.com.
  Aimed at the consumer, this magazine focuses on the creation of a healthy lifestyle within which chiropractic care is a central feature.
- *Clinical Chiropractic*, published by Elsevier Ltd., 1997– . Four times a year. ISSN: 1479-2354. www.elsevier.com/locate/clch.
  An international peer-reviewed journal, *Clinical Chiropractic* seeks to enhance the quality of chiropractic treatment by providing clinical information of interest to the practicing chiropractor. Articles focus on the developing of a professional chiropractic practice, on clinical skills and performance, and on the delivery of excellent care.
- *Dynamic Chiropractic*, published by MPA Media, 1983– . Biweekly. ISSN: 1076-9684. www.dynamicchiropractic.com/mpacms/dc/home.php.
  With 26 issues a year, this newsletter provides chiropractors with reliable news and information about their profession and their practices.
- *ICA Review: International Review of Chiropractic*, published by International Chiropractors Association, 1944– . Bimonthly. ISSN: 0899-9260. www.chiropractic.org/index.php?p=services/review_articles.
  The long-running *ICA Review* is a scholarly journal that publishes both scientific and general articles on chiropractic and health-related issues. It is especially known for its review articles that summarize recent relevant professional literature.
- *The Journal of Chiropractic Education*, published by the Association of Chiropractic Colleges, 1989– . Semi-annual. ISSN: 1042-5055. www.journalchiroed.com.
  Covering chiropractic education, this journal includes articles on educational theory, educational methods, and other topics relevant to the practice of chiropractic.
- *Journal of Chiropractic Humanities*, published by National University of Health Sciences, 1992– . Annual. ISSN: 1556-3499. www.journalchirohumanities.com.
  A peer-reviewed journal, the *Journal of Chiropractic Humanities* is devoted to publishing articles on the interaction of the chiropractic profession with the humanities. It covers such topics as history, philosophy, linguistics, literature, jurisprudence, ethics,

theory, sociology, comparative religion, and even the social sciences that examine historical or philosophical approaches.

- *Journal of Chiropractic Medicine*, published by Elsevier Inc., 1989– . Quarterly. ISSN: 1556-3707. www.elsevier.com/wps/find/journaldescription.cws_home/709855/description#description.
  This journal's purpose is to disseminate information related to the development of an emphasis on primary care within the profession of chiropractic. It publishes both practical and applied information for those practicing chiropractic.
- *Journal of Manipulative and Physiological Therapeutics*, published by Mosby Inc., 1978– . Nine times a year. ISSN: 0161-4754. www.elsevier.com/locate/jmpt.
  This journal is dedicated to the advancement of chiropractic health care by publishing current, peer-reviewed articles on developments in manipulative techniques, on physical therapy, and on other clinical methods.
- *Journal of the American Chiropractic Association*, published by American Chiropractic Association, 1930– . Monthly. ISSN: 1081-7166. www.amerchiro.org/level2_css.cfm?T1ID=11&T2ID=53.
  A major peer-reviewed journal of the practice chiropractic, this journal publishes articles on treatment procedures, current research, and developments in the field of chiropractic.
- *Today's Chiropractic Lifestyle*, published by Life University, 1972– . Bimonthly. ISSN: 1931-7085. www.todayschiropractic.com.
  Written for the practicing chiropractor, *Today's Chiropractic Lifestyle* covers news related to both clinical care and business management.

Chapter 7

Energy Medicine and Energy Healing

Background and History

Energy medicine and energy healing are difficult topics to summarize in a few paragraphs since the concept of "energy" has a wide variety of meanings and its scope can be great or limited, depending on the viewpoint of the individual. To many health care professionals, energy medicine means using electrical current as a therapeutic or diagnostic agent. This may include the use of electroencephalograms (EEGs), transcutaneous electrical nerve stimulation (TENS), or the use of magnetic resonance imaging (MRI). Even in the world of alternative medicine, energy medicine can take on many forms. For example, some consider electro-acupuncture, light therapy, magnets, and sound therapy as versions of energy medicine. Other health care practitioners, both conventional and alternative, may consider all therapies to be based on an understanding of energy because energy, according to physics, is the capacity or power of a system to do work, to put things into motion, or to create light, heat, or sound. All functions of the body including chemical reactions either require energy or release energy. Thus, the use of a pharmaceutical drug or an herbal remedy can be thought of as a use of energy to encourage healing. Similarly, the use of magnets may also be considered a method of energy medicine.

Energy medicine, according to the National Center for Complementary and Alternative Medicine of the National Institutes of Health, falls into two types. First is veritable, which can be measured and employs mechanical vibrations such as sound and electromagnetic forces such as visible light, lasers, and magnetism, and the second is putative, which have yet to be measured. Putative energy includes concepts such as qi from traditional Chinese medicine, prana from ayurveda, vital life force from homeopathy, and therapies such as hands-on healing, Reiki, polarity therapy, acupuncture, and even prayer.

The use of energy medicine, when both definitions are accepted, lies at the basis of most, if not all, healing. More specifically, however, the term "energy" is usually more narrowly used to describe the interrelationship between humans and their environment. The human body itself is seen as an energy system and interacts with the world through this system. As a result, the theory of the human energy system has been developed to a high degree of specificity in medical systems such as traditional Chinese medicine and ayurveda. Concepts such as qi, meridians, prana, chakras, and auras are the result. In overly simplistic terms, energy, known by a variety of terms including qi and prana, flows through channels and energy centers, often called the meridians and chakras, and manifest as the human aura through which the human body interfaces with the world. There is no standardized definition of the anatomy of the human energy system and no direct physical evidence of its existence, although several photographic techniques, including Kirlian photography, claim to be able to photograph the aura. The energy system has also been described by "intuitives" who can see or feel the chakras and aura.

Primary Uses and Actions

According to practitioners of energy healing, most illnesses, whether physical, mental, emotional, or spiritual, can be helped if not healed completely by therapies that use energy techniques. Illness results from disturbances or imbalances of the subtle energies of the body, and these disturbances can be seen or felt in the energy system of the client. When the subtle energy system is unbalanced or blocked, pain and disease may result.

By manipulating the flow of energy to clear an energetic block in the body or to balance the energy system, for example by cleansing an aura, repairing a chakra, or using needles on the acupuncture meridians, health can be restored to the subtle energetic system of the body, which will then, in turn, cause the physical body to return to a state of health. In many energy healing techniques, for example in Reiki and therapeutic touch, the practitioner will use his or her hands to channel or guide the energy flow. In other techniques, devices such as bells and crystals may be used to help direct the energy.

Training

There are no standards for the training of energy healers. Energy healing principles, however, form the basis of traditional Chinese medicine and ayurveda, which have rigorous training programs that can last several years. Others such as Reiki can be learned in a weekend. Several schools of energy healing, such as the Barbara Brennan School of Healing, require at least four years of part-time study.

Sources

Brennan, Barbara Ann. 1988, ©1987. *Hands of Light: A Guide to Healing through the Human Energy Field.* New York: Bantam Books.

Bruyere, Rosalyn L. 1994. *Wheels of Light: Chakras, Auras, and the Healing Energy of the Body.* New York: Simon & Schuster.

Scott-Mumby, Keith. 2005. *Virtual Medicine: A New Dimension in Energy Healing.* Orem, UT: Timpanogos.

See also Ayurveda; Eye Movement Desensitization and Reprocessing; Reiki; Spirituality, Religion, and Prayer; Traditional Chinese Medicine, Acupuncture, and Accupressure

Annotated Bibliography

Print Resources

- Andrews, Ted. 2006. *The Healer's Manual: A Beginner's Guide to Energy Therapies.* Woodbury, MN: Llewellyn. 250 pp. ISBN: 0875420079; 9780875420073.
  Aimed at the beginner, this is a general guide to using energy and vibrational healing techniques on oneself or on others. The author covers topics such as vibrational healing through touch, color, sound, flower and gem elixirs, and incense and oils. He also incorporates discussions of the human energy system and the meridians as a basis for understanding the theory of vibrational healing.

- Birla, Ghanshyam Singh, and Hemlin, Colette. 1999. *Magnet Therapy: The Gentle and Effective Way to Balance Body Systems*. Rochester, VT: Healing Arts Press. 146 pp. ISBN: 0892818417; 9780892818419.
  This small book is an excellent introduction to the use of magnet therapy to enhance the health of the body. The author covers the history of using magnets for health, the types of magnets, the properties of magnets, biomagnetism and its effect on the systems of the body, magnet therapy, and magnetized water. He also presents several case studies of using magnets in a clinical setting.
- Black, Stuart. 2007. *A Way of Life: Core Energetics*. Lincoln, NE: iUniverse. 108 pp. ISBN: 0595328857; 9780595328857.
  The author provides the basics of core energetics, including the dilemmas and the ways each of the character defenses uses to get out of the dilemmas. He also presents the concept of spirituality and God and how these concepts can be used to find pleasure and fulfillment in life.
- Bradford, Michael. 1993. *The Healing Energy of Your Hands*. Berkeley, CA: Crossing Press. 218 pp. ISBN: 0895947811; 9780895947819.
  Using stories from his own experiences in healing others, the author introduces the topic of using the hands to facilitate healing. After writing about his own introduction to hands-on healing, he discusses the concept of energy, sensing energy, understanding healing, and understanding illness. He then proceeds to the relationship between the mind and the healing process and then the role of the healer. Other chapters discuss the healing session itself and include both the interaction between the healer and the recipient and specific techniques that can be used.
- Brennan, Barbara Ann. 1988, ©1987. *Hands of Light: A Guide to Healing through the Human Energy Field*. New York: Bantam Books. 294 pp. ISBN: 0553345397; 9780553345391.
  This is a core work on energy healing written by one of the major teachers of energy work. The author provides a detailed introduction to the concepts of the human energy system, the chakras, and especially the aura. She then examines the psychodynamics of the human energy field, discusses the development of the perceptual abilities of the hands-on healer, delves into spiritual healing, and emphasizes self-healing and the development of one's healing capacities. If only one book on energy healing can be purchased, this is the book.
- Brennan, Barbara Ann. 1993. *Light Emerging: The Journey of Personal Healing*. New York: Bantam Books. 341 pp. ISBN: 0553354566; 9780553354560.
  Written for the healer who uses hands-on energy techniques, this book dives more deeply into the concept of using energy to heal, whether physically, emotionally, psychologically, or spiritually. After an overview of healing and the techniques of healing, the author examines the personal experience of healing, the creation of a healing plan, healing and relationships, and healing through our higher spiritual realities. A variety of exercises are used to enhance the experience of reading the text. For anyone interested in energetic healing, this is a must-read.
- Brownstein, Arthur H. 2005. *Extraordinary Healing: The Amazing Power of Your Body's Secret Healing System*. Gig Harbor, WA: Harbor Press. 367 pp. ISBN: 0936197498; 9780936197494.

In this interesting book, the author discusses the body's own healing system, a topic that is not often broached by medical doctors. Part 1 of the book describes this healing system, how it works, and specific techniques that can be used to strengthen it. Many of the suggestions are common sense, such as getting regular exercise, eating a nutritious diet, and maintaining bowel regularity. Others are less well known, such as the power of humor and laughter in strengthening the immune system, the use of stress reduction techniques, and breathing exercises. Although the book does not really break new ground, it does provide a refreshing way to look at taking charge of one's own health and offers many techniques to increase our resistance to a variety of ailments.

- Bruce, Robert. 2007. *Energy Work: The Secret of Healing and Spiritual Development.* Charlottesville, VA: Hampton Roads. 172 pp. ISBN: 1571745408; 9781571745408.
  This book is for anyone who wants to experience energy healing, whether for themselves or for others. Although the author covers the major concepts of energy anatomy, his focus is primarily on providing direct experience of doing the work through the use of a variety of exercises. Thus, the reader can quickly develop his or her abilities to run energy and to perform healing work on themselves or on others.

- Bruyere, Rosalyn L. 1994. *Wheels of Light: Chakras, Auras, and the Healing Energy of the Body*. New York: Simon & Schuster. 288 pp. ISBN: 0671796240; 9780671796242.
  For those wishing to learn more about the human energy system, this is an excellent introduction. Using a variety of historical images, the author covers the chakras and the auras associated with the healing energy of the body. Special attention is given to the first chakra, which sustains life. Of special note are the chapters on science and the chakras and on the role of the human energy system in disease and dysfunction.

- Chopra, Deepak. 2009. *Reinventing the Body, Resurrecting the Soul: How to Create a New You*. New York: Harmony Books. 287 pp. ISBN: 0307452336; 9780307452337.
  The author argues that the bond between body and soul must be restored so that joy and meaning can return to our lives. Through exercises such as a personal energy efficiency quiz and stories of individuals, Chopra guides the reader through ways to reinvent the body and resurrect the soul, such as his ten steps to wholeness, which can help restore balance and health.

- Co, Stephen, Robins, Eric B., and Merryman, John. 2002. *Your Hands Can Heal You: Pranic Healing Energy Remedies to Boost Vitality and Speed Recovery from Common Health Problems*. New York: Free Press. 297 pp. ISBN: 0743235622; 9780743235624.
  Designed to teach pranic energetic healing especially for use on oneself, this guide provides easy-to-follow instructions that take the reader through the process of pranic healing. The first two chapters focus on the energetic anatomy and the nature of the human mind, while the next ten chapters provide step-by-step directions on using the pranic healing techniques for self-healing. Next, the authors provide directions on using energetic healing techniques to work on 24 common health problems and setting up a daily routine for self-healing. The illustrations that accompany the directions assist in the learning of the techniques.

- Cross, John R. 2008. *Acupuncture and the Chakra Energy System: Treating the Cause of Disease*. Berkeley, CA: North Atlantic Books. 184 pp. ISBN: 1556437218; 9781556437212.

Basing his work on the chakras and the body's energy system, the author presents a technique for healing that incorporates acupuncture for the healing of disease. The first chapter delves into the subtle energy fields of the body, including the aura, while the second chapter provides an in-depth discussion of traditional Chinese medicine and the chakras. Other chapters cover the treatment of pain and chronic conditions, order of treatment, and treatment of ten different conditions. The final chapter presents case histories. The goal of the work is to provide a model for healing, not just treating symptoms.

➤ Dossey, Larry. 2001. *Healing Beyond the Body: Medicine and the Infinite Reach of the Mind*. Boston: Shambhala. 369 pp. ISBN: 1570628602; 9781570628603.
In the essays in this book, the author considers the concepts of mind and consciousness and their interaction with health and healing. To make his arguments, the book is divided into three sections: meaning, mind, and nonlocality. In the section on meaning, he argues that the meanings we perceive affect our minds and our health. The mind, surprisingly, is often ignored in medical education and even in neurology textbooks. In this section, the author reintroduces the mind and its actions to medicine. In the final section, nonlocality, topics such as spirituality, prayer, love, creativity, and immortality are addressed. Thus, for those interested in mind–body medicine, this book provides an easy-to-read foundation in its basic theories.

➤ Eden, Donna, with Feinstein, David. 2008. *Energy Medicine: Balancing Your Body's Energies for Optimal Health, Joy, and Vitality*. Updated and expanded ed. New York: Jeremy P. Tarcher/Penguin. 404 pp. ISBN: 1585426504, 9781585426508.
Designed for those who wish to learn to harness the body's natural energy as a healing modality, the author discusses both the theoretical and the practical aspects of energy medicine. The first part focuses on the concept of energy, on energy testing within the body, and on establishing a daily routine to keep the energy of the body in balance. Part 2 discusses the energetic anatomy of the body and includes chapters on the meridians, the chakras, the aura, the five rhythms, and the triple warmer and the radiant circuits. The last part examines illness, pain, and living within the energetic world. For those seeking an excellent introduction to the concept and principles of energy medicine, this is a wonderful book.

➤ Eden, Donna, and Feinstein, David. 2008. *Energy Medicine for Women: Aligning Your Body's Energies to Boost Your Health and Vitality*. New York: Jeremy P. Tarcher/Penguin. 326 pp. ISBN: 1585426474; 9781585426478.
Aimed specifically at women, the authors first introduce the concepts of vibration and energy. They then provide chapters on topics such as energy techniques for health and vitality, dancing with your hormones, reclaiming the wisdom of your menstrual time, sexuality and fertility, menopause and weight management. The appendix gives tips on examining your body's energies and energy testing.

➤ Emery, Marcia. 1999. *The Intuitive Healer: Accessing Your Inner Physician*. New York: St. Martin's Press. 231 pp. ISBN: 0312199023; 9780312199029.
Using a variety of exercises, the goal of this book is to develop the intuitive power of the reader, especially in regard to one's own health. The Mindshift Method as explained by the author permits one to use one's inner physician to help define a problem or issue and to ask for and receive diagnoses, remedies, and healing

insights. Tapping into the power of dreams and understanding what the intuitive body says can help us create perfect health, minimize stress, and increase wellness.

- Freston, Kathy. 2008. *Quantum Wellness: A Practical and Spiritual Guide to Health and Happiness*. New York: Weinstein Books. 282 pp. ISBN: 1602860181; 9781602860186.
  This is a guidebook to creating what the author calls quantum wellness, which unifies the body, the mind, and the spirit. Chapters discuss the eight pillars of wellness; clearing mental chatter; doing a cleanse; creating a supportive environment; the health, environmental, and spiritual implications of the foods we eat; eating consciously; personal energy management; becoming your own healer; and breaking bad habits.
- Gerber, Richard. 2001. *A Practical Guide to Vibrational Medicine: Energy Healing and Spiritual Transformation*. New York: Quill. 446 pp. ISBN: 0060959371; 9780060959371.
  Building on the author's other work on vibration medicine, this book provides practical advice and information to individuals who wish to learn more about a variety of alternative healing techniques. After a short introduction to vibrational medicine and its principles, the author examines topics such as the energetics of illness and wellness, the chakra system, homeopathy, acupuncture and traditional Chinese medicine, flower essences, color and light, magnetic healing, radionics and distant healing, hand-on healing, and spiritual healing.
- Gerber, Richard. 2001. *Vibrational Medicine: The #1 Handbook of Subtle-Energy Therapies*. 3rd ed. Rochester, VT: Bear & Co. 605 pp. ISBN: 1879181584; 9781879181588.
  Discussing the theory of vibrational, or energy medicine and healing, this is an integral book in seeking to understand this topic. The author synthesizes a wide variety of related topics into a readable book that addresses how vibrational or energy medicine works. He traces the historical perspectives on the art and science of medicine, examines the Einsteinian view of living systems, and discusses the birth of vibrational medicine, especially through the discovery and development of X-rays, CAT scanners, and MRIs. He then introduces the human subtle energy system, including the chakras, the auras, and the acupuncture meridians. He also examines such topics as psychic healing and the use of crystals for healing. The last chapters are devoted to exploring the personal and planetary evolution and recent developments in vibrational medicine.
- Gordon, Richard. 2004. *Your Healing Hands: The Polarity Experience*. Berkeley, CA: North Atlantic Books. 141 pp. ISBN: 1556435258; 9781556435256.
  The pencil drawings and clear directions of this book provide a very good introduction to the energy healing technique known as polarity balancing. After a brief introduction to polarity and to the energy system of the body, the author provides three lessons that lead the reader through the offering of a polarity healing session to others. He then builds on this basic session and discusses specific moves, the use of a polarity circle for healing, natural healing with life force energy, and science and life force. In summary, the book introduces the reader to this simple to learn yet powerful healing technique.

➤ Gordon, Richard. 2006. *Quantum-Touch: The Power to Heal.* 3rd ed. Berkeley, CA: North Atlantic Books. 222 pp. ISBN: 1556435940; 9781556435942.

Quantum-touch is a type of hands-on healing that uses a very light touch to accelerate the body's own healing response. It can be used on oneself or on others. In this book, the author addresses the principles of quantum touch, introduces the various techniques that can be used, and then provides examples of the application of the modality in healing others, oneself, and even animals. Photographs and drawings accompany the clear directions.

➤ Jonas, Wayne B., and Crawford, Cindy C., eds. 2003. *Healing, Intention and Energy Medicine: Science, Research Methods, and Clinical Implications.* New York: Churchill Livingstone. 408 pp. ISBN: 044307237X; 9780443072376.

The chapters in this edited book seek to answer basic questions on the efficacy of mental and spiritual healing techniques such as prayer, ritual, laying on of hands, and imagery. Specifically, the various authors examine the effects of these techniques as related by the scientific literature, the size of the effects, and the clinical impacts of such healing. In total, the authors examined over 2,200 published reports in books, journals, dissertations, abstracts, and other writings. The authors reviewed the correlation between health and spiritual and religious practices, healing or intercessory prayer, energy healing, therapeutic qigong, mental interactions, and mind–matter interaction. Overall, the results suggest that there may be some efficacy in mental and spiritual healing, but the effects are small. In addition, some studies suggest that chronically ill patients may benefit from such healing. For those interested in the effects of spiritual and energy healing, this book is a welcome addition to the literature.

➤ Lade, Arnie. 1998. *Energetic Healing: Embracing the Life Force.* Twin Lakes, WI: Lotus. 272 pp. ISBN: 0914955462; 9780914955467.

This book examines the subtle energy of the inner landscape. It includes discussions of birth, death, and rebirth; the psychoenergetic core; the meridians, qi, and fascia; healing concepts and meditation; Chinese medicine; and yoga and ayurveda.

➤ McCartney, Francesca. 2005. *Body of Health: The New Science of Intuition Medicine for Energy and Balance.* Novato, CA: Nataraj Publishing. 315 pp. ISBN: 1577314883; 9781577314882.

The goal of this book is to teach self-awareness and how to be healthy based on understanding the energetics of our lives. The author stresses that by paying attention to the messages from our bodies and our sensations, we can begin to appreciate our lives at a deeper level and, thus, we will view our worlds in a new way that can lead to a healthier life. Throughout this book, there are exercises and information that facilitate this exploration. Chapters discuss meditation, healing energy, the chakra system, the aura, and color as a healing agent. By the end of the book, readers will have a good understanding of the potential that energy healing can have in their lives.

➤ Myss, Caroline M. 1996. *Anatomy of the Spirit: The Seven Stages of Power and Healing.* New York: Three Rivers Press. 302 pp. ISBN: 0609800140; 9780609800140.

The author is a medical intuitive, one who can "read" a person's illness from their subtle energy. Building on her experiences, she presents a detailed study of the seven major chakras, the power centers of the body. After initial chapters on energy medicine, intuition, and spirituality in which she discusses the human energy field and the symbolic power of the chakras, the Christian sacraments, and the ten sefirot of kabbalah, Myss devotes a chapter to each chakra in which she explores its traditional meaning and its influence on our lives and health. In each chapter she also poses questions for self-examination. For those who wish to learn more about the chakras, this is a must-read.

- Myss, Caroline M. 1998, ©1997. *Why People Don't Heal and How They Can*. New York: Three Rivers Press. 263 pp. ISBN: 0609802240; 9780609802243.
  Divided into two parts, this book examines the twin topics of why people don't heal and how they can from the perspective of energy medicine. The first part addresses the cultural and personal reasons that prevent people from healing and includes chapters on woundology, the five myths about healing, and a review of the chakras. The second part focuses on healing and gives hints on finding the right path to healing, visualizing the chakras, and using the chakras for healing.

- Myss, Caroline M., and Shealy, C. Norman. 1998, ©1993. *The Creation of Health: The Emotional, Psychological, and Spiritual Responses That Promote Health and Healing*. New York: Three Rivers Press. 391 pp. ISBN: 0609803239; 9780609803233.
  Written as a collaboration of two of the most well known writers in the field of alternative and integrative medicine, this book discusses the relationships between emotional dysfunction and physical illness. It focuses primarily on the role that emotional disturbances and stress can play in the creation of common diseases and ailments, from colds to heart disease and cancer. In addition, the authors give many examples on how to create health, how to stay healthy, and how to become an elegant spirit. Throughout the work, case studies support the observations of the authors.

- Nelson, Dawn. 2006. *From the Heart through the Hands: The Power of Touch in Caregiving*. New rev. and updated ed. Findhorn, Forres, Scotland: Findhorn Press. 183 pp. ISBN: 1844090833; 9781844090839.
  Touch is a powerful way to relate to another human being. In this book, the author presents the efficacy of touch in a variety of situations but focuses primarily on care for those who are chronically ill or dying. She provides details on touch techniques, using touch on those in wheelchairs and beds, and establishing touch sessions. In addition, she introduces other complementary relaxation techniques and reviews effective communication skills for use during a touch session.

- Null, Gary. 1998. *Healing with Magnets*. New York: Carroll & Graf. 224 pp. ISBN: 0786705302; 9780786705306.
  This book seeks to detail the use of the power of magnetism to provide optimum health. The author presents the main issues related to using magnet therapy and how to use magnets for healing. He then gives both anecdotal reports from clinicians on how they use magnets and the experiences of patients who receive magnet therapy. The longest chapter of the book provides an annotated listing of peer-reviewed scientific studies on the healing effects of magnets.

- Oschman, James L. 2000. *Energy Medicine: The Scientific Basis*. New York: Churchill Livingstone. 275 pp. ISBN: 0443062617; 9780443062612.
  Based on the scientific literature, this book explores the concept of energy as applied to medicine and healing. It focuses primarily on the theoretical aspects of and the

actual research on the topic rather than on the techniques themselves. Thus, the author has produced a work that is of interest not only to practitioners of energy healing but also to physicians, therapists, patients, and anyone interested in the topic.

➤ Philpott, William H., Kalita, Dwight K., and Goldberg, Burton. 2000. *Magnet Therapy: An Alternative Medicine Definitive Guide*. Tiburon, CA: AlternativeMedicine.com Books. 245 pp. ISBN: 1887299211; 9781887299213.
In this guide, the authors suggest using magnets as a therapeutic tool to treat 35 health conditions, including addictions, asthma, colitis, infections, sleep disorders, and warts. The guide also presents the basics of using magnets to heal and discusses the importance of magnetic fields to health, the history of magnet therapy, how magnets heal, and how to use magnets therapeutically. In addition to the use of magnets, the authors also provide helpful diet and nutrition information for the treatment of the conditions included in the book.

➤ Pierrakos, John C. 2005. *Core Energetics: Developing the Capacity to Love and Heal*. 300 pp. ISBN: 0977439402; 9780977439409.
Written by the founder of Core Energetics, this work provides an excellent introduction to the concepts that underlie this technique. It addresses the physical, emotional, rational, and spiritual aspects of our lives so that we can understand ourselves better and live a more centered and fulfilling life.

➤ Scott-Mumby, Keith. 2005. *Virtual Medicine: A New Dimension in Energy Healing*. Orem, UT: Timpanogos. 256 pp. ISBN: 0935329021; 9780935329025.
Energy is all around us and even within us. This book examines the role that energy plays in health and in healing. After an overview of the history of energy medicine, the author discusses topics such as electro-acupuncture, bioresonance therapy, electrodermal computer screening, and light therapy. Using the concept of energy, the book also attempts to explain the workings of homeopathy, flower remedies, acupuncture, and other healing techniques.

➤ Seidman, Maruti. 2000. *Balancing the Chakras*. Berkeley, CA: North Atlantic Books. 177 pp. ISBN: 1556433395; 9781556433399.
The chakras lie at the heart of the human energy system, and each of the seven major chakras perform specific physical, emotion, and spiritual functions in the body. This guide is a good introduction to the chakras, the energies associated with them, and their use in healing and transformation. The author explores how to balance the chakras using polarity therapy and other modalities such as homeopathy, aromatherapy, herbs, and flower essences. For anyone with an interest in the chakras, this is a good introduction.

➤ Shumsky, Susan G. 2003. *Exploring Chakras: Awaken Your Untapped Energy*. Franklin Lakes, NJ: Career Press. 284 pp. ISBN: 1564146561; 9781564146564.
Although focusing primarily on the experience of the force known as kundalini, this book also uncovers the mysteries of the chakra system. After an initial section devoted to understanding subtle energy, the chapters focus on the individual chakras and on awakening the kundalini. In addition to the seven major chakras, the author discusses seven additional chakras that are related to the major chakras. The anatomy of the chakras is discussed as well as their physical, mental and spiritual manifestations.

- Siegel, Alan. 2006. *Polarity Therapy: Healing with Life Energy*. London: Masterworks International. 196 pp. ISBN: 0954445058; 9780954445058.
  Polarity therapy is rooted in the theory that the energy of the human body forms a pattern or matrix that the body can use to heal itself. In this book, the author seeks to teach how to manipulate or guide that energy to help others heal. Chapters discuss basic energy theory, the law of polarity, the five elements, the three modes of touch, and life energy balancing techniques. In addition, the author briefly examines yoga, diet and nutrition, and counseling.
- Sills, Franklyn. 2005. *The Polarity Process: Energy as a Healing Art*. Berkeley, CA: North Atlantic Books. 191 pp. ISBN: 1556434103; 9781556434105.
  This book is an excellent introduction to polarity therapy and its primary concepts. The author covers such topics as energetic anatomy, the five elements, health and the elements, food, and exercise. Although it is not a text on how to do polarity therapy, it provides deep insight into polarity therapy and will serve as a handy reference to those with an interest in energy healing techniques.
- Smith, Fritz Frederick. 1990, ©1986. *Inner Bridges: A Guide to Energy Movement and Body Structure*. Atlanta: Humanics Limited. 197 pp. ISBN: 0893340863; 9780893340865.
  In this book, the author seeks to build a bridge between Eastern and Western healing systems through a discussion of the human energy system and how it manifests in these disparate systems. He provides a good discussion of the chakra system and how it relates to the physical anatomy of the body. He also examines concepts such as using touch for evaluation of the human body, observing the therapeutic response, and diagnosing illness. Other topics discussed include energy and movement, homeostatic relationships, a new understanding of health and illness, complementary views of disease, and the unfolding life process.
- Stein, Diane. 2006. *Essential Psychic Healing: A Complete Guide to Healing Yourself, Healing Others, and Healing the Earth*. Berkeley, CA: Crossing Press. 191 pp. ISBN: 1580911730; 9781580911733.
  Designed to introduce psychic healing, this book will teach the reader how to get started. The chapters are designed to take the reader through the process of learning about and actually performing psychic healing and cover meditation, visualization, the chakras and aura, energy, spirit guides, hands-on healing, emotional release, crystal healing, distance healing, karma, soul retrieval, spirit attachments, and death.
- Villoldo, Alberto. 2000. *Shaman, Healer, Sage: How to Heal Yourself and Others with the Energy Medicine of the Americas*. New York: Harmony Books. 243 pp. ISBN: 0609605445; 9780609605448.
  Often when energy medicine or energetic healing is discussed, Asian techniques are the first to come to mind. This book shows that energy medicine can also be found in the Americas, especially among the Native American shamans of North and South America. Part 1 examines the belief system of the shamans and their clients on which the healing techniques are based. Part 2 helps the reader understand how the shaman views the world and how sacred and healing spaces are created. Finally, Part 3 describes some of the techniques that a master healer may use, such as working with release points and the chakras. This is not a text on how to use these techniques,

since most must be learned from a master through an apprenticeship, but a description that can open the reader to the myriad ways in which healing can occur.

- White, Ruth. 2003, ©2002. *Energy Healing for Beginners: A Step-by-Step Guide to the Basics of Spiritual Healing*. New York: Jeremy P. Tarcher/Putnam. 195 pp. ISBN: 1585422339; 9781585422333.
  In this book, the author, a transpersonal psychotherapist, seeks to demystify the practice of energy healing. Through stories of individuals, exercises, and a clear writing style, she helps the beginner explore the realm of energy healing and guides him or her toward employing many techniques to aid in their own health and in the health of others. Topics covered include getting started in healing, the meaning of disease, the chakras, the aura, the use of color and crystals to heal, and becoming a professional healer.

Internet Resources

- Barbara Brennan School of Healing, www.barbarabrennan.com.
  The Barbara Brennan School of Healing is one of the largest energy healing schools with over 500 students from around the world. Although the website is dedicated to the school, it also is a good introduction to this popular method of energy healing.
- Energetic Medicine Research, www.energetic-medicine.net.
  This site is one of the largest resources on energetic medicine. Pages include reviews and comparisons of bioenergetic devices used by practitioners, forums for discussion of topics related to energy medicine, information on researchers in the field, articles on bioenergetic medicine, a practitioners directory, and reviews of books.
- The Energy Medicine Institute, www.energymed.org.
  The Energy Medicine Institute is a nonprofit organization that seeks to advance the use of energetic therapies through education, professional training, advocacy, research, and the development of standards for the provision of energetic healing services.
- The International Society for the Study of Subtle Energies and Energy Medicine, www.issseem.org.
  The International Society for the Study of Subtle Energies and Energy Medicine is a respected and authoritative organization that is devoted to the exploration of subtle energies and their application to healing. The organization is interested in all aspects of subtle energy as understood in a broad array of disciplines including quantum physics, subtle energy therapies and healing, psychology, and consciousness. The society also publishes a peer-reviewed, scholarly journal that includes articles of interest to physicians, medical researchers, practitioners of energy medicine, and interested laypeople.
- Natural Healers, www.naturalhealers.com.
  This is an excellent guide to finding a school related to energy healing. Searching can be done by specialty such as acupuncture, homeopathy, or nutrition and by location, especially the United States and Canada.

Periodicals/Magazines/Journals

- *Energy & Consciousness: International Journal of Core Energetics*, published by Institute of Core Energetics, 1991– . Semi-annual. ISSN: 1050-5326. coreenergetics .org/archives/journal.

Including articles on the theory and clinical practice of core energetic psychotherapy, this journal is published by the leading institute focusing on core energetics. It also includes articles that report on current research reports and summarize the literature on this method of psychotherapy.

- *Kindred Spirit: The UK's Leading Guide for Body, Mind and Spirit*, published by Kindred Spirit, 1987– . Six times a year. ISSN: 0955-7067. www.kindredspirit.co.uk.
  Focusing on the body, mind, and spirit, this British magazine covers issues as diverse as spiritual growth, personal development, complementary and alternative medical therapies, travel, and healthful living. It seeks to be a source of positive change in both the lives of individuals and in the world.
- *Smart Life News*, published by Cognitive Enhancement Research Institute, 1992– . Ten times a year. ISSN: 1097-5055. www.ceri.com.
  Dedicated to improving mental performance, increasing energy, and alleviating the symptoms of aging, *Smart Life News* discusses topics such as dealing with Alzheimer's disease, Parkinson's disease, and other afflictions of older individuals.
- *Subtle Energies and Energy Medicine: An Interdisciplinary Journal of Energetic and Informational Interactions*, published by International Society for the Study of Subtle Energies and Energy, 1990– . Three times a year. ISSN: 1099-6591. www.issseem.org/journal.cfm.
  As a peer-reviewed journal, *Subtle Energies and Energy Medicine* is designed to provide scientifically valid and credible research on the healing effects of subtle energies and energy medicine. In addition, it publishes technical and theoretical papers, reports from the field, perspectives of practitioners and researchers, and other articles of interest to clinicians, healers, and laypersons.

Chapter 8

Eye Movement Desensitization and Reprocessing

Background and History

Eye movement desensitization and reprocessing (EMDR) was developed by psychologist Francine Shapiro in 1987. While walking in a park, Shapiro realized that her eye movements appeared to decrease the negative emotions associated with her own distressing memories. Since she assumed that these eye movements had a desensitizing effect, she experimented on others and found that they had the same response. Shapiro believed that eye movements alone could not create this desensitizing by themselves so she added other treatment methods, including a cognitive component, and developed a procedure that she called Eye Movement Desensitization (EMD). After conducting both a case study and a controlled study to test the effectiveness of EMD, she discovered that EMD did result in significant decreases of distress and significant increases of confidence in a positive belief as reported through self-ratings by the clients.

Shapiro continued to develop her approach and over time included a theory that she calls information processing theory into the treatment In 1991, the name of the therapy was changed to Eye Movement Desensitization and Reprocessing (EMDR). Information processing theory seeks to describe how traumatic events can affect the physiology and psychology of an individual. After a traumatic event such as combat, rape, or abuse, information processing about the event may generate strong negative emotions or dissociation, which can interfere with general information processing and prevent more adaptive information processing from occurring. EMDR seeks to help the client process such events so that he or she can return to a state of health.

EMDR has become an accepted therapy as recognized by the American Psychological Association. It has been shown in various studies to be an effective method for treating stress-related disorders such as post-traumatic stress disorder.

Primary Uses and Actions

Eye Movement Desensitization and Reprocessing generally takes place during a therapy session with a certified practitioner. First, the therapist assesses the client's readiness for EMDR treatment and develops a personalized treatment plan to address the issues for which the client has sought therapy. During the treatment itself, the client may be instructed to visualize a vivid image related to the memory of the issue being addressed. The client then focuses on that image, any negative thoughts or feelings, and body sensations while moving his or her eyes back and forth following the therapists fingers for 20 to 30 seconds. In place of the eye movements, some therapists may use another stimulus such as sound or tapping. Next, the client is told to let his or her mind go blank and to notice any thoughts, feelings, memories, or images that arise. The goal is to have the client process any reactions, whether physical, emotional, or mental, that may arise after the visualization and eye movement phase and to replace any negative reactions with a positive belief that has been determined at the beginning of the session. This process may be repeated several times in a session and in subsequent sessions.

Training

As a psychological treatment method, EMDR should be used only by those who have been certified as EMDR practitioners and are licensed mental health clinicians such as social workers, counselors, marriage and family therapists, psychologists, psychiatrists, psychiatric nurses, or graduate students under the supervision of a licensed clinician. The EMDR International Association grants certification only to those who have completed both parts of the basic training course, have at least two years experience in their field of practice as indicated by their licensure, certification, or registration, have conducted at least 50 EMDR sessions with no less than 25 clients, and have received at least 20 hours of consultation with an approved consultant in EMDR. It is estimated that over 60,000 individuals have been trained in EMDR.

Sources

The EMDR Institute, www.emdr.com.

Shapiro, Francine. 2001. *Eye Movement Desensitization and Reprocessing: Basic Principles, Protocols, and Procedures.* 2nd ed. New York: Guilford Press.

See also ENERGY MEDICINE AND ENERGY HEALING; NEURO-LINGUISTIC PROGRAMMING

Annotated Bibliography

Print Resources

- Hartung, John G., and Galvin, Michael D. 2003. *Energy Psychology and EMDR: Combining Forces to Optimize Treatment.* New York: W. W. Norton. 325 pp. ISBN: 0393703789; 9780393703788.
  In this book, the authors discuss the combined use of energy psychology (EP) and EMDR in the clinical setting. After an initial chapter that discusses the basics of both EP and EMDR, they present the research supporting both treatment methods, the methods of conducting therapy using EP or EMDR alone, using them together as complementary therapies, client self-use and phone consultations, self-care for the therapist, applying these therapies in special circumstances, and training for employing each therapy. Throughout the book, examples from actual case studies are used for illustrative purposes.
- Hensley, Barbara J. 2009. *An EMDR Primer: From Practicum to Practice.* New York: Springer. 305 pp. ISBN: 0826119867; 9780826119865.
  As a primer for clinicians who wish to expand their understanding of EMDR and sharpen their skills, this book gives a comprehensive review of the Adaptive Information Processing model and EMDR principles, protocols, and procedures.

- Lipke, Howard. 2000. *EMDR and Psychotherapy Integration: Theoretical and Clinical Suggestions with Focus on Traumatic Stress*. Boca Raton, FL: CRC Press. 152 pp. ISBN: 0849306302; 9780849306303.
  The focus of this book is the author's personal exploration of what he has learned about EMDR and its clinical use, especially with combat veterans. He provides a brief background of EMDR but emphasizes practical implications based on examples from his treatment of those who suffer from combat trauma.
- Maiberger, Barb. 2009. *EMDR Essentials: A Guide for Clients and Therapists*. New York: W. W. Norton. 230 pp. ISBN: 0393705692; 9780393705690.
  This is a good book to introduce the basics of EMDR therapy. The author, a practitioner of EMDR, presents the technique in a straightforward manner and uses stories of individuals who have undergone EMDR to illustrate how the therapy has helped them. Chapters provide an inside look at EMDR therapy and what happens in the therapeutic session as well as discussions of why the therapy works.
- Manfield, Philip, ed. 2003. *EMDR Casebook*. Expanded 2nd ed. New York: W. W. Norton. 360 pp. ISBN: 0393704165; 9780393704167.
  Containing 14 case reports, the purpose of this book is to encourage therapists to use EMDR in their practices for a broad range of cases. It also seeks to give illustrations of how EMDR can treat trauma and to demystify the use of EMDR. Furthermore, it can help newly trained EMDR clinicians begin to use EMDR effectively in their practices. The cases include those dealing with traumatic memories such as post-partum depression and guilt as well as those adults who suffer from childhood trauma or abuse.
- Parnell, Laurel. 2007. *A Therapist's Guide to EMDR: Tools and Techniques for Successful Treatment*. New York: W. W. Norton. 363 pp. ISBN: 0393704815; 9780393704815.
  In addition to reviewing the theoretical basis for EMDR, this book emphasizes ways to successfully utilize EMDR in the therapeutic setting. Citing case examples to illustrate the concepts discussed, the author focuses on tools and techniques for ego strengthening, case formulation, and target development. She also expands the procedural steps and techniques for processing difficulties during the EMDR session itself. The final section deals with specific clinical applications such as working with phobias, recent traumas, and care for the caregiver. Overall, this is a helpful book for the practicing EMDR therapist or student.
- Phillips, Maggie. 2000. *Finding the Energy to Heal: How EMDR, Hypnosis, TFT, Imagery, and Body-Focused Therapy Can Help Restore Mindbody Health*. New York: W. W. Norton. 276 pp. ISBN: 0393703266; 9780393703269.
  This book examines a variety of psychological techniques, including EMDR, hypnosis, thought field therapy, imagery, and body-focused therapy, and it discusses how they can be integrated into a model that can address the complex health needs of a client. Thus, the author introduces these techniques and provides her model of their integration, illustrating her techniques throughout with examples drawn from her own clinical experiences.
- Shapiro, Francine. 2001. *Eye Movement Desensitization and Reprocessing: Basic Principles, Protocols, and Procedures*. 2nd ed. New York: Guilford Press. 472 pp. ISBN: 1572306726; 9781572306721.

This book serves as the definitive guide to EMDR and is used as the textbook for the basic training course in EMDR. It is aimed at researchers, clinicians, and clinical graduate students, although others can readily understand the content. The author discusses the background and history of the technique and offers a model of why EMDR works in a therapeutic setting. She provides in-depth directions on the use of the technique with clients as well as protocols and procedures for using EMDR in special situations and with special populations such as sexual abuse victims and combat veterans.

- Shapiro, Francine, ed. 2002. *EMDR as an Integrative Psychotherapy Approach: Experts of Diverse Orientations Explore the Paradigm Prism*. Washington, DC: American Psychological Association. 441 pp. ISBN: 1557989222; 9781557989222.
  The goal of this book is to provide a better understanding of EMDR and its place in psychological treatment. Aimed at practicing clinicians and others interested in psychotherapy, it includes chapters written by experts from a broad array of psychotherapeutic orientations, including cognitive-behavioral therapy, schema-focused therapy, hypnosis, experiential psychotherapy, feminist therapy, family systems therapy, and transpersonal psychology. The various authors show that EMDR can be integrated into other styles of treatment to produce more robust treatment of psychological trauma.

- Shapiro, Francine, and Forrest, Margot Silk. 2004. *EMDR: The Breakthrough "Eye Movement" Therapy for Overcoming Anxiety, Stress, and Trauma*. Updated ed. New York: Basic Books. 311 pp. ISBN: 0465043011; 9780465043019.
  Designed as a overview of the clinical use of EMDR, this book introduces both the general and the specialist reader to EMDR. The authors take the reader through the process of discovery of EMDR, its development, and its use as a psychotherapeutic technique. Chapters discuss many of the uses of EMDR, including the treatment of post-traumatic stress disorder from combat and sexual assault, phobias, sleep disorders, grief, and addiction.

- Shapiro, Robin, ed. 2005. *EMDR Solutions: Pathways to Healing*. New York: W. W. Norton. 360 pp. ISBN: 039370467X; 9780393704679.
  This book consists of 16 solutions for clinical problems and provides step-by-step instructions on using them with clients. Thus, the work is directed toward practicing EMDR therapists and students. A variety of groups or types of behaviors are addressed, including dissociative identify disorder, phantom limb pain, addictions and dysfunctional behavior, codependence and procrastination, trauma, binging, abuse, anxiety, couples therapy, and children.

- Shapiro, Robin, ed. 2009. *EMDR Solutions II: For Depression, Eating Disorders, Performance, and More*. New York: W. W. Norton. 514 pp. ISBN: 0393705889; 9780393705881.
  Building on her previous work, the editor has compiled a collection of solutions that can assist the therapist in effectively using EMDR to treat a range of issues. Topics covered include using EMDR to treat problems such as depression, eating disorders, and multiple chemical sensitivities, and the book gives assistance in strengthening therapeutic skills.

Internet Resources

- The EMDR Institute, www.emdr.com.
  The website of the EMDR Institute, this site provides almost anything you may want to know about EMDR. It includes pages on efficacy, finding an EMDR clinician, training information, and references to articles about EMDR.
- The EMDR International Association, www.emdria.org.
  The EMDR International Association is the professional association of EMDR clinicians. The association promotes training, research, and the sharing of clinical information about EMDR. The site includes information for clinicians, researchers, and clients.
- The EMDR Network, www.emdrnetwork.org.
  The EMDR Network provides information for clients and clinicians. Pages include a description of EMDR, cautions for clients and clinicians, links for training in EMDR, and resources on marriage and family and on war and disaster.

Periodicals/Magazines/Journals

- *Journal of EMDR Practice and Research*, published by Springer Publishing Company, 2007– . Quarterly. ISSN: 1933-3196. www.springerpub.com/journal.aspx?jid=1933-3196.
  This peer-reviewed scholarly journal is devoted to publishing case studies, research studies, clinical contributions, and review articles about EMDR.
- *What's Happening Now...*, published by EMDR Humanitarian Assistance Programs, 2004– . Three issues per year. No ISSN. www.emdrhap.org/news/archives/php.
  Produced by the EMDR Humanitarian Assistance Programs, this newsletter includes news about EMDR from around the world, the availability of EMDR training, and the use of EMDR for treating trauma and PSTD.

Chapter 9

Feldenkrais Method

Background and History

The Feldenkrais Method was developed by Dr. Moshe Feldenkrais, an atomic physicist, athlete, judo black belt, and educator who was born in the Ukraine but emigrated to Palestine in 1918. He moved to Paris in 1928 and received his Doctor of Science degree from the Sorbonne. In the years before World War II he worked in the field of nuclear science in the laboratory of Nobel Prize winner Frédéric Joliot-Curie of the Curie Institute. He escaped from Nazi occupied Paris and went to England, carrying with him research notes on nuclear fission, plans for bombs, and heavy water that were later used in the Manhattan Project, which resulted in the development of the atomic bomb. Working for the British Admiralty during the war, he also helped develop sonar and other means of detecting submarines.

When Feldenkrais was a young man in Palestine, he injured his knee playing soccer. Although the injury seemed to heal over many months, it was aggravated during a bus accident in England. After surgeons could not offer him a good chance of successful surgery to repair the damage to his knee, Feldenkrais became increasingly interested in movement, health, and healing. Through his study and the application of the ideas he was developing, his knee healed and he discovered that the key to healing was becoming more aware of what one is doing. Then, he successfully applied his techniques to a friend who had severe and chronic back pain. By working with one person at a time, Feldenkrais developed a technique that he called "functional integration." He then began to teach his method to classes and called the class "awareness through movement."

The method that he developed, now called the Feldenkrais Method, uses somatic, or body, education in which the "teacher" uses gentle movement and directed attention to teach the "student" how to improve his or her movement, thereby enhance functioning. The method can help increase range of motion, improve flexibility and coordination, and increase the body's own innate capacity for graceful and efficient movement. These improvements and the awareness that they instill may also improve other aspects of life.

Primary Uses and Actions

The Feldenkrais Method is especially recommended for those with back pain, muscle pain, sports injuries, and neuromuscular conditions, including cerebral palsy and multiple sclerosis. It is also recommended for those with learning disabilities, those who have trouble focusing their attention, those who wish to improve their athletic or musical performance, and for others who simply want to experience improved physical and mental health.

The goal of the Feldenkrais Method is to learn to move with less effort. Since movement and thought are intrinsically related, the method teaches that we can improve our daily lives, our creativity, and our mental awareness by learning to move properly. To learn to move more efficiently and effectively requires that we become aware of our habitual patterns of movement that have been ingrained in our bodies throughout our lifetimes.

Feldenkrais work is offered in two formats. The first format, called Awareness through Movement, is done in group classes in which the teacher will lead the class through sequences of movements in basic positions, including reaching, sitting, lying on the floor, standing, and sitting in a chair. The movements will gradually change from easy and comfortable to ones with greater range and complexity. The classes are usually 30 to 60 minutes in length and may last for four to six weeks. The goal of Awareness through Movement is for the student to learn which movements work better and to increase awareness of the movement. This awareness helps the student recognize habitual patterns and develop new methods of moving that will result in greater flexibility and coordination.

The second format, called Functional Integration, consists of private lessons tailored to the specific needs of each student. During Functional Integration, the teacher uses touch and manipulation to guide the movements of the student who remains clothed throughout the session. Functional Integration seeks to help the student quickly understand their patterns of movement and to develop new movement patterns.

Training

To become a certified Feldenkrais practitioner, one must complete 740–800 hours of training over a three- to four-year period. The trainings consist of participating in Awareness through Movement and Functional Integration lessons, lectures, discussions, group process, and videos of Dr. Feldenkrais teaching. The next step requires that the novice practitioner teach Awareness through Movement and Functional Integration under supervision by a certified practitioner.

In the United States, the Feldenkrais Guild of North America maintains the responsibility of granting certification to practitioners of the Feldenkrais Method by establishing professional practice guidelines and educational requirements.

Sources

Feldenkrais, Moshe. 1990. *Awareness through Movement: Health Exercises for Personal Growth*. San Francisco: HarperSanFrancisco.

Feldenkrais Guild of North America, www.feldenkrais.com.

See also THE ALEXANDER TECHNIQUE; CHIROPRACTIC; THERAPEUTIC MASSAGE AND BODYWORK

Annotated Bibliography

Print Resources

- Baniel, Anat. 2009. *Move into Life: The Nine Essentials for Lifelong Vitality*. New York: Harmony Books. 304 pp. ISBN: 0307395294; 9780307395290.
  Based both on the work of Moshe Feldenkrais and her own method, the author gives the nine essential skills the brain uses in order to thrive. She devotes a chapter to each skill and includes exercises that permit anyone to incorporate them into their everyday

activities. She calls the skills movement with attention, the learning switch, subtlety, variation, slow, enthusiasm, flexible goals, imagination and dreams, and awareness.

- Feldenkrais, Moshe. 1990. *Awareness through Movement: Health Exercises for Personal Growth.* San Francisco: HarperSanFrancisco. 173 pp. ISBN: 0062503227; 9780062503220.
Written by the father of the Feldenkrais Method, this is a good introduction to the principles of the method. Part 1 presents the background and principles of the method. Part 2 gives 12 practical lessons, including lessons on good posture, breathing, pelvic movements, carrying the head, and the relationship between movement of the eyes and movement of the body. The main weakness of the book is that there are only a few illustrations to help in performing the exercises.

- Feldenkrais, Moshe. 2002. *The Potent Self: A Study of Spontaneity and Compulsion.* Berkeley, CA: Frog. 240 pp. ISBN: 1583940685; 9781583940686.
Published posthumously, this work by Feldenkrais serves as an introduction to his thoughts on the human condition and to his method of improving human functioning. He explicates the relationship between faulty posture, pain, and the emotions that can lead to compulsive and dependent behavior. He discusses correct posture and his techniques to teach proper posture while providing several exercises as examples of how to develop proper posture.

- Nelson, Samuel H., and Blades-Zeller, Elizabeth. 2002. *Singing with Your Whole Self: The Feldenkrais Method and Voice.* Lanham, MD: Scarecrow Press. 171 pp. ISBN: 0810840499; 9780810840492.
Although aimed at the singer, this is very good introduction to the Feldenkrais Method in general. The chapters include discussions of the feet and legs, pelvis, breathing, upper trunk, shoulder girdle and arms, head and neck, head and mouth, and the eyes. Within each chapter, the authors have incorporated exercises taken from Feldenkrais's *Awareness through Movement.*

- Plonka, Lavinia. 2004. *What Are You Afraid Of? A Body/Mind Guide to Courageous Living.* New York: Jeremy P. Tarcher/Penguin. 174 pp. ISBN: 1585422851; 9781585423934.
Based on the teachings offered by the Feldenkrais Method, the author tackles dealing with fear. By working with movement directly, the habits associated with physical or psychological issues can be addressed. In this book, she shows how such issues, especially fear, are manifested in our bodies and how they can be addressed by examining the body landscape, thoughts, and posture. She provides exercises that can help correct the way we hold our bodies which, in turn, can relieve the stress related to fear and other physical and psychological issues.

- Rywerant, Yochanan. 2003, ©1983. *The Feldenkrais Method: Teaching by Handling.* North Bergen, NJ: Basic Health. 221 pp. ISBN: 1591200229; 9781591200222.
This book is designed to provide a framework for understanding the Feldenkrais Method, which yields change in the mind and body through guiding changes in the movement of the body. It is especially aimed at those who wish to increase their efficiency through better coordination and at those who address such problems in their professions such as dancers, music teachers, physical education teachers, actors, psychologists, and medical professionals. The book focuses exclusively on Functional Integration and not on the Awareness through Movement lessons.

- Shafarman, Steven. 1997. *Awareness Heals: The Feldenkrais Method for Dynamic Health*. Reading, MA: Addison-Wesley. 216 pp. ISBN: 0201694697; 9780201694697.
  In this excellent book the author uses a variety of exercises to take the reader through the basics of the Feldenkrais Method. In addition to sections on the history and background of the method, the book provides six specific lessons based on the teachings of Feldenkrais: bending and breathing, turning and twisting, leaning and lifting, uninhibited breathing, effortless sitting, and elegant walking. Ample illustrations assist in helping the reader perform the simple exercises. After doing just a few of the exercises, the reader will be able to tell differences in his or her body.
- Wildman, Frank. 2006. *Feldenkrais, The Busy Person's Guide to Easier Movement: 50 Ways to Achieve a Healthy, Happy, Pain-Free and Intelligent Body*. Berkeley, CA: Intelligent Body Press. 188 pp. ISBN: 1889618772; 9781889618777.
  This book presents exercises used in the Feldenkrais Method with the purpose of helping the reader achieve pain-free, easy movement. It is divided into eight sections, each dealing with specific activities or areas of the body. The sections include sitting in a chair; reducing tension in the jaw, mouth, face, and neck; driving; back pain; walking; the physical act of thinking; improving breathing; and stress relief. The directions and illustrations for each of the 50 exercises are easy to follow.

Internet Resources

- Feldenkrais Guild of North America, www.feldenkrais.com.
  The website of the Feldenkrais Guild, the official organization of practitioners and teacher of the Feldenkrais Method as established by Moshe Feldenkrais, provides information on the Feldenkrais Method, a directory of practitioners and classes, a listing of classes and related events, resources and publications, and membership information for the Feldenkrais Guild of North America.
- The International Feldenkrais Federation, feldenkrais-method.org.
  The coordinating organization of Feldenkrais Guilds, associations, and Feldenkrais professional organizations worldwide, the International Feldenkrais Federation seeks to coordinate efforts of the international Feldenkrais community to promote the Feldenkrais Method.

Periodicals/Magazines/Journals

- *The Feldenkrais Journal*, published by the Feldenkrais Guild, 1985– . Annual. No ISSN. www.feldenkrais.com/resources/feldenkrais_journal.
  Published annually, *The Feldenkrais Journal* provides articles that seek to increase the understanding of the Feldenkrais Method and its practice as well as photos, drawings, and poetry by Feldenkrais practitioners.
- *SenseAbility Newsletter*, published by the Feldenkrais Educational Foundation of North America, 1987– . Quarterly. No ISSN. www.feldenkrais.com/resources/senseability.
  SenseAbility is distributed to the public by Guild Certified Feldenkrais Practitioners and by the Feldenkrais Guild of North America and is available freely online. The newsletter provides good discussions of the Feldenkrais Method and its use as a therapeutic technique.

Chapter 10

Flower Therapies (Bach Flower Remedies and Flower Essences)

Background and History

Discovered by Dr. Edward Bach, an English physician, bacteriologist, and homeopath, Bach flower remedies use subtle energy to heal. After studying his patients, Dr. Bach came to believe that the emotional states of his patients were related to their diseases. Emotions such as despair or fear were harmful and could eventually lead to the development of disease. To find a cure that could heal such mental and emotional states, he left his medical practice and devoted six years in his search for a simple, natural treatment that did not result in the destruction or altering of the remedy itself.

Dr. Bach was a very spiritual man who believed in his power of intuition or inner knowing. He also had a dream of discovering and developing cures for diseases while simultaneously believing that the medicine of his day was not moving in the correct direction since new illnesses continued to rise and some medicines were becoming useless. Relying on his intuition and through the experimentation that he conducted primarily on himself, he discovered that remedies based on flowers could help heal specific mental states or emotions that he recognized as being the basis of most diseases.

One day, while walking through a field in Wales, he saw the dew sparkling on the flowers and wondered if the dew might be energized with the healing power of the flowers through the action of sunlight. He placed some dew on his tongue and immediately felt the powerful effects, both mentally and physically. He also found that the dew that was not in direct sunlight lacked the power of the dew that was in sunlight. With this as his starting point, he sought to duplicate the process. Thus, he gathered a single type of flower, placed it in a bowl filled with fresh stream water, and left the bowl in the sun for two to three hours. When he tested the water, he felt the same effects as he had with the dew. Over the next couple years, he created the remedies that are known as the Twelve Healers, his first remedies.

After testing and seeing the results of the Twelve Healers on his patients, he published papers and lectured on his new healing technique. He also continued his research and developed the Four Helpers for patients with either persistently negative states of mind or feelings of helplessness. He still felt that there were more remedies to be discovered, and by the end of his life he had discovered 38 remedies.

Since the time of Dr. Bach, others have continued his research into flower essences, and more flowers with healing properties have been found. Of special importance is the Flower Essence Society, which has added 103 North American flower essences to the original 38 discovered by Dr. Bach.

Primary Uses

According to Dr. Bach, the flower remedies work because they raise one's vibrational level and permit the spiritual virtue that one needs to flood throughout our being. Thus, instead of directly treating a disease, Bach flower remedies are used to treat the mental and emotional states that can cause disease. Dr. Bach, in his own writings, classed his remedies under seven headings, specifically remedies for fear, uncertainty, insufficient interest in present circumstances, loneliness, oversensitivity to influences and ideas, despondency or despair, and overcare for the welfare of others. For example, if a patient has a fear of worldly things or a fear of being alone, he or she may be prescribed mimulus. People who are confident that they are right and seek to convert others around them to their ideas may need vervain, while others who feel that they are not quite clean may need crab apple.

Prescribing the correct remedy is an act of intuition and insight into the needs of the patient, with special attention given to the state of mind of the patient. Since several remedies may be indicated, a close analysis of the severity or importance of the symptoms and states of mind must be made. Several remedies may need to be tried before the correct one is found. Usually the remedy is diluted in a small amount of water and sipped during the day. The remedy can also be taken directly on the tongue, added to a bath, or rubbed onto the skin.

The flower remedies themselves, since they are a dilute form of the energy of the flowers, will not cause harm if an overdose is taken. They will also not interact with ordinary prescription medicines.

Training

There is no specific certification or training program required to administer Bach flower remedies or other flower essences. The Flower Essence Society, the Bach Foundation, and a variety of other organizations, institutions, and schools regularly sponsor classes, both in person, by correspondence, or online for those interested in learning about the use of Bach Flower Remedies and other flower essences. The Bach Foundation also maintains a list of practitioners who have completed the foundation's registration process. Many books are available that provide detailed information on the personal use of Bach flower remedies and other flower essences.

Sources

Bach, Edward, and Wheeler, F. J. 1997. *The Bach Flower Remedies*. New Canaan, CT: Keats Publishing.

Scheffer, Mechthild. 2001. *Encyclopedia of Bach Flower Therapy*. Rochester, VT: Healing Arts Press.

See also AROMATHERAPY AND ESSENTIAL OILS; HOMEOPATHY

Annotated Bibliography

Print Resources

- Bach, Edward, and Wheeler, F. J. 1997. *The Bach Flower Remedies*. New Canaan, CT: Keats Publishing. 182 pp. ISBN: 0879838698; 9780879838690.

This small work includes two seminal works by Dr. Edward Bach, *Heal Thyself* and *The Twelve Healers* in addition to *The Bach Remedies Repertory* by F. J. Wheeler. Together these works provide the basic theory that underlies the use of Bach remedies and give a repertory of the moods with their suggested Bach flower remedies.

➤ Ball, Stefan. 2005, ©1998. *The Bach Remedies Workbook.* London: Vermilion. 190 pp. ISBN: 0091906520; 9780091906528.
The aim of this book is to give the reader enough information and practical exercises to help them use the Bach remedies effectively. The book is arranged so that it can be completed in seven days, with each day devoted to a specific topic. For example, day 1 discusses mood remedies while day 5 focuses on healing yourself. Throughout the text, the author intersperses bits of history, details about the various Bach remedies, and even case histories. Each day also has exercises that allow the reader to check his or her understanding of the material. By the end of the book, the reader will have an excellent grasp of the use of the different Bach remedies.

➤ Blome, Gotz. 1999. *Advanced Bach Flower Therapy: A Scientific Approach to Diagnosis and Treatment.* Rochester, VT: Healing Arts Press. 389 pp. ISBN: 089281828X; 9780892818280.
For the individual who is already familiar with the Bach flower remedies, this book permits a deeper understanding of each of the 38 remedies discovered by Dr. Bach. The first section gives a detailed discussion of each remedy, including the characteristics for which the remedy should be used, the emotional or psychological area of use, the causes and symptoms of the syndrome associated with the remedy, the effects of the remedy, psychotherapeutic notes, and common combinations with other essences. The second section delves into new combinations of remedies and their specific uses. The final section is a repertory of symptoms and their associated remedies.

➤ Bradford, Nikki. 2007. *Heal Yourself with Flowers and Other Essences.* London: Quadrille. 304 pp. ISBN: 1844004287; 9781844004287.
Copiously illustrated with photographs of many of the flowers discussed, this book gives a very short introduction to flower essences and arranges the flower essences by their use—for example, relaxation, energy, confidence, joy, sex, purification, letting go, and intuition. Other sections include emergencies, an index to symptoms, and where to buy essences. For each essence, the author provides indications for its use and its effects.

➤ Chancellor, Philip M., comp. and ed. 2005. *Illustrated Handbook of the Bach Flower Remedies: An Authoritative Guide to Natural Healing with Flower Essences.* London: Vermilion. 256 pp. ISBN: 0091906482; 9780091906481.
This is a useful compendium of the Bach flower remedies. The work is divided into two sections. The first describes the method of prescribing the flower remedies for others, for oneself, for pregnancy and childbirth, for children, for mental distress, for animals, and for plants. The bulk of the book is devoted to the 38 remedies themselves, with each remedy being given several pages. For each remedy, keywords are given for its use and then a fuller description of the use of the remedy is presented. The highlights of the chapters for each remedy are the case studies that describe a patient, the reasons the remedy was prescribed, and the result of using the remedy.

- Craydon, Deborah, and Bellows, Warren. 2005. *Floral Acupuncture: Applying the Flower Essences of Dr. Bach to Acupuncture Sites.* Berkeley, CA: Crossing Press. 128 pp. ISBN: 1580911692; 9781580911696.

  In this book, the authors combine the use of the Bach flower remedies with acupuncture. Instead of needles, however, the authors use the flower remedies themselves on the acupuncture points. The chapters present cursory overviews of the flower essences and their uses and of acupuncture and the meridians. The third chapter discusses how to apply the flower essences to the acupuncture points. The final chapter presents the flower essences in alphabetical order and details the specific acupuncture points to use with each remedy.

- Devi Stone, Lila. 2007. *The Essential Flower Essence Handbook: For Perfect Well-Being.* 4th ed. Nevada City, CA: Crystal Clarity Publishers. 336 pp. ISBN: 1565890817; 9781565890817.

  A guidebook to the 20 spirit-in-nature essences, this work provides in-depth information on each essence made from such common plants as lettuce, cherry, peach, corn, apple, strawberry, and grape. The author includes chapters on the origin of the essences, how they work, and producing the essences. She also provides case studies on their use and recipes. The work concludes with an index to positive and negative qualities and conditions along with the suggested essence.

- Harvey, Clare G. 2007. *The New Encyclopedia of Flower Remedies: The Definitive Practical Guide to All Flower Remedies, Their Making and Uses.* London: Watkins Publishing. 428 pp. ISBN: 1842931784; 9781842931783.

  Divided into three parts, this book is a rich compendium of useful information on flower essences. Part 1 discusses using flowers in healing, energy fields, the effects of stress and pollution, and the healing action of flower essences. Part 2, the bulk of the work, discusses flower essences divided by region of the world and their use with babies and children and with pets and animals. Brief descriptions of the properties and therapeutic benefits of over 2,000 essences, combinations, mists, and creams are provided. Part 3 includes an ailment chart to determine appropriate remedies, recipes for combining essences, and advice to practitioners.

- Howard, Judy Ramsell. 2005, ©1992. *Bach Flower Remedies for Women: A Woman's Guide to the Healing Benefits of the Bach Remedies.* London: Vermilion. 184 pp. ISBN: 0091906547; 9780091906542.

  This book focuses specifically on using the Bach flower remedies to treat issues of relevance to women. Chapters discuss a woman's view of herself, especially of her body and her sexuality, menstruation and the reproductive cycle, fertility and infertility, pregnancy and childbirth, unwanted pregnancy or loss of a baby, work and health issues, screening for cervical and breast cancer, and advancing years. Within each chapter, appropriate Bach remedies are suggested to help deal with the issues raised.

- Howard, Judy Ramsell. 2005. *The Bach Flower Remedies Step by Step: A Complete Guide to Selecting and Using the Remedies.* London: Vermilion. 78 pp. ISBN: 0091906539; 9780091906535.

  This short book provides a good introduction to the Bach flower remedies. The author gives an introduction to Dr. Bach and his 38 remedies, and she discusses how to choose the appropriate remedy for others, for oneself, for children, and for animals and plants.

- Hyne Jones, T. W. 2005. *Dictionary of the Bach Flower Remedies: Positive and Negative Aspects.* New ed. London: Vermilion. 88 pp. ISBN: 0091906490; 9780091906498.
  This is a simple dictionary that permits users of the Bach flower remedies to choose an appropriate remedy quickly. Arranged alphabetically by the Bach flower remedy name, each entry gives the negative and the positive aspects of the remedy along with the keywords associated with the remedy.
- Kaminski, Patricia, and Katz, Richard. 2004. *Flower Essence Repertory: A Comprehensive Guide to North American and English Flower Essences for Emotional and Spiritual Well-Being.* Nevada City, CA: Flower Essence Society. 306 pp. ISBN: 0963130684; 9780963130686.
  Aimed at both professional and home use of flower essences, this book is encyclopedic in scope. Part 1 discusses the purpose of flower essence therapy, the properties of flower essences, and the selection and use of flower essences for healing. The second part delves into issues that can be addressed by using flower essences. This section is arranged by specific terms, such as *avoidance*, *confidence*, *guilt*, *perseverance*, and *shame*, and then selected essences are listed with their specific uses related to the term. The third part provides in-depth profiles on 142 different flower essences. For each essence is listed its positive qualities, the patterns of imbalance that it can treat, cross-references to terms from Part 2, and a short discussion of its use.
- Krämer, Dietmar. 1995. *New Bach Flower Therapies: Healing the Emotional and Spiritual Causes of Illness.* Translated by H.-G. Bakker. Rochester, VT: Healing Arts Press. 156 pp. ISBN: 0892815299 9780892815296.
  The author presents his reclassification of the Bach flower remedies that he derived after working with his patients. His classifications include outer flowers that treat negative emotions that arise from external influences and inner flowers that treat internally derived emotions. He further divides the inner flowers into 12 groups or tracks, each of which has one communication flower, one compensation flower, and one decompensation flower. The chapter on discovering the appropriate remedy is very useful and contains a questionnaire that can be of great help during the interview of a patient. This is a companion volume to *New Bach Flower Body Maps.*
- Krämer, Dietmar. 1996. *New Bach Flower Body Maps: Treatment by Topical Application.* Translated by H.-G. Bakker. Rochester, VT: Healing Arts Press. 285 pp. ISBN: 0892815310; 9780892815319.
  Building on his work with his patients, Krämer presents his system of using the Bach flower remedies on the skin to affect healing. He maps 242 areas of the body for their use in healing. The book includes over 200 diagrams that will assist the reader in diagnosing conditions and selecting the appropriate remedy for treatment. This is a companion volume to *New Bach Flower Therapies.*
- McCabe, Vinton. 2007. *The Healing Bouquet: Exploring Bach Flower Remedies.* Laguna Beach, CA: Basic Health Publications. 452 pp. ISBN: 1591200725; 9781591200727.
  This is an excellent introduction to the Bach flower remedies. Part 1 presents a good history of the flower remedies and compares them to homeopathic and allopathic remedies. Part 2 is a reference guide to the 38 Bach remedies, arranged by the seven moods, or emotional states, as identified by Bach. The author provides an in-depth discussion of each remedy, including botanical and general information, negative

and positive qualities of the individual who can benefit from the remedy, use of the remedy for children and adults, and specific issues that suggest use of the remedy. The final part describes the use of the remedies in a healing practice, especially taking cases, combining remedies, and using the remedies themselves.

- PallasDowney, Rhonda. 2007. *The Healing Power of Flowers: Bridging Herbalism, Homeopathy, Flower Essences, and the Human Energy System*. Orem, UT: Woodland Publishing. 446 pp. ISBN: 1580541755; 9781580541756.
  Using ideas derived from herbalism, homeopathy, and Bach flower remedies, the author combines the dimension of the human energy system as represented by the chakras with the use of flower essences. She provides a good discussion of each of the seven major chakras, providing the functions of the chakra and the flower essences that affect it. She also includes the symptoms and patters of imbalance within the chakra and how to treat it with flower essences and with plants of specific colors. A major portion of the book is devoted to a materia medica of 48 different flower essences that lists the plant's common and botanical names, the primary quality associated with the essence, where the plant can be found in nature, the traditional use of the plant, the positive healing patterns that the recipient wishes to gain when taking the essence, suggestions for taking the remedy, and case studies in its use.
- Salmon, Philip, and Jeoffroy, Anna. 2006. *Dr. Bach's Flower Remedies: Tapping into the Positive Emotional Qualities of the Chakras*. Berkeley, CA: North Atlantic Books. 120 pp. ISBN: 1556436408; 9781556436406.
  The authors combine the use of Bach flower remedies with an understanding of the action of the chakras. After a general discussion of Dr. Bach and the chakras, the book is arranged by the seven major chakras. Within each of these chapters, a brief overview of the qualities of the chakra is given followed by a discussion of the remedies associated with that chakra.
- Scheffer, Mechthild. 1988. *Bach Flower Therapy: Theory and Practice*. Translated by A. R. Meuss. Rochester, VT: Healing Arts Press. 240 pp. ISBN: 0892812397; 9780892812394.
  This is a good book for those who are interested in learning about the Bach flower remedies since it combines both the theory and the practice of using the remedies. Of special note is the chapter that provides detailed discussions of each of the 38 different Bach flower remedies.
- Scheffer, Mechthild. 2001. *Encyclopedia of Bach Flower Therapy*. Rochester, VT: Healing Arts Press. 343 pp. ISBN: 0892819413; 9780892819416.
  One of the best general books on the Bach flower remedies, this volume covers all aspects of the history, theory, and use of the remedies for both self-healing and for the healing of others. The chapter on the remedies themselves presents an excellent photograph of each flower and begins with a quote from the writings of Dr. Bach. A detailed discussion of each remedy is given, including the key symptoms for which the remedy can be used, behavior patterns that may indicate the need for the remedy, the positive potential that the remedy can instill, and empowering statements that can be used with the remedy. Other chapters assist the reader in finding the correct Bach remedy, in helping others through the use of the remedies, and in using the remedies in a therapeutic practice. A set of questionnaires and a checklist of symptoms helps the practitioner decide on the appropriate remedy to suggest.

- Scheffer, Mechthild. 2009. *Bach Flowers for Crisis Care: Remedies for Emotional and Psychological Well-Being*. Rochester, VT: Healing Arts Press. 245 pp. ISBN: 1594772967; 9781594772962.
  This book focuses specifically on using the Bach flower remedies for managing psychological and emotional crises. The author presents 50 case studies of common crisis situations, such as divorce, losing one's job, and the death of a loved one and the Bach flower remedies that can be used to provide relief.
- Vennells, David F. 2001. *Bach Flower Remedies for Beginners: 38 Essences That Heal from Deep Within*. St. Paul, MN: Llewellyn Publications. 287 pp. ISBN: 0738700479; 9780738700472.
  For the individual who desires to learn about the Bach flower remedies, this is a good work with which to start. The author provides an interesting account of Dr. Bach's life and work, a good description of preparing and using the remedies, and a brief introduction to each of the 38 remedies. Also included are chapters on using the Bach remedies on animals and on meditation.
- Williamson, Vivien. 2000. *Bach Remedies and Other Flower Essences*. New York: Lorenz Books. 96 pp. ISBN: 075480626X; 9780754806264.
  Copiously illustrated, this book introduces both Bach flower remedies and other flower essences. Although the section on the essences themselves does not provide as much information as some other sources, the explanations for the use of each essence is clear and concise. The strength of this book is its section on prescribing flower essences, which delves into how to conduct a flower essence consultation, how to diagnose which essence to prescribe, and how to treat oneself, children, and animals.

Internet Resources

- Bach Flower Research Programme, www.edwardbach.org.
  A noncommercial site, the Bach Flower Research Programme supports the development of healing herbs, especially the use of the Bach Flower Remedies. The site has links to documents, books, images of flowers, and legal judgments.
- Bach Original Flower Remedies, www.bachremedies.com.
  Provided by Nelsons, a company specializing in the production of homeopathic and flower remedies, this website is devoted to the Bach flower remedies. Nelsons is the official producer of the remedies for the worldwide market. The site provides excellent information about the remedies and their properties, incorporates an interactive remedies chooser, and has information on training programs.
- Bachflower.com, www.bachflower.com.
  Bachflower.com is a retailer of the Original Bach flower remedies. Although this is a commercial website, it does include useful information on the Bach flower remedies, articles on the remedies, a handy questionnaire that can help determine the proper remedies, and descriptions of each remedy drawn from the writings of Dr. Bach.
- The British Flower and Vibrational Essences Association, bfvea.com.
  Although this website has a British slant and its directory lists primarily British practitioners, the pages provide excellent information on flower essences and Bach flower remedies, the history of essences, and their effects on health.

- Dr. Edward Bach Centre, www.bachcentre.com.
  The Dr. Edward Bach Centre is located in Mount Vernon, Oxfordshire, England. Mount Vernon was the home of Dr. Bach during the last years of his life and is where he completed his research into his flower remedies. The center provides excellent information on the remedies themselves and their uses, on training, and on Dr. Bach himself. This is the best single site for the Bach flower remedies.
- Flower Essence Services, www.fesflowers.com.
  Although Flower Essence Services is a commercial site that sells flower essences, the site also provides a wealth of information on the use of flower essences and Bach flower remedies, including frequently asked questions about flower essences and photographs of the flowers used in the essences.
- The Flower Essence Society, www.flowersociety.org.
  The Flower Essence Society (FES) is an international organization composed of health practitioners, researchers, students, and others who maintain an interest in flower essence therapy. The FES was founded in 1979 and is a nonprofit organization that promotes research on the therapeutic uses of flower essences, conducts training and certification programs for flower essence practitioners, and provides information on flower essence therapy to practitioners and to the general public. FES also maintains a referral network of practitioners who employ flower essences in their therapeutic work.

Periodicals/Magazines/Journals

- *The Bach Centre Newsletter*, published by the Bach Centre, 1950– . Three times a year. No ISSN. www.bachcentre.com/centre/nletter.htm.
  As its official newsletter, this publication seeks to present the work of the Bach Centre to the general public and to increase the understanding of the remedies discovered by Dr. Edward Bach. Each issue provides an in-depth description of a particular remedy and its associated mood or personality type. It also presents case histories and success stories drawn from practitioners from around the world.
- *Calix: International Journal of Flower Essence Therapy*, published by the Flower Essence Society, 2004– . No frequency stated. No ISSN. us.fesflowers.com/fes_books.htm#calix.
  Calix presents research on the use of flower essences, including their use in clinical settings. It includes articles on plant studies and scientific reports of flower essence therapy from around the world.
- *Essence: The Journal of the British Flower and Vibrational Essences Association*, published by the British Flower and Vibrational Essences Association, 1998– . Quarterly. ISSN: 1465-8704. bfvea.com/index.php?pr=Essence.
  Available to members of the British Flower and Vibrational Essences Association, this magazine includes articles on research into all aspects of flower essences.
- *Flower Essence Healing Arts Newsletter*, published by the Flower Essence Society, 1981– . Irregular. No ISSN. www.bachflowersusa.com/newsletters.php.
  This newsletter includes articles not only on flower essences but also on other healing arts. Each issue also provides details on a specific flower essence.

- *Vibration Magazine*, published by the World Wide Essence Society, 1998– . Monthly. No ISSN. www.floweressencemagazine.com/blog.
  Available only on the Internet as a blog, *Vibration Magazine* covers all aspects of vibrational remedies, especially flower remedies. It includes articles on single essences, case examples, and special applications of the essences.

Chapter 11

Herbs, Vitamins, Minerals, and Nutritional Supplements

Background and History

The use of plant products for healing probably goes back to the beginning of humankind. The records of using herbs, or plants, as medicines can be traced to the beginning of writing in Sumeria. The ancient medical systems of India (ayurveda) and China (traditional Chinese medicine) have as one of their major bases the use of herbs as medicines. In ancient Egypt, Greece, and Rome, herbs were regularly used for their medicinal purposes. In the Americas, the native peoples all used herbs to treat illness. It is only in recent history that synthetic drugs have replaced herbs from their place as the major sources of healing remedies.

The active constituents of these plant-based remedies were not known until recent times. Medical science, especially beginning in the nineteenth century, began to study medicinal plants and slowly revealed their secrets. As knowledge of the human body and its biochemistry expanded, vitamins and other nutrients were discovered. Such discoveries led to recommendations on the amount of these key ingredients of life that were needed for the proper functioning of the body. Such work continues today as even more vitamins and nutrients are discovered. Thus, the use of supplements to support health has become a multi-billion-dollar business.

The most frequently used terms for employing herbs as medicine are herbalism or herbology, although other terms such as botanical medicine, medical herbalism, herbal medicine, and phytotherapy are also used. Often, the field of herbalism, especially in many traditional medical practices such as traditional Chinese medicine, may include the use of fungi and bee products, minerals, and parts of animals.

Primary Uses and Actions

The action and uses of herbs, vitamins, and other supplements are often equal or superior to that of other remedies, including allopathic drugs. The active ingredients in many modern drugs are actually derived from herbs that have been used traditionally to treat similar problems. It is only in the past century that the active ingredients in herbs have been identified, although many herbalists argue that the whole plant is superior for effective treatment rather than just the active ingredient due to the chemical complexity of most plants. Thus, herbs and other nutrients may be used to treat a wide variety of illnesses and complaints.

Training

There is no standard training for a practitioner of herbalism or for those who recommend the use of vitamins and supplements. For those who practice ayurveda, traditional

Chinese medicine, and naturopathy, a thorough knowledge of the medicinal use of herbs is required and is an integral part of their professional education. With the increase in interest in integrative medicine, some medical schools now offer courses on herbology or include additional information about herbs, vitamins, and supplements in other classes. Other sources of education on herbs, vitamins, and nutritional supplements abound, especially correspondence courses, online programs, and weekend classes. Many health food stores offer consultations on the use of herbs, vitamins, and supplements and some provide classes in their use as well.

Sources

Fritchey, Philip. 2004. *Practical Herbalism: Ordinary Plants with Extraordinary Power.* Warsaw, IN: Whitman Publications.

Miller, Lucinda G., and Murray, Wallace J. 1998. *Herbal Medicinals: A Clinician's Guide.* Binghamton, NY: The Haworth Press.

Tierra, Michael. 1998. *The Way of Herbs: Fully Updated—With the Latest Developments in Herbal Science.* New York: Pocket Books.

See also AROMATHERAPY AND ESSENTIAL OILS; AYURVEDA; HOMEOPATHY; NATUROPATHY AND NATURAL MEDICINE; TRADITIONAL CHINESE MEDICINE, ACUPUNCTURE, AND ACUPRESSURE

Annotated Bibliography

Print Resources

➤ Angier, Bradford, and Foster, David K. 2008. *Field Guide to Medicinal Wild Plants.* 2nd ed. Mechanicsburg, PA: Stackpole Books. 258 pp. ISBN: 0811734935; 9780811734936.
Providing detailed information on over 120 wild plants, this guide is essential for those who wish to find and use medicinal herbs in forests and fields. For each plant, the authors give a color drawing, the plant family, common names, characteristics, area where found, and uses.

➤ Aronson, J. K. 2009. *Meyler's Side Effects of Herbal Medicines.* Amsterdam; London: Elsevier. 303 pp. ISBN: 0444532692; 9780444532695.
After a short introduction to herbal medicines in general, the bulk of this work is a listing of herbal medicines, from acanthaceae to zygophyllaceae, and their possible side effects as drawn from the scientific literature, clinical case studies, expert analysis, and case reports. This is an extremely useful book for medical practitioners, for pharmacists, and for those who wish to use herbal medicines in combination with prescription drugs.

➤ Awang, Dennis V. C., and Robbers, James E. 2009. *Tyler's Herbs of Choice: The Therapeutic Use of Phytomedicinals.* 3rd ed. Boca Raton, FL: CRC Press. 269 pp. ISBN: 0789028107; 9780789028105.
Covering the basics of the use of medicinal herbs as well as the scientific literature, the goal of this work is to provide health care professionals and those with an interest in herbs with a useful compendium of information that can be applied in the treatment of patients. The authors provide a good introduction to the basic principles of

using herbal medicines and to the regulation of these agents. The bulk of the book is devoted to discussing the use of herbal medicines for the treatment of specific health problems organized by bodily system. Other resources provide more information on the herbs themselves, but this one excels in emphasizing their uses.

- Barnes, Joanne, Anderson, Linda A., and Phillipson, J. David. 2007. *Herbal Medicines*. Chicago: Pharmaceutical Press. 710 pp. ISBN: 085369656X; 9780853696568.
  Covering over 150 of the most commonly used medicinal herbs, this resource provides comprehensive monographs on each herb complete with its phytochemical, pharmacological, and clinical aspects such as uses, dosage, efficacy, adverse effects, contraindications, and drug interactions.

- Barrett, Marilyn, ed. 2004. *The Handbook of Clinically Tested Herbal Remedies*. Binghamton, NY: The Haworth Press. 1435 pp. ISBN: 0789010682; 9780789010681.
  These two volumes cover over 160 herbal products made from 32 different herbs and 10 multiherb formulas that have been tested in over 360 clinical studies. Part 1 presents the fundamentals of herbal medicine, including the history and regulation of botanical medicines in the United States, the efficacy and safety of herbal remedies, and the process of conducting clinical trials on herbal remedies and supplements. Part 2 details the methods used in the clinical trials, and Part 3 includes the actual product and clinical trial information. The standard presentation for each herb provides the preparations used in the reviewed clinical studies, a summary table of the studies, adverse reactions, information from a variety of pharmacopaeial monographs, and details on the various related herbal products and their clinical studies. Thus, this is a comprehensive source of information on these commonly used herbs.

- Basch, Ethan M., and Ulbricht, Catherine E. 2005. *Natural Standard: Herb & Supplement Handbook: The Clinical Bottom Line*. St. Louis, MO: Elsevier Mosby. 963 pp. ISBN: 0323029930; 9780323029933.
  Although designed for the medical and health clinician, this work is a wonderful reference resource that provides excellent, scientifically based information on 91 different herbs and supplements that are commonly used. The entry for each herb or supplement gives related terms, background, uses based on scientific evidence with a grade for the strength of that evidence, dosing directions, safety, interactions, and selected references from the medical and scientific literature. Two appendixes on interactions and conditions complete the work. The conditions table is especially helpful since it lists 160 specific illnesses and diseases followed by herbs and supplements rated by their levels of scientific evidence. Thus, this is one of the best general reference works on herbs and supplements due to its reliance on evidence-based practice.

- Blake, Steve. 2008. *Vitamins and Minerals Demystified*. New York: McGraw-Hill. 342 pp. ISBN: 0071489010; 9780071489010.
  For those who need to develop a better understanding of the role of vitamins and minerals in heath, this is a helpful work. Each of the vitamins and minerals needed by the body is thoroughly discussed, including the foods that supply the vitamin or mineral, the amount needed, and its biochemical function within the body. A variety of charts, graphs, and illustrations enhances the text. A quiz on the material concludes each chapter, and a longer test is provided for each part of the book.

- Blumenthal, Mark, ed. 2003. *The ABC Clinical Guide to Herbs*. Austin, TX: American Botanical Council. 480 pp. ISBN: 1588901572; 9781588901576.
  Produced by the American Botanical Council, this is an authoritative guide to the clinical use of 29 of the most commonly used herbs. For each herb it gives an overview of the herb and its historical use, a description of the plant, primary uses, other potential uses, dosages, duration of administration, chemistry, pharmacological actions, mechanisms of action, contraindications, adverse effects, drug interactions, safety rating, regulatory status worldwide, clinical review, branded products, and references to clinical studies. In addition, a chart of the clinical studies that includes the study design, duration, herbal dosage and preparation, and results is given at the end of each chapter. Although the number of herbs covered is much less than many other resources, this is a highly useful guide, especially for those with an interest in the clinical efficacy of herbal products.
- Bohager, Tom. 2009. *Everything You Need to Know about Enzymes: A Simple Guide to Using Enzymes to Treat Everything from Digestive Problems and Allergies to Migraines and Arthritis*. Austin, TX: Greenleaf Book Group Press. 315 pp. ISBN: 1608320197; 9781608320196.
  In this book, the author explains how to use enzymes for good health and to treat specific ailments. Chapters give a general introduction to enzymes and their effects on health, their place in the digestive process, and the use of enzymes for better health. The second part of the work provides information on treating 140 different ailments, from acne and age spots to viral infections and yeast infection.
- Boon, Heather, and Smith, Michael. 2009. *55 Most Common Medicinal Herbs: The Complete Natural Medicine Guide*. 2nd ed., newly expanded and rev. Toronto: R. Rose. 413 pp. ISBN: 0778802159; 9780778802150.
  The authors, both pharmacists, have scoured the scientific literature to produce this work, which covers 55 of the most common medicinal herbs found in pharmacies or health food stores. For each herb they give a sketch of the herb, the medicinal qualities of the herb, its therapeutic value in treating health conditions, current research, and dosage recommendations. There is also a quick reference guide to health conditions and explanations of FDA regulations.
- Bratman, Steven, and Girman, Andrea M. 2003. *Mosby's Handbook of Herbs & Supplements and Their Therapeutic Uses*. St. Louis, MO: Mosby/Healthgate. 1334 pp. ISBN: 0323020151; 9780323020152.
  Designed for the health care provider, this handbook has two sections that can assist providers in discussing potential treatments with their patients. The first covers 76 common medical conditions and the second provides information on 163 commonly used herbs and supplements. For each medical condition, the entry lists principal natural therapies that can be proposed for use, approach to the patient that gives clinical evidence of efficacy of the herbal treatments, other natural therapies that can be tried, and potential drug interactions. For the herbs and supplements, the entries provide the commons uses, approach to the patient, mechanism of action, dosage, safety issues, and drug interactions.
- Capasso, Francesco, Gaginella, Timothy S., Grandolini, Giuliano, and Izzo, Angelo A. 2003. *Phytotherapy: A Quick Reference to Herbal Medicine*. New York: Springer. 424 pp. ISBN: 3540000526; 9783540000525.

Designed for health care professionals, this reference guide provides excellent and scientifically based information on a wide variety of medicinal herbs. The first section of the book discusses phyotherapy in general and includes such topics as the safety of herbal medicines, the scientific research on their use, parts of the plants used, active principles, and regulation of herbal products. The second section is the heart of the book and gives information on the use of medicinal plants with specific systems of the body. For each plant presented, the entry includes the botany and key constituents, the mode of action, clinical efficacy, adverse reactions and contraindications, and preparations and dosage.

- Chevallier, Andrew. 2000. *Encyclopedia of Herbal Medicine*. 2nd American ed. New York: DK Publishing. 336 pp. ISBN: 0789467836; 9780789467836.

  Featuring more than 550 plants, this one-volume encyclopedia seeks to combine the traditional and the folkloric use of plants with discussions of their active constituents and pharmacology. The entries include each plant's history, traditions, folklore, parts used, habitat and cultivation, key constituents, key actions, preparations and their uses, and a research summary, although the studies themselves are not cited. The chapter on the home use of herbal remedies provides cultivation advice as well as instructions on making preparations such as infusions, decoctions, tinctures, syrups, ointments, and poultices. A listing of common problems suggests herbs that can be used as remedies.

- Chevallier, Andrew. 2007. *Herbal Remedies*. New York: DK Publishing. 288 pp. ISBN: 0756628660; 9780756628666.

  A wealth of color photographs enhance this guide to over 140 medicinal herbs. In addition, the author provides good background on the use and safety of herbal medicines. The entries for the individual herbs give the parts used, the actions, and the systems and problems that they address. Key information about the herb is given in a highlighted box that relates the safety and research of the herb as well as the best way to take the herb, its dosage, and any cautions.

- Chillemi, Stacey, and Chillemi, Michael. 2007. *The Complete Herbal Guide: A Natural Approach to Healing the Body*. Morrisville, NC: lulu.com. 487 pp. ISBN: 1430328746; 9781430328742.

  Encyclopedic in scope, this reference work is divided into two parts. The first part lists 60 different conditions and the herbal remedies that can treat them. The conditions vary from acne and anxiety to liver disease and diabetes. For each condition, the entry gives background information and suggests treatments that may include diet, nutritional supplements and vitamins, and herbs and essential oils that can be used. The second section is a listing of over 100 different herbal remedies. Under each herb, the authors give a overview of the herb, a description of the plant, a history of its use, medical uses, dosages, and precautions.

- Combs, Gerald F. 2008. *The Vitamins: Fundamental Aspects in Nutrition and Health*. 3rd ed. Boston: Elsevier Academic Press. 583 pp. ISBN: 012183493X; 9780121834937.

  This is a key text on the vitamins, their biochemistry, and physiological effects for students, health professionals, and anyone interested in learning more about nutrition. Divided into three parts, the book addresses all aspects of vitamins. Part 1 examines the concept of vitamins, their discovery, their chemical and physiological properties, and vitamin deficiency. Part 2 provides detailed information on the individual vitamins, including their sources, absorption, transport, metabolism, excretion, metabolic functions, deficiency, toxicity, and case studies. The final part is practical and focuses on sources of vitamins, assessing vitamin status in humans, quantifying the needs for vitamins, and examining vitamin safety. This work can be considered an encyclopedia of the vitamins.

- Connors, Martha Schindler, and Altshuler, Larry. 2009. *The Everything Guide to Herbal Remedies: An Easy-to-Use Reference for Natural Health Care.* Avon, MA: Adams Media. 292 pp. ISBN: 1598699881; 9781598699883.
  For the general reader, this is a good source that explains the background and practical usage of herbs and herbal preparations. Individual chapters cover topics as broad as healing foods, herbs for specific conditions, herbs for men and women, and herbs for older adults and children. It is especially useful for using herbs to strengthen the immune system and to treat common ailments. The appendixes cover common health concerns and popular herbs.
- Davis, W. Marvin. 2006. *Consumer's Guide to Dietary Supplements and Alternative Medicines: Servings of Hope.* Binghamton, NY: The Haworth Press. 532 pp. ISBN: 0789030411; 9780789030412.
  Written by a long-time professor of pharmacology, this is an excellent overview of both the good and the bad of supplements and their uses. Using a clear writing style that is accessible to any reader, the author examines the truth, the fiction, and the hype surrounding many supplements, including vitamins, minerals, and herbal products. He also discusses the interactions of supplements with prescription drugs and the potential dangers from using supplements incorrectly. This is an important book that provides information that will be of interest to anyone who takes nutritional supplements.
- Duke, James A. 1997. *The Green Pharmacy: New Discoveries in Herbal Remedies for Common Diseases and Conditions from the World's Foremost Authority on Healing Herbs.* Emmaus, PA: Rodale Press. 507 pp. ISBN: 0875963161; 9780875963167.
  Arranged by ailment, the entries suggest a variety of herbal remedies. For example, the suggested remedies for arthritis include ginger, pineapple, red pepper, stinging nettle, oregano, and willow. For each herb, a short description of its action is given and often the dosage or use recommendation, such as brewing a tea, is given. This is a handy, easy to use primer on treating over 120 conditions using herbs.
- Duke, James A. 2002. *The Green Pharmacy Herbal Handbook: Your Everyday Reference to the Best Herbs for Healing.* New York: St. Martin's Paperbacks. 391 pp. ISBN: 0312981511; 9780312981518.
  Covering 180 medicinal herbs that are readily available, this is a wonderful compilation of information. For each herb, the author gives the common and scientific name, a brief discussion of the herb, its therapeutic uses, its medicinal properties, any prescription counterparts, dosage options, a safety rating, and precautions for its use. The major drawback is the lack of illustrations, although most of these herbs are available in health food stores in prepared, usually capsule, form.
- Duke, James A. 2009, ©2008. *The Green Pharmacy Guide to Healing Foods: Proven Natural Remedies to Treat and Prevent More Than 80 Common Health Concerns.* Emmaus, PA: Rodale. 400 pp. ISBN: 1594867135; 9781594867132.

In this book, the author examines the use of food to treat and prevent a variety of health concerns such as high cholesterol, hot flashes, back pain, and the common cold. For each ailment, he gives suggested foods that may prove helpful in treating the ailment and rates the remedies based on his evaluation of scientific studies and anecdotal reports.

- Ebadi, Manuchair S. 2007. *Pharmacodynamic Basis of Herbal Medicine.* 2nd ed. Boca Raton, FL: CRC/Taylor & Francis. 699 pp. ISBN: 0849370507; 9780849370502.
  This is a wide ranging book whose scope is broader than the title indicates. In addition to herbal medicines, the author covers topics such as alternative therapies, vitamins and diet, dietary antioxidants, food–drug and herb–drug interactions, and the use of natural products as a resource to create new drugs. The majority of the book, however, is devoted to examining a wide variety of herbs and related substances, from aloe to chocolate and from algae to yogurt. The focus is the pharmacodynamics of the substance; that is, its actions and effects on the body. The sources of the substance, its chemical constituents, a history of its use, and its efficacy are generally given. Although at times highly technical, this resource gives unique information not found in most other discussions of herbs.

- Editors of Prevention Magazine. 2008. *Healing with Vitamins: The Best Nutrients to Slow, Stop, and Reverse Disease.* Rev. and updated ed. New York: Rodale. 597 pp. ISBN: 1594868069; 9781594868061.
  Designed for the general reader, this guide provides ways to use vitamins and minerals to help heal 90 common health concerns, such as allergies, depression, high blood pressure, high cholesterol, insomnia, and migraines. The recommendations are based on recent research in nutrition science.

- Ernst, Edzard, ed. 2000. *Herbal Medicine: A Concise Overview for Professionals.* Boston: Butterworth-Heinemann. 120 pp. ISBN: 0750645407; 9780750645409.
  Written for health professionals but accessible to the educated layperson, this short work seeks to cover many topics related to herbal medicine. Chapters cover phyto-pharmacology, the quality and standardization of herbal products, the efficacy of herbal drugs, safety issues, and regulation of herbal medicinal products.

- Fiedler, Chrystle. 2009. *The Complete Idiot's Guide to Natural Remedies.* New York: Alpha Books. 452 pp. ISBN: 1592577482; 9781592577484.
  Divided into two main parts, this work provides both background information on natural remedies as well as specific recommendations to treating over 50 different ailments, from acne to weight loss. In addition to functional foods and herbs, it also presents a variety of other alternative therapies that can be used to treat common ailments.

- Foster, Steven, and Duke, James A. 2000. *A Field Guide to Medicinal Plants and Herbs of Eastern and Central North America.* 2nd ed. Peterson Field Guide Series. Boston: Houghton Mifflin. 411 pp. ISBN: 0395988144; 9780395988145.
  For those who wish to find medicinal herbs in the fields and forests of the eastern and central United States, this book is a must-purchase. Covering 500 medicinal plants, this book is a true field guide with excellent photographs that make identification easier. The entry for each plant includes the part of the plant used, a description of

the plant, where it is found, its uses, and warnings about its use. Special symbols are used to indicate if the plant is poisonous, if there are specific cautions, if it is known to cause allergic reactions in some individuals, if it is known to cause dermatitis in some people, and if it is used in modern American medicine.

- Foster, Steven, and Hobbs, Christopher. 2002. *A Field Guide to Western Medicinal Plants and Herbs*. Peterson Field Guide Series. Boston: Houghton Mifflin. 442 pp. ISBN: 0395838061; 9780395838068.
  This volume of the Peterson Field Guide Series covers almost 500 species of medicinal plants and herbs found in the western United States. Color photographs of each plant help in their identification. For each plant the guide provides the common and scientific names, the parts used, a description of the plant, where it can be found, medicinal uses, and warnings, if any. Most of the medicinal uses of the plants are derived from Native American traditions. For those who wish to find medicinal herbs and plants in the wild, this is an essential tool.
- Foster, Steven, and Johnson, Rebecca L. 2006. *Desk Reference to Nature's Medicine*. Washington, DC: National Geographic Society. 416 pp. ISBN: 0792236661; 9780792236665.
  Wonderfully illustrated, this book focuses on healing plants from around the world. Arranged alphabetically, 150 medicinal plants are included. For each plant, the entry includes traditional and current medicinal uses, common names, Latin name, description, habitat, range maps, cultivation and preparation, research, and cautions. A sidebar gives additional interesting information that varies by plant. Separate essays discuss the plants of Africa, Australia and New Zealand, Central and South America, China, Europe, India, North America, the Middle East, and Oceania.
- Fritchey, Philip. 2004. *Practical Herbalism: Ordinary Plants with Extraordinary Power*. Warsaw, IN: Whitman Publications. 444 pp. ISBN: 1885653220; 9781885653222.
  An excellent reference for the practicing herbalist or for those with an interest in natural medicine, this book provides a complete introduction to herbalism, its history, the plants themselves, and the conditions that can be treated using herbs. After a discussion of the evolution of herbal medicine complete with timelines, the author gives a brief review of preparing and preserving herbs. He then devotes a chapter to 48 different herbal actions, such as antacids, anticatarrhals, cholagogues, emetics, lithotriptics, and vulneraries. The bulk of the rest of the book is devoted to descriptions of 46 commonly used herbal remedies, from birch bark to passion flower, from gravel root to yellow dock. For each herb, he gives the scientific and common names, a good photograph of the plant, physical features, historical information, growing range, parts used, cultivation/wildcrafting tips, primary constituents, actions, special considerations, notes, energetics, and tissues, organs, and body systems affected. Then, in chart form he details preparations and dosages, both internal and external, and indicated usages. This is a wonderfully accessible book that will prove to be very valuable to library patrons.
- Gaby, Alan. 2006. *A – Z Guide to Drug–Herb–Vitamin Interactions: Improve Your Health and Avoid Side Effects When Using Common Medications and Natural Supplements Together*. Rev. and expanded 2nd ed. New York: Three Rivers Press. 338 pp. ISBN: 0307336646; 9780307336644.

For almost any library, this is an essential purchase. Since many herbs and nutritional supplements may interact with prescription medicines, and since many individuals do not tell their physicians all of the supplements that they take, it is important to be able to identify possible interactions that may affect a person's health. The book is organized by generic drug type and gives the following categories of interactions: depletion or interference, adverse interaction, side effect reduction/prevention, supportive interaction, and reduced drug absorption/bioavailability. In total, over 4,500 interactions are reviewed. A special appendix lists drug interactions by herb or supplement.

➤ Garran, Thomas Avery. 2008. *Western Herbs According to Traditional Chinese Medicine: A Practitioner's Guide*. Rochester, VT: Healing Arts Press. 257 pp. ISBN: 159477191X; 9781594771910.

This work approaches Western herbs from the Chinese medical perspective and provides a materia medica to these herbs arranged by their action according to traditional Chinese medicine. For example, the materia medica includes chapters such as herbs that resolve the exterior, herbs that clear heat, herbs that drain dampness, and herbs that rectify qi. The book also provides directions to create one's own herbal preparations, tinctures, poultices, and suppositories. Thus, it is an excellent introduction to using herbs in the treatment of common disorders.

➤ Gottlieb, Bill. 2002, ©2000. *Alternative Cures: The Most Effective Natural Home Remedies for 160 Health Problems*. Emmaus, PA: Rodale. 716 pp. ISBN: 1579545920; 9781579545925.

Covering 160 different ailments in an A to Z format, this work suggests remedies for common illnesses as well as serious health problems. For each ailment, a variety of remedies may be suggested including food, fatty acids, vitamins and minerals, herbs, flower essences, or aromatherapy and therapies such as acupressure, massage, homeopathy, breathing exercises, and diet changes. In addition, the author provides one to two page summaries of 22 different healing techniques from acupressure and affirmations to vitamin and mineral therapy. For those who want a simple reference to ailments and their remedies, this is a useful resource.

➤ Graedon, Joe, and Graedon, Teresa. 2002. *The People's Pharmacy Guide to Home and Herbal Remedies*. New York: St. Martin's Press. 608 pp. ISBN: 0312981392; 9780312981396.

This book is specifically designed for those with no medical background and includes a wealth of time-tested home remedies, such as eating raisins soaked in gin to relieve arthritis and drinking ginger tea to relieve the symptoms of a cold. The book is divided into two sections. The first section lists almost 60 common ailments, from allergies to warts, that can be treated using herbal and home remedies. The second section focuses on the herbal therapies themselves and includes detailed information on 50 common herbs, including active ingredients, uses, doses, special precautions, adverse effects, and possible interactions.

➤ Green, James. 2000. *The Herbal Medicine-Maker's Handbook: A Home Manual*. Berkeley, CA: Crossing Press. 384 pp. ISBN: 0895949903; 9780895949905.

For those who wish to make their own herbal medicines, this is a good place to start. The author takes the reader through the process of finding or growing herbs, extracting their essences, distilling hydrosols, creating tinctures and infusions, making ointments and lotions, preparing poultices, and even making herb gelatins. Although there are very few illustrations, the directions are clear and easy to follow. In all, this is a wonderful resource that is different from most books on herbs since its emphasis is on preparing and using the herbs personally.

➤ Griffith, H. Winter. 1998. *Vitamins, Herbs, Minerals, & Supplements: The Complete Guide*. Rev. ed. Tucson, AZ: Fisher Books. 504 pp. ISBN: 1555611656; 9781555611651.
Providing information in easy to use charts, this reference work is truly encyclopedic in scope. It covers vitamins, minerals, amino acids and nucleic acids, other supplements, and medicinal herbs. Each entry provides information such as natural sources, reasons to use, deficiency symptoms, dosage and usage, warnings and precautions, overdose/toxicity, adverse reactions or side effects, and interactions with medicines, vitamins, or minerals.

➤ Hershoff, Asa, and Rotelli, Andrea. 2001. *Herbal Remedies: A Quick and Easy Guide to Common Disorders and Their Herbal Remedies*. New York: Avery. 352 pp. ISBN: 0895299496; 9780895299499.
The authors, both naturopaths, have done an admirable job in distilling a huge amount of information into this useful book. Part 1 discusses how to use herbs including herbal actions, effects, sources, and quality. Part 2 focuses on the systems of the body and how they interact with herbal remedies. Part 3 is the heart of the book and lists 76 conditions and the herbs that can alleviate them. Part 4 presents the herbs themselves as well as their sources, dosage, and safety.

➤ Higdon, Jane. 2003. *An Evidence-Based Approach to Vitamins and Minerals: Health Benefits and Intake Recommendations*. New York: Thieme. 253 pp. ISBN: 1588901246; 9781588901248.
It is estimated that over half the population of the United States currently uses some type of dietary supplement. Thus, it is imperative that health professionals become aware of the best scientific information available on vitamins and minerals that are often used as nutritional supplements. This book provides evidence-based information on 13 vitamins and 14 nutritionally important minerals. The chapters for each vitamin and mineral discuss the function of the nutrient, signs and symptoms of deficiency, role in disease prevention, usefulness in disease treatment, sources, safety, and references to the clinical literature. Although designed for the clinician, this work is also a very good reference source for scientifically based information on vitamins and minerals.

➤ Hobbs, Christopher. 1998. *Herbal Remedies for Dummies*. Foster City, CA: IDG Books. 352 pp. ISBN: 0764551272; 9780764551277.
This is a good introduction to herbal remedies. The first part covers the use of herbs as medical remedies, choosing the best herbal products, and aromatherapy. The second part focuses on growing and making herbal remedies at home. It includes a variety of recipes for oils, compresses, poultices, teas, and syrups. The symptom guide is a practical reference to a variety of complaints and illnesses and gives both a medical description and the holistic understanding of the symptom, suggested herbal remedies and formulas, and healthy habits that can prevent or lessen the symptom. The herb guide lists over 100 herbs with their descriptions, uses, and recommended dosages.

- Hobbs, Christopher, and Haas, Elson. 1999. *Vitamins for Dummies*. Foster City, CA: IDG Books Worldwide. 334 pp. ISBN: 0764551795; 9780764551796.
  Although the title mentions only vitamins, this book also covers minerals, amino acids and proteins, fats and oils, hormones, supplements, and herbs as well as lifestyle. Written in an accessible style that also provides a great deal of useful information, the work will be helpful to most readers. Part 5 provides healing programs for common diseases and symptoms and gives suggestions for supplements to take to restore health to the body.
- Hoffman, David. 2003. *Medical Herbalism: The Science and Practice of Herbal Medicine*. Rochester, VT: Healing Arts Press. 666 pp. ISBN: 0892817496; 9780892817498.
  Intended for practitioners and students of medical herbalism, the goal of this book is to provide foundational information for the skilled use of herbs to treat a variety of ailments. Part 1 is an introduction to the principles and practices of herbal medicine, including its scientific basis and the chemistry and pharmacology of herbs. Part 2 gives practical treatment approaches arranged by body systems. Thus, it is helpful to anyone who wishes to learn more about the use of herbs to treat medical conditions.
- Kuhn, Merrily A., and Winston, David. 2008. *Winston & Kuhn's Herbal Therapy and Supplements: A Scientific and Traditional Approach*. 2nd ed. Philadelphia: Wolters Kluwer/Lippincott Williams & Wilkins Health. 560 pp. ISBN: 1582554625; 9781582554624.
  This pocket guide covers 115 herbal remedies and 14 nutritional supplements commonly used in the United States and Canada. The entry for each item includes detailed information on pharmacology, traditional and current uses, side effects, contraindications and toxicities, safety, use in pregnancy/lactation/children, and a bibliography of related research and references.
- Lieberman, Shari, and Bruning, Nancy. 2007. *The Real Vitamin and Mineral Book: The Definitive Guide to Designing Your Personal Supplement Program*. 4th ed. New York: Avery. 424 pp. ISBN: 158333274X; 9781583332740.
  The goal of the authors in writing this book is to provide readers with guidelines that can help them create their own supplement program based on what they call the ODI, optimum daily intake. Each of the vitamins and the major minerals are all covered in individual chapters. Other supplements, including coenzyme Q10, essential fatty acids, and flavonoids are also discussed. The chapters provide such information as the functions and uses of the nutrient in the body, deficiency, food sources, the optimum daily intake, and toxicity and adverse effects. The appendixes include a worksheet for determining personal ODIs for supplements and summaries of the research literature on the various nutrients discussed.
- MacWilliam, Lyle Dean. 2007. *NutriSearch Comparative Guide to Nutritional Supplements*. 4th ed. Vernon, BC: Northern Dimensions Publishing. 191 pp. ISBN: 097325386X; 9780973253863.
  This resource provides comparative data on over 1,500 U.S. and Canadian supplements. Each supplement is evaluated using a health support profile consisting of 18 criteria such as completeness in health support, potency, bone health, metabolic health, and potential toxicities. Charts are presented for 300 different products and provide graphical representations of the nutrients included in the supplement and

the ratings on the health support profile. Other charts list all 1,500 supplements and give each a rating of 1 to 5 stars so that the supplements can be compared. Since so many supplements are available today, it is difficult to judge their quality. This source provides some such comparison.

- Marian, Mary, Williams-Mullen, Pamela, and Bowers, Jennifer Muir, eds. 2007. *Integrating Therapeutic and Complementary Nutrition*. Boca Raton, FL: CRC/Taylor & Francis. 634 pp. ISBN: 084931612X; 9780849316128.
  This work is designed for both consumers and health care professionals who wish to use dietary supplements and other nutrition-related practices. Although ayurveda receives its own chapter, the rest of the work is devoted to specific groups (infants, women, adolescents, and men) and to diseases related to specific systems of the body. For example, the chapter on promoting small and large bowel health discusses the role of nutrition in colon cancer, diverticulosis and diverticulitis, irritable bowel disease, inflammatory bowel disease, and celiac disease. Information such as incidences, etiology, signs and symptoms, and interventions using nutritional and other alternative therapies is given. Due to its comprehensive nature and its basis in evidence-based research, this is an exceptional book that will provide good guidance to physicians and their patients.
- McIntyre, Anne. 2006. *The Top 100 Herbal Remedies: Safe, Effective Remedies for 100 Common Ailments*. London: Duncan Baird. 128 pp. ISBN: 1844832538; 9781844832538.
  This small book provides information on 50 common herbs and 100 different conditions that can be treated by them. For each herb, the parts used, the properties/actions, the indications, and a color photograph are given. For each ailment, several useful herbs and other treatments are suggested. Although only basic information is given, this is a useful book due to its size and the brevity of its entries.
- McVicar, Jekka. 2002. *New Book of Herbs*. New York: DK Publishing. 288 pp. ISBN: 0789489422; 9780789489425.
  Highly illustrated with color photographs, this book looks at herbs from a variety of viewpoints, including using them in gardening, cooking, and remedies. The first section on the garden details analyzing the soil, preparing the bed for planting, designing the herb garden, and harvesting. The second section focuses on the kitchen, especially using herbs in cooking. Herbs in the home is the theme of the third section and includes using herbs for first aid and relaxation. The final section is a catalog of 100 herbs and gives information on how to use herbs in cooking, for medicinal remedies, and around the home.
- Meckling, Kelly Anne, ed. 2007. *Nutrient–Drug Interactions*. Boca Raton, FL: CRC/Taylor & Francis. 336 pp. ISBN: 157444915X; 9781574449150.
  Although this book is not a comprehensive study of the interactions between herbal remedies, supplements, and pharmaceutical drugs, it does provide a wealth of highly detailed information written by experts in their respective fields. The goal of the book is to focus on the chemical constituents of herbs and food and how these constituents relate to chronic disease development and treatment and specifically how these constituents affect response to prescribed drugs. Thus, the work is aimed at health care professionals. Individual chapters focus on diabetes, high cholesterol, cancer, neurodegenerative disorders, depression, anesthesiology, and cardiovascular

disease. Although limited in scope, the work does break new ground in its depth of coverage and its basis in pharmacological research.

- Miller, Lucinda G., and Murray, Wallace J. 1998. *Herbal Medicinals: A Clinician's Guide*. Binghamton, NY: The Haworth Press. 382 pp. ISBN: 0789004666; 9780789004666.
  Using case studies, this edited work seeks to address potential interactions between conventional medicines and herbal remedies. This is necessary since up to a third of American adults use alternative and herbal remedies in addition to conventional treatments. Chapters include topics such as renal and hepatic effects of herbal remedies and the use of herbal medicines to treat colds and flu, gastrointestinal problems, arthritis, diabetes, hypertension, atherosclerosis, asthma, cancer, and gynecological and obstetric issues. The final chapter covers the history of herbs in the United States, including legal and regulatory perspectives.

- Mills, Simon, and Bone, Kerry. 2000. *Principles and Practice of Phytotherapy: Modern Herbal Medicine*. New York: Churchill Livingstone. 643 pp. ISBN: 0443060169; 9780443060168.
  A textbook that includes more than 4,000 citations, this work is aimed at students and practitioners of phytotherapy and covers topics such as the principles of herbal pharmacology, the principles of herbal treatment, safety, dosage, herbal prescribing, and herbal approaches to pathological states and system dysfunctions. The final section is a materia medica and covers 45 commonly used herbs. For each of these herbs, the entry gives synonyms, a description of the plant, effects, traditional view, actions, use, preparations, dosage, duration of use, an assessment of safety, and technical data such as the pharmacodynamics, pharmacokinetics, clinical trials, contraindications, and interactions.

- Mills, Simon, and Bone, Kerry. 2005. *The Essential Guide to Herbal Safety*. St. Louis, MO: Elsevier Churchill Livingstone. 684 pp. ISBN: 0443071713; 9780443071713.
  Since so many people use herbal products, often with little understanding of their proper use, this book is a welcome addition to the literature on herbs. It provides an extensive discussion of the major issues related to the safety of herbs and their use, including topics such as adverse effects of herbal remedies, adverse herb–drug interactions, and allergic reactions to herbal medicines. In addition, it contains reviews of the published literature on the safety of 125 common herbs, from aloe to zizyphus seed.

- Mitchell, Deborah R. 2009. *The Complete Book of Nutritional Healing: The Top 100 Medicinal Foods and Supplements and the Diseases They Treat*. New York: St. Martin's Paperbacks. 339 pp. ISBN: 0312945116; 9780312945114.
  This is an A-to-Z listing of the top 51 health challenges, more than 80 medicinal foods, and major supplements. It includes good information on each of the foods and supplements while giving suggestions for their safe and effective use. Often, healthy recipes are given.

- Murray, Michael T. 2004. *The Healing Power of Herbs: The Enlightened Person's Guide to the Wonders of Medicinal Plants*. 2nd ed., rev. and expanded. New York: Gramercy Books. 410 pp. ISBN: 051722321X; 9780517223215.
  Written for anyone who wishes to learn more about the medicinal use of herbs, this book provides a brief introduction to herbal medicine, a materia medica of 37

commonly used herbs, and 34 health conditions that can be treated using herbs. The entries in the materia medica provide basic information on each herb including a general description, key uses, chemical composition, historic and folk uses, pharmacology, clinical applications, dosage, and toxicity. The section on health conditions suggests herbs and dosages that can be used to treat the condition.

- Navarra, Tova. 2007. *The A to Z of Vitamins, Minerals and Supplements.* 2nd ed. New York: Checkmark Books. 353 pp. ISBN: 0816069344; 9780816069347.
  This reference work includes over 900 entries related to vitamins. In addition to entries on individual vitamins, minerals, and supplements, the encyclopedia includes entries on herbs, therapies, individuals, and ailments. For the entries on the vitamins, minerals, and supplements, the author gives background information, signs of deficiency, dietary sources, supplements, dosages, and toxicity. Although many of the entries are rather short, they provide basic information that will answer many questions.
- *PDR for Nonprescription Drugs, Dietary Supplements, and Herbs.* 2009. 31st ed., 2010 ed. Montvale, NJ: Thomson Healthcare. 618 pp. ISBN: 1563637502; 9781563637506.
  Produced annually, this book is designed as an aid to health care professionals in providing safe management of the drugs, supplements, and herbs used by their patients. The section on nonprescription drugs is arranged by therapeutic category and indication, such as smoking cessation, acid indigestion, and aches and pains. Dietary supplements and herbal medicines are arranged by brand name. Indexes to product category and active ingredients help find the desired entries. Although the data provided for supplements and herbs is much less than that provided in other reference works, this is a standard reference work that should be included in most reference collections.
- Pedersen, Mark. 1998. *Nutritional Herbology: A Reference Guide to Herbs.* Rev. and expanded ed. Warsaw, IN: Wendell W. Whitman. 336 pp. ISBN: 1885653077; 9781885653079.
  This book is predicated on the belief that herbs or plants can serve as both food and medicine. Thus, specific herbs can be used as a food to treat specific ailments. The author has compiled a wealth of information and presents it in a logical, useful manner. After introducing the concept of nutritional herbology, he gives good background on the classification of herbs and the wide variety of nutrients that are present in herbs and other foods. He then presents the nutritional and use profiles of 93 different herbs. The following chapters are devoted to the systems of the body, including the circulatory, digestive, glandular, immune, nervous, respiratory, structural, and urinary systems, and herbal therapies that can be useful for treating conditions involving each system. This work is especially useful since it approaches the use of herbs from their nutritional contribution to health in addition to their purely medicinal properties.
- Pressman, Alan H., and Buff, Sheila. 2007. *The Complete Idiot's Guide to Vitamins and Minerals.* 3rd ed. New York: Penguin. 422 pp. ISBN: 1592576095; 9781592576098.
  Covering the full range of vitamins in addition to selected minerals and other supplements, this book provides good, clear information to those who want an easy to read, current source of information. Separate chapters are devoted to each vitamin and to the major minerals. Each chapter includes charts of the RDAs for various

groups of people, food sources, signs of deficiency, and the functions of the vitamin or mineral. The section on supplements focuses on amino acids, essential fatty acids, antioxidants, flavonoids, coenzyme Q10, hormones, and fiber. This is an inexpensive source that will see a lot of use.

- Reavley, Nicola. 1999. *New Encyclopedia of Vitamins, Minerals, Supplements, & Herbs.* New York: M. Evans and Co. 792 pp. ISBN: 0871318970; 9780871318978.
  This is a complete handbook to a wide array of substances that many individuals use to enhance their health. All of the major vitamins and minerals plus a variety of other nutrients necessary for health, such as essential fatty acids, flavonoids, and glucosamine, are included. The entries include what the substance does in the body, how it is absorbed and metabolized, symptoms of deficiency, sources, the daily recommended dietary intake, toxic effects of excess intake, interactions, therapeutic use, and cautions in its use. Brief information, including uses and cautions, is given for 88 different common herbs. Additional chapters cover optimum health and specific health problems and recommend supplements that can be beneficial.

- Richter, Rowena K. 2003. *Herbal Medicine: Chaos in the Marketplace.* Binghamton, NY: The Haworth Press. 220 pp. ISBN: 0789016192; 9780789016195.
  In this well-written book, the author evaluates the situation of herbal medicines in the United States from a public health perspective. In particular, she examines the role of governmental regulation of the supplement industry and how this affects the health of Americans. Many areas of the world, especially Europe and Asia, use herbal remedies much more frequently than in the United States, primarily because many physicians in those areas prescribe herbal medicines to their patients. The author argues for a more coherent regulatory policy for the use of these substances so that they are more available to American consumers.

- Sarubin-Fragakis, Allison, and Thomson, Cynthia. 2007. *The Health Professional's Guide to Popular Dietary Supplements.* 3rd ed. Chicago: American Dietetic Association. 682 pp. ISBN: 0880913630; 9780880913638.
  Produced by the American Dietetic Association, the goal of this reference work is to provide to health care professionals essential information on over 100 popular dietary supplements. The entries cover both the scientific evidence about the efficacy or lack thereof for the supplements as well as the claims made by manufacturers and consumer media. For each supplement, the guide provides details on safety, drug/supplement interaction, food sources, dosage information/bioavailability, and relevant research. Although written for health care professionals, the writing is understandable to anyone interested in finding reliable information on dietary supplements.

- Skidmore-Roth, Linda. 2010. *Mosby's Handbook of Herbs & Natural Supplements.* 4th ed. St. Louis, MO: Mosby Elsevier. 746 pp. ISBN: 0323057411; 9780323057417.
  Covering 300 commonly used herbal products and natural supplements, this is an excellent resource for those seeking information on such products. Each profile includes the common and scientific names, origin, uses, dosages, precautions such as contraindications and side effects, interactions with drugs and other herbs, client considerations, pharmacology, actions, and references. Although designed for health care professionals, this book will serve as an authoritative reference source for many questions on medicinal herbs and other nutritional supplements.

- Smith, Pamela Wartian. 2008. *What You Must Know about Vitamins, Minerals, Herbs, & More: Choosing the Nutrients That Are Right for You.* Garden City Park, NY: Square One Publishers. 433 pp. ISBN: 0757002331; 9780757002335.
  Divided into three parts, this is a good introduction to nutritional supplements. Part 1 includes chapters on vitamins, minerals, fatty acids, amino acids, selected herbs, and other major nutrients. Part 2 presents over 100 different health conditions and the nutrients and herbs that can be used to treat them. Part 3 discusses maintaining health and topics such as enhancing energy, liver health, and weight loss.
- Stargrove, Mitchell Bebel, Treasure, Jonathan, and McKee, Dwight L. 2008. *Herb, Nutrient, and Drug Interactions: Clinical Implications and Therapeutic Strategies.* St. Louis, MO: Mosby/Elsevier. 932 pp. ISBN: 0323029647; 9780323029643.
  Although technical in nature, this reference work should be in most libraries. Due to the number of individuals who use herbal remedies and nutritional supplements, health care professionals need to be aware of possible interactions with prescription drugs. The authors provide a comprehensive evaluation of the interactions of 30 of the most commonly used herbs with drugs as well as of the interactions between drugs and vitamins, minerals, amino acids, and selected supplements, including coenzyme Q10, DHEA (dihydroepiandrosterone), and probiotics. For the herbs, the entry gives basic information such as the parts used, common forms of the herb, and the use of the herb in clinical practice. The heart of each entry is the interactions review that examines the clinical literature and rates the types of interactions that may occur. Similar data is also provided for the vitamins, minerals, amino acids, and supplements but also includes the chemistry and forms of the nutrient, its affect on physiology and function, clinical uses, deficiency symptoms, and dietary sources.
- Stein, Diane. 2009. *Healing Herbs A to Z: A Handy Reference to Healing Plants.* Berkeley, CA: Crossing Press. 239 pp. ISBN: 1580911927; 9781580911924.
  The author provides an alphabetical reference to 200 medicinal plants and discusses their healing attributes, how they should be used, potential side effects, and contraindications in their use.
- Talbott, Shawn M. 2003. *A Guide to Understanding Dietary Supplements.* Binghamton, NY: The Haworth Press. 713 pp. ISBN: 0789014564; 9780789014566.
  Written by an expert in sports nutrition and performance, this book not only provides detailed information on over 140 supplements, it also examines the supplement industry, discusses the product development process for dietary supplements, and provides a critical evaluation of dietary supplements in general. The supplements themselves are arranged by their primary action, such as weight loss, bone health, heart health, and immune system support. For each supplement, the author provides a brief description of the supplement, any claims made for its use, the theory behind its functions, scientific support, safety, value, dosage, and a listing of works consulted. This is an excellent resource on supplements that provides balanced, scientifically based, useful information.
- Talbott, Shawn M., and Hughes, Kerry. 2007. *The Health Professional's Guide to Dietary Supplements.* Philadelphia: Lippincott Williams & Wilkins. 444 pp. ISBN: 0781746728; 9780781746724.

The goal of this book is to provide health professionals with the background information needed so that they can discuss the clinical evidence on supplements with their patients and clients. Over 120 supplements are arranged into 12 chapters corresponding to their primary use, such as for weight loss or immune support. For each supplement, the entry gives an overview, comments scientific support, safety/dosage, and references to clinical research. In addition, up to five stars can be awarded to the supplement based on the strength of the scientific evidence for its major effects.

➤ Tierra, Michael. 1988. *Planetary Herbology: An Integration of Western Herbs into the Traditional Chinese and Ayurvedic Systems.* Twin Lakes, WI: Lotus Press. 485 pp. ISBN: 0941524272; 9780941524278.

By combining Western herbalism with traditional Chinese and ayurvedic understanding of the actions of herbs and methods of diagnosis and treatment, this book will benefit anyone interested in using herbs to treat disease and ailments. Part 1 provides an excellent background to the nature, preparation, and use of medicinal herbs and compares and contrasts the Western, ayurvedic, and Chinese traditions and uses of herbs. Part 2 is a materia medica of herbs, primarily of Western origin, but the arrangement differs from many other works in that the herbs are classified by their actions, such as laxatives, heat-clearing herbs, stimulants, tonics, and sedatives and nervines. The general index is helpful in finding specific herbs when the action is not known.

➤ Tierra, Michael. 1998. *The Way of Herbs: Fully Updated—With the Latest Developments in Herbal Science.* New York: Pocket Books. 375 pp. ISBN: 0671023276; 9780671023270.

For those interested in learning more about herbal remedies, this is one of the best introductory books. The author discusses the theory of using herbs, various herbal therapies, methods of application, the properties of herbs, diagnosis and treatment using herbs, obtaining and storing herbs, and making your own herbal formulas. Several chapters are devoted to the herbs themselves and give the common names, family, parts used, energy and flavors, systems affected, biochemical constituents, properties, uses, and notes that includes common and traditional uses as well as cautions. Other topics presented include diet, using herbs for specific ailments and for cancer treatment, and using magnet therapy.

➤ Tillotson, Alan Keith, Tillotson, Nai-shing Hu, and Abel, Robert. 2001. *The One Earth Herbal Sourcebook: Everything You Need to Know about Chinese, Western, and Ayurvedic Herbal Treatments.* New York: Twin Streams, Kensington Publishing Corp. 596 pp. ISBN: 1575666170; 9781575666174.

Combining information from the major herbal traditions, this book provides an excellent introduction to the use of herbs as healing agents. The first section covers the basics of herbal medicine, including how herbal remedies are grown, manufactured, and stored; how to evaluate information on herbs; how to assess the safety of herbs; and how herbs can be safely used. The second section covers 96 commonly used herbs from around the world. The final section focuses on herbs that are useful for treating ailments of specific systems within the body while also addressing such issues as nutrition, lifestyle, and longevity.

➤ Ulbricht, Catherine, and Basch, Ethan M., eds. 2005. *Natural Standard Herb & Supplement Reference: Evidence-Based Clinical Reviews.* St. Louis, MO: Elsevier Mosby. 1012 pp. ISBN: 0323029949; 9780323029940.

Seeking to provide reliable, clinically based information, this source presents the scientific data on 98 herbs and supplements. The entries vary from less than two pages to 35 pages in length. Entries generally give, depending on the available information, synonyms/common names/related substances, a summary of the clinical research, dosing and toxicology guidelines, adverse effects/precautions/contraindications, interactions, mechanism of action, history of use, a discussion of the evidence, and a list of references. An appendix lists conditions and suggested remedies along with a grade for the quality of the evidence available for the remedies.

➤ Watson, Ronald R., ed. 2001. *Vegetables, Fruits, and Herbs in Health Promotion*. Boca Raton, FL: CRC Press. 341 pp. ISBN: 084930038X; 9780849300387.
The goal of this book is to provide an overview of the use of vegetables, nutrient supplementation, fruits, and herbs in the promotion of health, the increase of longevity, and the reduction of the risk of cancer and heart disease. Based on the scientific literature, each chapter focuses on a specific topic, such as tomatoes and health promotion, nutrients and vegetables in skin protection, garlic and health, and nutrition and stress management. Although not as comprehensive as some other resources, this is a helpful volume for those seeking scientifically based research on the effects of herbs, vegetables, and fruit on health.

➤ Williamson, Elizabeth M., Driver, Samuel, and Baxter, Karen. 2009. *Stockley's Herbal Medicines Interactions: A Guide to the Interactions of Herbal Medicines, Dietary Supplements and Nutraceuticals with Conventional Medicines*. Chicago: Pharmaceutical Press. 423 pp. ISBN: 0853698651; 9780853698654.
Due to the growth of the use of herbal medicines and dietary supplements, it is extremely important to know how these products interact with conventional medicines. This is an excellent, professional level reference work on herb–drug, herb–supplement, herb–food, and herb–laboratory test interactions. References are given to all data included. Thus, this is a must-have reference resource.

➤ Wood, Matthew. 2004. *The Practice of Traditional Western Herbalism: Basic Doctrine, Energetics, and Classification*. Berkeley, CA: North Atlantic Books. 289 pp. ISBN: 1556435037; 9781556435034.
Combining concepts drawn from herbal medicine, homeopathy, and Native American medicine, the author presents a different way to approach health and the treatment of ailments through the use of herbal medicines. Specifically, the author returns to the use of the concepts of humors, qualities, and tissue states to describe pathology rather than the conventional medical views of lesions within the body. Herbs can then be used to restore the self-regulation of the body, which will lead to health. Part 1 of the book discusses these topics, which the author calls "forgotten energetics." In Part 2, he uses a traditional classification of medicinal plants, such as sedatives, relaxants, and astringents, to present information about a variety of herbs.

Internet Resources

➤ Dietary Supplements, U.S. Food and Drug Administration, www.fda.gov/Food/DietarySupplements/default.htm.
The FDA has the responsibility to regulate dietary supplements within the United States. This site provides consumer information, alerts, and information on dietary supplement ingredients, regulations, and labeling.

- Drugs, Supplements, and Herbal Information, U.S National Library of Medicine, www.nlm.nih.gov/medlineplus/druginformation.html.
  Provided by the National Library of Medicine, the information on this webpage covers not only drugs but all types of supplements and herbal products. Arranged alphabetically, complete information is available for over 80 specific major supplements and herbs. The entry for each supplement or herb includes a background on its use, evidence from scientific evidence to its efficacy, dosing information, safety concerns, and interactions with other herbs and dietary supplements.
- The Herb Research Foundation, www.herbs.org.
  The Herb Research Foundation offers accurate, science-based information on the health benefits and safety of herbs, yet the foundation provides very little information online. It produces information packets on over 200 herbs, specific health conditions, and related topics, which must be purchased individually.
- HerbMed, www.herbmed.org.
  HerbMed is an interactive, public herbal database of scientific data on 30 of the most popular herbs used for medical purposes. A more complete database of 221 herbs is available by subscription.
- HerbNET, www.herbnet.com.
  Maintained by the Herb Growing and Marketing Network, this site is a cornucopia of things herbal. It includes links to herbal associations, information on gardens and herbs, links to sources of herbal products, educational opportunities, and practitioners.
- Office of Dietary Supplements, National Institutes of Health, ods.od.nih.gov/index.aspx.
  One of the best sources of scientific information on dietary supplements, the ODS is an excellent resource for those trying to learn about or use dietary supplements properly. The site covers the use and safety of dietary supplements, provides recommendations for the use of a variety of nutrients, and lists research and training programs run by the ODS. In addition, the ODS links to a variety of NIH databases, especially International Bibliographic Information on Dietary Supplements (IBIDS). IBIDS is the preeminent database of the scientific literature on dietary supplements, including vitamins, herbs, nutrients, and other supplements.
- Reference Guide for Herbs, www.realtime.net/anr/herbs.html.
  This guide to herbs covers almost 100 common herbs, from albizzia bark to yerba mate leaf. Each entry gives brief information that is regularly updated.
- Review of Natural Products, online.statref.com/titleinfo/fxid-15.html.
  This site includes more than 300 monographs of natural products and is updated monthly. Each monograph includes the scientific names, common names, source, history, chemistry, uses and pharmacology, dosing, pregnancy/lactation, interactions, adverse reactions, toxicology, and references. There is also a “Clinical Overview” box within each monograph that summarizes the use, dosing, contraindication, pregnancy/lactation, interaction, adverse reaction, and toxicology information for the product.
- Vitamins, U.S. National Library of Medicine, www.nlm.nih.gov/medlineplus/vitamins.html.

Produced by the National Library of Medicine, this is an authoritative and comprehensive overview of vitamins. The site covers the basics of vitamins, specific conditions related to vitamins, research, as well as specific information related to children, teenagers, and seniors.

- The Vitamins and Nutrition Center, www.vitamins-nutrition.org.
  Although sponsored by a maker of multivitamin products, this site does provide a wealth of information on vitamins and other supplements, such as creatine, ginseng, and omega 3 fatty acids. The entry for each supplement gives an overview, benefits, natural sources, cautions, symptoms of deficiency and overdose, side effects, and interactions.
- VitaminsDiary.com, www.vitaminsdiary.com.
  Covering vitamins, minerals, herbs, herbal remedies, amino acids, and other supplements, this is an excellent source of comprehensive and relevant information. For vitamins and minerals, the entries provide an overview, the recommended daily allowance, benefits, deficiency symptoms, and rich food sources. For herbs and other supplements, the entries provide less information but usually include a photograph, benefits, and conditions that can be treated using the herb or supplement.

Periodicals/Magazines/Journals

- *American Herb Association Newsletter*, published by American Herb Association, 1981– . Quarterly. No ISSN. www.ahaherb.com/newsletter.html.
  Written by professional herbalists, this newsletter covers current news, legal issues, and events related to medicinal plants.
- *American Journal of Clinical Nutrition*, published by American Society for Nutrition, 1952– . Monthly. ISSN: 0002-9165. www.ajcn.org.
  Containing original scientific research, this journal also contains reviews, reports of meetings and conferences, and special articles about clinical nutrition.
- *Better Nutrition*, published by Active Interest Media, 1938– . Monthly. ISSN: 0405-668X. www.betternutrition.com.
  This consumer magazine aims to educate readers on living naturally and achieving optimal health and longevity through the use of natural products such as herbs and supplements.
- *Canadian Journal of Herbalism*, published by Ontario Herbalists Association, 1979– . Quarterly. ISSN: 0848-9629. www.herbalists.on.ca/journal.html.
  Covering not only herbal medicine but also other forms of complementary health care, this journal includes herbal monographs, case studies, and articles about the use of herbs for treating disease and enhancing health.
- *Critical Reviews in Food Science and Nutrition*, published by Taylor & Francis Inc., 1970– . Eight times a year. ISSN: 1040-8398. www.tandf.co.uk/journals/titles/10408398.asp.
  As an academic journal, *Critical Reviews in Food Science and Nutrition* seeks to provide critical articles on food science and human nutrition. It focuses on scientific research related to nutrition, food safety, and food technology.
- *Environmental Nutrition: The Newsletter of Food, Nutrition and Health*, published by Belvoir Media Group, LLC, 1977– . Monthly. ISSN: 0893-4452. www.environmentalnutrition.com.

A newsletter designed for the consumer, each issue of *Environmental Nutrition* examines current research and information on supplements. The newsletter also provides guidance for the purchase of supplements and healthy foods.

- *The Herb Companion*, published by Ogden Publications, 1988– . Bimonthly. ISSN: 1040-581X. www.herbcompanion.com.
  Written with the consumer in mind, this publication covers all aspects of growing herbs for use in cooking, healing, and daily life. Issues include gardening tips, recipes, and other uses for herbs.
- *Herb Quarterly*, published by EGW Publishing Co., 1978– . Quarterly. ISSN: 0163-9900. www.herbquarterly.com.
  Celebrating the use of herbs in all aspects of live, this magazine includes articles on gardening with herbs, the medicinal use of herbs, and recipes for incorporating herbs into recipes.
- *HerbalGram: The Journal of the American Botanical Council*, published by American Botanical Council, 1983– . Quarterly. ISSN: 0899-5648. www.herbalgram.org/herbalgram/index.html.
  Produced by the American Botanical Council, this journal covers all aspects of herbs, including their use as medicines. Special attention is given to the legal and regulatory use of herbs.
- *Herbarist*, published by the Herb Society of America Inc., 1935– . Annual. ISSN: 0740-5979. www.herbsociety.org/public.php.
  This annual publication blends the latest scholarly research findings on herbs and other medicinal plants with popular articles that will be of interest to all who seek information on herbs, their uses, and their cultivation.
- *International Journal for Vitamin and Nutrition Research*, published by Verlag Hans Huber AG, 1930– . Bimonthly. ISSN: 0300-9831. www.verlag-hanshuber.com/zeitschriften/journal.php?abbrev=VIT.
  Since 1930 this scholarly journal has reported on important research on vitamins and nutrition.
- *Journal of Herbal Pharmacotherapy: Innovations in Clinical & Applied Evidence-Based Herbal Medicinals*, published by Taylor & Francis, 2001– . Quarterly. ISSN: 1522-8940. www.informaworld.com/smpp/title~content=t792304015~db=all.
  The peer-reviewed and scientifically based articles in this journal provide original research that can help in understanding the effects and uses of herbal medications.
- *Journal of Herbs, Spices & Medicinal Plants*, published by Taylor & Francis, 1991– . Quarterly. ISSN: 1049-6475. www.informaworld.com/smpp/title~db=jour~content=t792306868.
  This journal features both original research-based articles and short reviews on the production and development of herbs, spices, and medicinal plants.
- *Journal of Human Nutrition and Dietetics*, published by Wiley-Blackwell Publishing Ltd., 1988– . Bimonthly. ISSN: 0952-3871. www.wiley.com/bw/journal.asp?ref=0952-3871.
  An international peer-reviewed journal, the *Journal of Human Nutrition and Dietetics* publishes original research in applied nutrition and dietetics. Other areas of interest

include clinical nutrition, therapeutic dietetics, public health nutrition, health promotion, and the psychology of eating behavior and the sociology of food.

- *The Journal of Nutrition*, published by American Society for Nutrition, 1928– . Monthly. ISSN: 0022-3166. jn.nutrition.org.
  One of the longest published scholarly journals in the field of nutrition, *JN* covers all aspects of nutrition research.
- *Journal of Nutrition for the Elderly*, published by Routledge, 1980– . Quarterly. ISSN: 0163-9366. www.tandf.co.uk/journals/WJNE.
  Focusing specifically on the elderly, this journal publishes research studies on nutritional issues affecting older adults. Topics include preventive nutrition, nutritional interventions for the treatment or control of chronic diseases, changes in nutritional requirements due to age, dietary behaviors, the use of supplements, and nutrition in long-term care.
- *Journal of the American Dietetic Association*, published by Elsevier Inc., 1925– . Monthly. ISSN: 0002-8223. www.elsevier.com/locate/jada.
  A major journal in the field of nutrition, *JADA* is a scholarly journal that publishes research on all aspects of dietetics. Of special concern are nutrition, diet therapy, medical nutritional therapy, public health, and food science.
- *Journal of the American Herbalists Guild*, published by the American Herbalists Guild, 2000– . Biannual. ISSN: 1538-7496. americanherbalistsguild.com/journal_ samples.
  A peer-reviewed journal, *JAHG* publishes research produced by prominent herbalists and by scientists working in the field of botanical medicine. The articles include herbal monographs, reports on botanical therapeutics, case histories, and safety issues.
- *Natural Products Marketplace*, published by Virgo Publishing Inc., 1995– . Monthly. ISSN: 1948-4151. www.naturalproductsmarketplace.com.
  A trade magazine serving the dietary supplement industry, especially store owners and manufacturers, it provides news, market information, analyses, and new product information.
- *Nutrition: The International Journal of Applied and Basic Nutritional Science*, published by Elsevier Inc., 1985– . Monthly. ISSN: 0899-9007. www.nutritionjrnl.com.
  This scholarly journal publishes articles relating current research and practice in the field of applied and basic nutrition. It emphasizes new technologies and current data needed in clinical nutrition practices.
- *Nutrition Research*, published by Elsevier Inc., 1981– . Monthly. ISSN: 0271-5317. www.elsevier.com/locate/nutres.
  Nutrition Research provides articles on basic and applied research on all aspects of basic and applied nutrition. It also covers relevant topics from food science and other social sciences. One main focus of the journal is the publication of articles that advance the understanding of how nutrients and other constituents in food help improve human health.
- *Nutrition Research Newsletter: Technical Insights*, published by Frost & Sullivan, 1983– . Monthly. ISSN: 0736-0037. www.marketresearch.com/product/display.asp?productid =1207951.

This newsletter covers all aspects of nutrition. It summarizes the research on nutrition found in hundreds of journals so that the most important developments can be presented in the 20 concise summaries provided each month.

- *Nutrition Research Reviews*, published by Cambridge University Press, 1988– . Biannual. ISSN: 0954-4224. journals.cambridge.org/action/displayJournal?jid=NRR.
  Offering a comprehensive overview of current nutritional science today, *NRR* publishes in depth, state of the art research articles in all aspects of nutritional science.
- *Nutrition Reviews*, published by International Life Sciences Institute, 1942– . Monthly. ISSN: 0029-6643. www.ilsi.org/Pages/NutritionReviews.aspx.
  An international refereed journal, *Nutrition Reviews* publishes significant research in all areas of nutrition science, dietetics, food science, and nutrition policy.
- *Nutritional Outlook*, published by Canon Communications LLC, 1998– . Nine times per year. ISSN: 1098-1179. www.nutritionaloutlook.com.
  A trade magazine loaded with information for nutritional supplement and vitamin manufacturers, this publication also includes much helpful information on supplements, health foods and beverages, and vitamins.
- *Research Journal of Medicinal Plant*, published by Academic Journals Inc., 2006– . Quarterly. ISSN: 1819-3455. scialert.net/jindex.php?issn=1819-3455.
  This academic journal focuses on publishing peer-reviewed scientific research from fields as diverse as chemistry, pharmacology, and the use of medicinal plants and their derivatives. The goal is to provide access to significant new findings related to medicinal plants.
- *Today's Diet & Nutrition*, published by Great Valley Publishing Company Inc., 2005– . Quarterly. ISSN: 1559-5110. www.tdn-digital.com.
  As a magazine aimed at the general consumer, *Today's Diet & Nutrition* covers topics related to food, nutrition, herbs, supplements, and fitness.
- *Vitamin Retailer: The Dietary Supplement Industry's Leading Magazine*, published by Vitamin Retailer Magazine Inc., 1993– . Monthly. ISSN: 1537-503X. www.vitamin retailer.com.
  Although this is a trade magazine designed for store managers, it does contain useful information on vitamins, minerals, herbs, supplements, natural remedies, and other related products.

Chapter 12

Homeopathy

Background and History

Homeopathy is based on the principle that "like cures like," also known as the law of similars. The law states that any substance that can re-create in a healthy person the symptoms being experienced by someone who is ill will help cure the sick individual. This law was formulated by Dr. Samuel Hahnemann (1755–1843), considered to be the father of homeopathy. Hahnemann sought a more gentle approach to healing than was available in the medicine of his time, which included bloodletting, the use of poisons such as mercury, and induced vomiting. Most important, however, Hahnemann believed in human experimentation to discover the effects of potential therapeutic agents. Thus, he began to systematically test various substances on himself and on other willing physicians who diligently recorded the effects that the substances caused. When the effects matched the symptoms of an ill patient, he would then give that particular substance to the patient and observed the results. Hahnemann called this process of experimentation "proving" and developed stringent procedures in which to perform such experimental trials.

Within his method of proving the efficacy of substances, Hahnemann specified that healthy subjects be given various dosages of the substance to determine the effects. The substances studied could be derived from plants, minerals, animals, allopathic medicines, or even disease products. Various subjects would receive toxic doses of the substances, others hypotoxic doses, while others received highly diluted "potentized" doses and their reactions to these doses recorded. Since many of the substances were highly toxic, Hahnemann used highly diluted doses and found that the subjects still reacted to them. He continued to dilute the substances through succussion, a vigorous shaking of the substance in water or another solvent. To his surprise, the diluted substance yielded even stronger reactions, showing that the potentized formulation was more powerful than the original. When tested on ill patients, these potentized remedies actually worked better. According to Hahnemann's thought, the process of potentizing a remedy through succussion released the energy within the substance and this energy was then contained in the solution itself. Hahnemann, during his lifetime, oversaw the proving of approximately 100 remedies. Since his time, provings have continued until there are now several hundred remedies listed in the various versions of the repertories of homeopathic materia medica.

Homeopathic remedies, therefore, are highly diluted. Through the potentizing process of repeated dilution and succussion, little if any of the original substance is present in the final remedy. The process of creating such a remedy follows a multistep process. First, the substance is cleaned and often chopped into smaller pieces. It is then put into a glass jar with alcohol, water, or a combination of the two. The jar is sealed and the mixture stands for several weeks and is regularly shaken. Next, the mixture is strained to separate out the tincture. One drop of the tincture is then added to 99 drops of alcohol, water, or an alcohol/water solution and shaken vigorously (succussed). This process is repeated, with 1 drop of the resulting mixture being diluted over and over. Then a few drops of the final diluted solution is added to lactose powder or tablets that are stored in an airtight, dark glass bottle away from direct sunlight. The normal dilution ratio is either 1 drop of the tincture to 9 parts of an alcohol/water mixture (referred to as 1X) or 1 drop to 99 parts (referred to as 1C). This process is repeated until the desired potency is reached, from 10X to 30C with the more diluted mixtures considered to be the most powerful.

Primary Uses

Hahnemann believed that his remedies worked by interacting with some subtle energy inherent in all individuals, which he called the vital force. The energies of the remedies captured by the potentizing process interacted with this vital force to assist the body in healing itself—all the body needed was the gentle nudge provided by the remedy. Since illness manifests on the three levels of a human being (mental/spiritual, emotional/psychic, and physical), homeopathic remedies can heal on all three levels. Thus, homeopathy can be used to treat both acute and chronic illnesses, although chronic illness may be harder to treat due to the breadth of their symptoms.

When an individual visits a homeopath for treatment, the homeopath will generally ask the person to tell his or her life story, including the chief complaint for which the person is seeking assistance. Since the homeopath is looking for a complete picture of the individual and his or her symptoms, various questionnaires including a complete family history may be administered. The questionnaires may include questions concerning the various body systems, personality and temperament traits, food preferences, fears, and general features of lifestyle such as exercise and time of day that symptoms get better or worse. The homeopath will then use all of this information to try to understand the overall manifestation of disease so that the proper remedy can be provided. In general, homeopathy prefers a single remedy instead of a combination of remedies. Thus, a detailed analysis of the person's symptoms and lifestyle are necessary. Then, a repertory of remedies is consulted to determine the best remedy that will address the array of highly specific symptom displayed by the patient. Follow-up visits are often necessary so that the homeopath can evaluate the efficacy of the remedy or change the potency or frequency of dosage.

Often a patient will get worse after starting a remedy and then begin to get better. In homeopathy, this is called "the healing crisis." The healing crisis is usually signaled by a worsening of the symptoms soon after beginning the treatment. The symptoms then begin to lessen, sometimes within a few minutes. If the symptoms persist or get unbearable, a different remedy may be indicated, and the homeopath should be consulted immediately.

The efficacy of homeopathic remedies can be lessened through the interference of other substances such as coffee, many pharmaceutical medicines, and allergens. Even such diagnostic techniques as X-rays and MRI scans can negatively affect the homeopathic remedy.

Training

Although homeopathy was popular in the eighteenth and nineteenth centuries, its use declined in the early twentieth century with the rise of allopathic medicine. Since the

1960s it has again begun to grow in use, especially in Europe and India. Many countries, including England, France, Germany, the Netherlands, India, Argentina, Brazil, and Mexico have homeopathic medical schools and homeopathic hospitals. Around the world, there is a growing interest and use of homeopathy with a growing number of allopathic physicians prescribing homeopathic remedies in addition to pharmaceutical medicines.

In the United States and Canada, homeopathy is just beginning its comeback. The Council on Homeopathic Education (CHE), founded in 1982, serves as an independent agency to assess and accredit homeopathic training programs in the United States and Canada. Currently, only two schools are accredited by CHE. Many other schools offer programs in homeopathy but have not received accreditation from the CHE. Other programs are available through weekend programs and by correspondence courses. In the United States there is no overall regulation of homeopathic practitioners. Homeopathic remedies, on the other hand, are regulated by the Food and Drug Administration, but they are not regulated as medicines. Thus, efficacy does not have to be demonstrated.

Sources

Carlston, Michael. 2003. *Classical Homeopathy*. New York: Churchill Livingstone.
Hahnemann, Samuel. 1982. *Organon of Medicine*. 6th ed. Blaine, WA: Cooper Pub.
Vithoulkas, George. 1980. *The Science of Homeopathy*. New York: Grove Press.

See also ENERGY MEDICINE AND ENERGY HEALING; FLOWER THERAPIES

Annotated Bibliography

Print Resources

- Boericke, William. 2007. *Boericke's New Manual of Homeopathic Materia Medica with Repertory*. 3rd rev. and augmented ed. New Delhi: B. Jain Publishers. 1137 pp. ISBN: 813190184X; 9788131901847.
  For the practice of homeopathy, a homeopathic materia medica is a required reference since it lists the available homeopathic remedies and presents the symptoms that were demonstrated during the proving of a remedy. Thus under each remedy is a general description of the symptoms experienced by those who participated in the proving. This is followed by a more detailed list of symptoms categorized by their location, such as mind, head, face, stomach, abdomen, urine, female, respiratory, back, extremities, skin, and fever. Usually, other remedies that are similar are given and the appropriate dose is cited. A repertory of symptoms arranged by body system lists remedies associated with that particular symptom.
- Carlston, Michael. 2003. *Classical Homeopathy*. New York: Churchill Livingstone. 182 pp. ISBN: 0443065659; 9780443065651.
  Aimed at health care professionals and students, this text seeks to provide a basic understanding of homeopathy, its history, principles, and research on its efficacy. It does not address specific illnesses or discuss specific remedies.
- Feingold, Ellen. 2008. *The Complete Self-Care Guide to Homeopathy, Herbal Remedies & Nutritional Supplements: Everything You Need to Know about These Essential Natural Alternatives for Health*. Albany, NY: Whitston. 383 pp. ISBN: 0878755632; 9780878755639.

This is a comprehensive introduction to the use of homeopathy, herbal remedies, and nutritional supplements for personal health care. The book can be used in two ways. First, it is a good way to learn the basics of these three types of remedies. Second, it can be used to find ways to treat a specific ailment, condition, or disease. The first part of the book focuses on homeopathy and is divided into chapters that discuss specific conditions and their associated homeopathic remedies. Part 2 is much briefer and provides useful information on 16 major herbs that are commonly used. A separate chapter discusses women's health and includes 8 additional herbs. The final part discusses nutritional supplements including vitamins and minerals, antioxidants, and nutritional supplements for the heart, for weight control, and for the immune system. Due to its breadth of coverage this will be a well-used book in the library's collection.

- Griffith, Colin. 2007. *The New Materia Medica: Key Remedies for the Future of Homoeopathy*. London: Watkins Publishing. 561 pp. ISBN: 1905857276; 9781905857272.
  In this work, the author discusses 36 new homeopathic remedies made from crystal, botanical, and animal sources. The entry for each remedy describes the original source of the remedy, its traditional and medical uses throughout history, its relationship to the chakras and their associated glands and organs, the symptoms that can be treated by the remedy (including physical, mental, and emotional symptoms), related remedies, and case notes that give clinical evidence of the efficacy and use of the remedy. Thus, practitioners of homeopathy are the intended audience.

- Griffith, Colin. 2008. *The Practical Handbook of Homeopathy: Safe, Effective Home Prescriptions for Common Conditions*. New rev. ed. London: Watkins. 386 pp. ISBN: 1905857608; 9781905857609.
  This guide is designed for use in the home. It has several goals, among which are teaching the reader to think "homeopathically" when approaching physical illness, helping recognize when the help of a practitioner is needed, recognizing when symptoms or illness require emergency assistance, and providing assistance in choosing the correct homeopathic remedy for common ailments and first aid. The bulk of the book discusses selecting remedies for conditions, such as fever, influenza, headaches, sleep problems, hormone imbalances, or traveling abroad. The final section presents 50 remedies that should be kept in a home first-aid kit.

- Hahnemann, Samuel. 1982. *Organon of Medicine*. 6th ed. Translated by Alain Naudé. Blaine, WA: Cooper Pub. 270 pp. ISBN: 0963631209; 9780963631206.
  This book can be considered the bible of homeopathy. Hahnemann, as the father of homeopathy, is responsible for most of its basic tenets. In this work, he recorded his theories of homeopathy in a very orderly fashion so that they could be learned and applied methodically. Even today, this is the standard work on homeopathy.

- Haller, John S. 2005. *The History of American Homeopathy: The Academic Years, 1820–1935*. Binghamton, NY: The Haworth Press. 444 pp. ISBN: 0789026600; 9780789026606.
- Haller, John S. 2009. *The History of American Homeopathy: From Rational Medicine to Holistic Health Care*. New Brunswick, NJ: Rutgers University Press. 191 pp. ISBN: 078903641X; 978078903641.
  These two books trace the history of homeopathy in America through its many changes of fortune, beginning with its introduction into the United States until today.

- Hershoff, Asa. 2000. *Homeopathic Remedies: A Quick and Easy Guide to Common Disorders and Their Homeopathic Treatments.* Garden City Park, NY: Avery. 319 pp. ISBN: 089529950X; 9780895299505.
  This is a handy and useful book on homeopathic remedies. The first section discusses how to use homeopathy to treat illness and provides information on how homeopaths view symptoms, the life force, disease, healing, and remedy prescribing and preparation. The second section briefly examines the systems of the body and diseases related to those systems. The final section is a listing of over 100 ailments and the homeopathic remedies associated with them. The entries for the remedies guide the reader in selecting the appropriate remedy to use. Due to its arrangement and ease of use, this will be a frequently used resource.

- Jonas, Wayne B., and Jacobs, Jennifer. 1998. *Healing with Homeopathy: The Doctors' Guide.* New York: Warner Books. 349 pp. ISBN: 0446673420; 9780446673426.
  Written for doctors as well as for the general reader, the goal of the book, according to the authors, is to give an overview of homeopathy in addition to providing information for using homeopathy for common, minor health problems. Thus, there is a good, balanced discussion of the history and development of homeopathy and the research that supports the use of homeopathy. The chapters on common illnesses and injuries suggest specific remedies for children and babies, acute respiratory illness, women's health problems, digestive problems, skin problems, headaches and toothaches, musculoskeletal problems, and acute emotional problems and insomnia.

- Kayne, Steven B. 2006. *Homeopathic Pharmacy: Theory and Practice.* 2nd ed. New York: Elsevier Churchill Livingstone. 386 pp. ISBN: 0443101604; 9780443101601.
  Aimed at those practicing homeopathy and pharmacists, yet of interest to those who have an interest in homeopathy, Kayne has created a book that focuses on the homeopathic remedy and its proving. He offers details on the potencies and scales of homeopathic remedies, how they are made, their history, legislation, and standards.

- Kayne, Steven B. 2008. *Homeopathic Practice.* Chicago: Pharmaceutical Press. 360 pp. ISBN: 0853697264; 9780853697268.
  This book is designed for those who have a goal of practicing homeopathy. Coverage includes the theory of homeopathy, the proving of homeopathic drugs, the use of homeopathic medicines by health care providers around the world, and using the homeopathic materia medica.

- Kent, James Tyler. 2004. *Repertory of the Homeopathic Materia Medica.* 6th ed. (reprinted). New Delhi: B. Jain. 1542 pp. ISBN: 8131902315; 9788170210597.
  For anyone with a deep interest in homeopathy, a good repertory is a necessity. This one is based on Kent's original from the nineteenth century, but it is still a preferred version due to its depth. The repertory lists symptoms associated with a region of the body and remedies associated with these symptoms. Thus, the use of the repertory is a major step on the path to finding the correct remedy to treat the symptoms of a patient. Kent's repertory includes symptoms associated with 648 remedies.

- McCabe, Vinton. 2000. *Practical Homeopathy: A Comprehensive Guide to Homeopathic Remedies and Their Acute Uses.* New York: St. Martin's Griffin. 592 pp. ISBN: 0312206690; 9780312206697.

Although the author provides a very good introduction to the theory and philosophy of homeopathy, his goal is to provide a book that is useful for the treatment of acute illness. Thus, the focus is on the practical use of homeopathy. To this end, the book stresses the importance of the accurate diagnosis of symptoms, including states of being, states of mind, appearance of the face, indicators from the skin, and discharges from the body. Once the symptoms have been determined, the section on acute remedies and their uses can be consulted. This section is divided into wounds, injuries, emergencies, general aches and pains, ailments, and chronic complaints. The author also includes a materia medica of 60 major remedies that are useful for the treatment of acute illness. Of special note is the glossary of homeopathic terms, which can be very useful in negotiating the materia medica and other repertories of symptoms.

- McCabe, Vinton. 2005. *Household Homeopathy: A Safe and Effective Approach to Wellness for the Whole Family*. North Bergen, NJ: Basic Health Publications. 390 pp. ISBN: 1591200709; 9781591200703.
  The goal of this book is to provide practical information on how homeopathic remedies can be used in the home to treat acute situations such as wounds, bruises, injuries, emergencies, colds, and flu. Although the author briefly discusses the history and theory of homeopathy, he focuses primarily on case taking, the most frequently used remedies that can be keep in a homeopathic first aid kit, and the application of these remedies to treat a variety of common ailments and injuries.
- Owen, David. 2007. *Principles and Practice of Homeopathy: The Therapeutic and Healing Process*. Philadelphia: Churchill Livingstone Elsevier. 436 pp. ISBN: 0443100896; 9780443100895.
  Written by a homeopath who has been practicing for over 25 years, this is a comprehensive textbook on homeopathy, yet it is suitable for many general readers who seek a detailed understanding of the science and application of homeopathy. The text covers five themes: philosophy, materia medica (the remedies used in homeopathy), taking the case, analyzing the case, and managing the case. Case studies are regularly presented to help clarify specific issues.
- Panos, Maesimund B., and Heimlich, Jane. 1980. *Homeopathic Medicine at Home: Natural Remedies for Everyday Ailments and Minor Injuries*. New York: Jeremy P. Tarcher/Putnam. 287 pp. ISBN: 0874771951; 9780874771954.
  After a brief introduction to homeopathy and the work of the homeopathic physician, the authors delve directly into how homeopathy can be used in the home to treat minor illnesses and injuries. The chapters focus on preventing and treating colds, coughs, and earaches; on remedies for stomach and bowel problems; on creating a happier baby; on treating women and children; and on pet care. The appendixes provide useful information such as the remedies and their standard abbreviations, a mini-repertory of symptoms and their remedies, and a materia medica of the most frequently used remedies.
- Robins, Natalie S. 2005. *Copeland's Cure: Homeopathy and the War between Conventional and Alternative Medicine*. New York: Knopf. 330 pp. ISBN: 0375410902; 9780375410901.
  Using the life and work of Royal Copeland as a backdrop, this is the story of the struggle between homeopathy and conventional, allopathic medicine in the early

twentieth century. Copeland, who was an eye doctor, surgeon, mayor, dean, and United States senator, was a proponent of homeopathy and was responsible for the inclusion of homeopathic remedies in the Federal Food, Drug, and Cosmetic Act of 1938. In addition to Copeland's life and work the author covers the story of homeopathy in the United States before and after Copeland.

- Rowe, Todd. 1998. *Homeopathic Methodology: Repertory, Case Taking, and Case Analysis: An Introductory Homeopathic Workbook*. Berkeley, CA: North Atlantic Books. 158 pp. ISBN: 1556432771; 9781556432774.
  Designed for the student, beginning homeopath, or any interested individual with a basic knowledge of homeopathy, this workbook seeks to clarify the taking of cases from patients, the analysis of these cases, and the use of the homeopathic repertory to find appropriate remedies to prescribe. The author has succeeded in producing an easy-to-use, clear workbook that guides the reader through case taking and repertory use. A quiz for each lesson tests the knowledge learned in that lesson.
- Shalts, Edward. 2006. *Easy Homeopathy: The 7 Essential Remedies You Need for Common Illnesses and First Aid*. New York: McGraw-Hill. 267 pp. ISBN: 0071457585; 9780071457583.
  This book begins with an excellent introduction to the basic principles of homeopathy. The next seven chapters are devoted to remedies that should be found in every home: aconitum, arnica, belladonna, chamomilla, gelsemium, ignatia, and nux vomica. With only those seven remedies, many illnesses can be easily treated at home. The final section of the book examines common ailments and recommends homeopathic remedies to treat them.
- Shelton, Jay W. 2004. *Homeopathy: How It Really Works*. Amherst, NY: Prometheus Books. 319 pp. ISBN: 159102109X; 9781591021094.
  Although not a textbook about homeopathy, the author, a physicist, provides an in-depth assessment of homeopathy by delving into almost all aspects of homeopathy in his quest to understand the scientific basis of its workings. He discusses topics such as remedy potency, provings, the selection of the appropriate remedy for a patient, the administration of the remedy, and clinical effectiveness. He leans toward the explanation that homeopathy works due to its placebo effect and argues that homeopathy should be tested in a manner consistent with contemporary scientific method.
- Skinner, Sidney. 2001. *An Introduction to Homeopathic Medicine in Primary Care*. Gaithersburg, MD: Aspen Publishers. 473 pp. ISBN: 0834216760; 9780834216761.
  Written specifically for doctors, nurse practitioners, and physician assistants, this book is designed to introduce homeopathy and homeopathic remedies into the arsenal available to primary care providers. Although written for health care professionals, the educated reader will be able to understand and use this work. The first chapter gives an overview of homeopathy, its fundamentals, and the proper use of homeopathic remedies. Part 2 gives detailed information on 15 essential homeopathic remedies, from arnica montana to sulphur. The third section, "Clinical Prescribing," details how to prescribe remedies for common illnesses and diseases, arranged primarily by organ system. The final section discusses the history and future of homeopathy.

- Vithoulkas, George. 1980. *The Science of Homeopathy*. New York: Grove Press. 331 pp. ISBN: 0802151205; 9780802151209.
  Although slightly dated, this book remains one of the best general introductions to homeopathy by one of its leading practitioners. The author provides a detailed discussion of the basics of homeopathy including the laws and principles of cure and the practical application of homeopathy. Thus, excellent discussions are presented on the interaction of the human being and the environment, on the three levels of human existence (the mental, emotional, and physical planes), on the vital force, and on the outbreak of disease. The practical application section details how proving a remedy is accomplished, how medicines are prepared, how cases are taken, how symptoms are evaluated, how prescriptions are given, and how long-term care is provided.
- Wauters, Ambika. 2007. *The Homeopathy Bible: The Definitive Guide to Remedies*. New York: Sterling. 400 pp. ISBN: 1402745478; 9781402745478.
  Although other sources on homeopathy are more complete, this is a useful work for understanding homeopathy and using homeopathic remedies to help treat common ailments. The work includes a homeopathic materia medica as well as a section on treating acute and chronic conditions. The final section expands the scope by examining other adjunct therapies and essences.

Internet Resources

- ABC Homeopathy, abchomeopathy.com.
  Originally designed as a homeopathic remedy finder, the site has grown greatly and provides a good introduction to homeopathy and excellent discussions of 36 frequently used homeopathic remedies. In addition, the site now provides a homeopathic remedy store that offers over 50,000 products from a variety of providers.
- American Institute of Homeopathy, www.homeopathyusa.org.
  The AIH is a trade association that includes medical and osteopathic physicians, dentists, nurse practitioners, and physician assistants who incorporate homeopathy in their medical practices. The site is a good source of information on evidence based homeopathy. The AIH publishes the *American Journal of Homeopathic Medicine*.
- Classical Homeopathy, www.homeopathy-cures.com.
  Providing general information on homeopathy, this site seeks to disseminate information on a variety of problems that can be helped by homeopathic remedies including attention deficit disorder or attention deficit/hyperactivity disorder, allergies, asthma, bipolar disorder, candida and yeast infections, chronic fatigue, depression, ear infections, fibromyalgia, headaches and migraines, insomnia, menstrual problems, rheumatoid arthritis, temporomandibular joint problems, and more. There is also a directory of homeopaths.
- Council for Homeopathic Certification, www.homeopathicdirectory.com.
  Since 1991, the Council for Homeopathic Certification has certified homeopaths who have completed specific educational and clinical requirements and passed the certification exam. The site has a directory of certified homeopaths by state.
- The Homeopathic Academy of Naturopathic Physicians, www.hanp.net.
  HANP represents naturopathic physicians who incorporate homeopathy into their practices. In addition to publishing the journal *Simillimum*, HANP hosts conferences,

offers seminars and continuing education, and offers specialty certification in homeopathy for naturopathic physicians.

- Homeopathic Educational Services, www.homeopathic.com.
  This website seeks to be an all-encompassing resource center for homeopathic books, research, remedies, software, and correspondence courses for both the general public and the health care professional. The site also provides good general information on homeopathy and homeopathic remedies.
- Homeopathy for Everyone, www.hpathy.com.
  Based in India but with a worldwide coverage, this site offers information both for the professional and for the general public. Resources include full-text homeopathy books such as Hahnemann's *Organon of Medicine* and *Chronic Diseases*, Allen's *Materia Medica*, and Boericke's *Homeopathy Repertory*. Other resources include book reviews, clinical cases, recent papers, an online repertory and materia medica, and tools for the promotion of health.
- Homeopathy Home, www.homeopathyhome.com.
  Offering such resources as directories of homeopathic organizations, practitioners, pharmacies, and courses; references such as full-text books, articles, and other research information; and services such as links to providers of remedies and other supplied, Homeopathy Home provides a wealth of information although it is often embedded with advertising.
- The National Center for Homeopathy, homeopathic.org.
  One of the best resources for finding information on homeopathy, this site is useful to both the general public and the practicing homeopath. The site includes helpful articles on a wide variety of topics and provides additional links to professional associations, educational programs, products and services, and listings of homeopaths.
- North American Network of Homeopathic Educators, www.homeopathyeducation.org.
  NANHE is dedicated to providing excellence in homeopathic education and to increasing the awareness of homeopathy among the general public. The site provides a directory of sources for homeopathic education around the United States.
- North American Society of Homeopaths, www.homeopathy.org.
  The North American Society of Homeopaths seeks to set standards of competency and to certify individuals in the practice of classical homeopathy. Of special note is the section on current research in homeopathy, which provides full-text or scanned images of articles on topics such as AIDS, cancer, clinical studies, government reports, homeopathic drugs, and study design.

Periodicals/Magazines/Journals

- *The American Homeopath*, published by the North American Society of Homeopaths, 1994– . Annual. No ISSN. www.homeopathy.org/journal.html.
  Representing professional homeopaths in the United States and Canada, this journal includes interviews, scholarly feature articles, case studies, and studies on homeopathic materia medica. Its goal is to publish relevant information on classical homeopathy that can be used in the practice of homeopathy.

- *American Journal of Homeopathic Medicine*, published by American Institute of Homeopathy, 1846– . Quarterly. ISSN: 1934-2454. www.homeopathyusa.org/journal.
  A venerable peer-reviewed scientific journal, AJHM publishes research reports, case studies, book reviews, position papers, seminar summaries, and articles on the history of homeopathy.
- *Health and Homeopathy*, published by British Homeopathic Association, 1980– . Quarterly. ISSN: 0965-1292. www.trusthomeopathy.org/trust/tru_hh.html.
  Designed for both homeopathic doctors and those interested in a holistic approach to their health, this British magazine covers all aspects of homeopathy.
- *Homeopathy*, published by Churchill Livingstone, 1911– . Quarterly. ISSN: 1475-4916. www.elsevier.com/locate/homp.
  An international, peer-reviewed journal, *Homeopathy* seeks to publish articles based on clinical and basic research in addition to clinical studies and evidence-based practices in homeopathy. It also aims to increase the understanding of homeopathy and its practice among practitioners of both traditional medicine and complementary practices.
- *Homeopathy in Practice*, published by the Alliance of Registered Homeopaths, 2001– . Three times a year. ISSN: 1475-8555. www.a-r-h.org/Publications/Journal.htm.
  As its name states, this journal focuses on the practice of homeopathy. Articles include news features, interviews, reports of developments in homeopathic practice, and book reviews.
- *Homeopathy Today*, published by National Center for Homeopathy, 1980– . Bimonthly. ISSN: 0886-1676. homeopathic.org/media/homeopathy_today.
  Published six times a year, *Homeopathy Today* is included with membership in the National Center for Homeopathy. Its articles stress topics such as treatments for common ailments, the homeopathic treatment process, the philosophical foundations of homeopathy, and the use of specific remedies for the treatment of disease. Other features include discussions on homeopathic education, recent legislation that may impact homeopathic practice, updates on conferences and workshops, and reviews of new books.
- *Simillimum*, published by Homeopathic Academy of Naturopathic Physicians, 1988– . Quarterly. ISSN: 1526-1964. www.hanp.net/volumes/current.
  A peer-reviewed journal for practitioners of homeopathy, *Simillimum* presents case studies using both traditional and contemporary methods of analysis, information from the materia medica, and discussions on homeopathic philosophy. It also includes interviews with influential teachers and leaders, reviews new homeopathic publications and seminars, and discusses issues related to the practice of homeopathy and case management.

Chapter 13

Iridology and Sclerology

Background and History

Iridology is the study of the iris of the eye, especially its color and structure, as an aid in the diagnosis of the health of an individual. According to iridology, the iris, the colored portion of the eye surrounding the pupil, is a mirror of the body, its functions, and its dysfunctions. Thus, inflammation and inherent bodily weaknesses will be apparent in the iris, sometimes even before obvious symptoms are being exhibited. Sclerology is a related discipline that studies the red lines in the white of the eyes, known as the sclera. The sclerologist interprets these red lines as a way of determining how the body is attempting to maintain its healthy balance in response to the stress present in life.

Although there are claims that iridology is much older, its modern history can be traced to nineteenth-century Europe. Two individuals stand out as discoverers of iridology: Dr. Ignatz von Peczely and Rev. Nils Liljequist. In 1837 in Hungary, as the traditional story goes, von Peczely, then aged 10, captured an owl, which broke its leg in an attempt to get free. As soon as the break happened, von Peczely saw that a spot developed in the iris of the owl. Many years later, von Peczely noticed a similar spot in the iris of a man who had also broken his leg. Von Peczely remembered his earlier experience with the owl. After studying medicine, von Peczely began a practice in which he utilized iridology to assist in the diagnosis of disease. To assist his diagnoses, he created a chart of the irides (the plural form of iris) showing the location of major organ systems that are affected by disease or illness.

At about the same time in Sweden, Liljequist noticed that his irides were becoming discolored as a result of medications he was taking during a severe illness. He also noticed that the color of his eyes began to return to normal when he stopped taking the medications. He continued to observe his own irides and those of others and eventually created a chart of the irides that showed remarkable similarities to the chart created by von Peczely.

Iridology was introduced into Germany by Erdmann Leopold Stephanus Emanuel Felke, a clergyman. The Felke Institute continues to operate and promote iridology in Germany. Iridology came to the United States through the work of Dr. Henry Edward Lane, an Austrian physician. Lane, in turn, taught iridology to Dr. Henry Lindlahr, who promulgated the use of iridology through his many writings. The most important contemporary proponent for iridology was Dr. Bernard Jensen, a chiropractor and nutritionist. Jensen wrote extensively about iridology and taught workshops and classes around the world until he died in 2001 at the age of 92.

Primary Uses and Actions

Iridology and sclerology are generally considered tools in the arsenal of techniques used by a holistic health practitioner. Such a practitioner seeks to treat the whole person, not just the disease. Iridology and sclerology permit the practitioner to examine and analyze the overall health of an individual and search for areas of inflammation or weaknesses that may signal a threat to the individual's health. The irides also show healing so that the course of treatment can be traced. The iridologist examines the color of the eye, spots that may be located in the iris, and the arrangement of the fibers that compose the iris. Iridology must not be confused with ophthalmology, which treats diseases and dysfunctions of the eye, or with optometry, which examines and treats errors of vision using optical lenses. Iridologists will not diagnose diseases since only a licensed medical doctor can legally diagnose.

Iridologists usually employ highly detailed charts that map the body onto each of the irides. Although the charts are similar for each iris, they are not identical since some organs are more prominent in one iris than in the other. For example, the heart is represented in the left iris, but not in the right. Similarly, the spleen maps onto the left iris while the liver maps onto the right. Special reverse charts are available for examining your own eyes since they show the maps arranged to match your eyes as they appear in a mirror. At one time, iridologists had to perform their analyses using lights and magnifying glasses. Today there are special cameras, microscopes, and viewing systems to assist them in their work.

Sclerologists also use specific eye charts to help them determine the areas of stress in the body. They prefer to work using natural light and will chart the sclera from the top of the eye in a clockwise manner.

Training

There is no standard education or training for the practice of iridology or sclerology, and most practitioners of both techniques are self-taught through personal reading, attendance at workshops, and web-based courses. Founded in 1982, the International Iridology Practitioners Association seeks to increase knowledge concerning iridology. The association has also developed educational criteria for becoming a certified iridologist, manages the certification examinations, and offers classes in iridology. The International Sclerology Institute promotes the use of sclerology and provides certification for sclerologists.

Sources

Jensen, Bernard. 1995, ©1952. *The Science and Practice of Iridology: A System of Analyzing and Caring for the Body through the Use of Drugless and Nature-Cure Methods.* Escondido, CA: Bernard Jensen International.

Tips, Jack. 2007. *Sclerology, The Foundational Program: A Course on the Art & Science of Sclerology*. Austin, TX: Apple-a-Day Press.

See also ALTERNATIVE DIAGNOSIS TECHNIQUES

Annotated Bibliography

Print Resources

➤ Bamer, Donald R. 1996. *Practical Iridology and Sclerology*. Pleasant Grove, UT: Woodland Publishing. 216 pp. ISBN: 1885670028; 9781885670021.

Aimed at both the layperson and the professional, this book provides an introduction to iridology and sclerology. Both techniques can be used by the individual or a health professional to identify healthy and unhealthy trends in lifestyle. Major concepts from iridology and sclerology are illustrated through the use of black and white drawings and color photographs of the eye. In addition, the author suggests herbal remedies that are indicated by the readings of the eye.

- Jensen, Bernard. 1995, ©1952. *The Science and Practice of Iridology: A System of Analyzing and Caring for the Body through the Use of Drugless and Nature-Cure Methods.* Escondido, CA: Bernard Jensen International. 372 pp. ISBN: 1885653239; 9781885653239.
  A complete introductory text to the study and practice of iridology by one of the world's leading authorities, this book can be considered the bible of iridology. Divided into six parts, all aspects of iridology are covered. Part 1 provides the historical and theoretical bases of iridology while also discussing the concepts of healing and cure. Part 2 instructs the reader in how to perform an iris reading, compares the normal and the abnormal iris, and presents the ten general field areas that map onto the iris. The interpretation of iris manifestations of illness, disease, toxicity, and other health problems is the focus of Part 3, while Part 4 provides black and white and color illustrations of iris manifestations. Part 5 gives case histories according to iridology, while Part 6 introduces advanced research in iridology.
- Jensen, Bernard, and Bodeen, Donald V. 1992. *Visions of Health: Understanding Iridology.* Garden City Park, NY: Avery Publishing Group. 176 pp. ISBN: 0895294338; 9780895294333.
  One of the best introductions to iridology, this book provides both an overview of the field and an examination of iridology in action. The authors cover the history of iridology, its use in analyzing health, and the basics of doing a reading of the iris. A variety of illustrations help the beginner to understand the concepts being discussed.
- Navratil, Frank 2001. *For Your Eyes Only: A Fascinating Look at the Art and Science of Iris Diagnosis, the Diagnostic Method of the New Millennium.* Prague, Czech Republic: Frank Navratil; Woodstock, NY: Distributed by Beekman Publishers. 158 pp. ISBN: 8023872206; 9788023872200.
  This is an excellent introduction to the study of iridology. Color photographs accompany the text and provide excellent support for learning to diagnose using the irides. The author includes chapters that both introduce the practice of iridology and delve into the specific body systems as shown in the irides. Case histories also give additional support to the text.
- O'Brian, Betty Sue, and Tips, Jack. 2007. *Causations: Using Sclerology to Clarify Iridology.* Austin, TX: Apple-a-Day Press. 126 pp. ISBN: 0929167325; 9780929167329.
  Based on the naturopathic philosophy of health and healing, this book presents the use of sclerology as an adjunct to the diagnosis of illness using iridology. Through case histories and photographs of eyes, the authors present sclerology and iridology as methods for examining the health issues of clients and for determining the proper therapies to administer.
- Tips, Jack. 2007. *Sclerology, The Foundational Program: A Course on the Art & Science of Sclerology.* Austin, TX: Apple-a-Day Press. 444 pp. ISBN: 0929167333; 9780929167336.
  Providing a detailed introduction to sclerology, this work can serve as a desk reference for the practicing alternative health provider. The author discusses how to use sclerology properly for diagnostic purposes and how to identify illness and disease in

specific tissue zones. The work is well illustrated and includes detailed case histories of clients.

- Tips, Jack, and Richardson, Mark. 1999. *Insights in the Eyes, An Introduction to Sclerology: How to Interpret the Red Lines in the White of the Eye*. Austin, TX: Apple-a-Day Press. 77 pp. ISBN: 0929167112; 9780929167114.
  This small book can serve as a brief sclerology, the interpretation of the red lines in the whites of the eyes. In addition, the authors discuss using sclerology to help fight candida and fungus infection and for determining the gender of the unborn child.

Internet Resources

- The International College of Iridology, americancollegeofiridology.org/index.html.
  Dedicated to the education of iridologists worldwide, the International College of Iridology provides continuing education programs and conferences for both students of iridology and the practicing iridologist. The ICI also seeks to advance iridology through research and clinical practice.
- The International Iridology Practitioners Association, www.iridologyassn.org.
  The International Iridology Practitioners Association seeks to increase the knowledge of iridology and to provide a forum for the exchange of information and research on iridology. It also promotes international standards for the practice of iridology.
- International Sclerology Institute, www.sclerology-institute.org.
  The goal of the International Sclerology Institute is to promote the use of sclerology as a method for assisting in the diagnosis and treatment of health-related issues. The institute seeks to promote education and research in the use of sclerology.

Periodicals/Magazines/Journals

- *Advanced Iridology Research Journal*, published by John Andrews, 2000– . Semi-annual. ISSN: 1471-3926. www.johnandrewsiridology.net/index.htm.
  This journal seeks to publish iridology research from around the world.
- *International Journal of Iridology and Integrative Healthcare*, published by the International College of Iridology, 2004– . Three times a year. No ISSN. americancollegeofiridology.org/index.html.
  Covering both iridology and the integration of alternative therapies into general health care, this journal is published by the International College of Iridology, the major professional association of iridologists.

Chapter 14

Meditation

Background and History

Meditation is often associated with Hinduism and Buddhism, yet meditation or quiet contemplation is found in many world religions. The origins of meditation in India can be traced back for over 5,000 years. Sometimes considered to be a form of prayer, meditation is a method through which the mind is quieted so that the one who is meditating may experience a state of deep relaxation or higher awareness of the world, of himself or herself, or of the divine. The goal of meditation is to free the mind of its conditioning or habitual ways of thinking and observing the world so that a higher state of consciousness can be obtained.

Different meditation techniques offer their practitioners different goals. Some practitioners wish to quiet the mind and commune with the divine, while others may seek to find answers to major life questions. Still others seek increased self-awareness or simple relaxation. Mindfulness meditation focuses on heightening the experience of one's own perceptions and may involve concentration on routine tasks. Some meditation involves the practitioner's concentration on a specific object, such as the flame of a candle. During this style of meditation, the intense focus quiets the mind and frees it of its conditioned thoughts. Meditation can be done sitting, lying, standing, or even walking. Sometimes prayers or mantras—that is, a specific sound or phrase—may be repeated during the meditation in order to help the mind focus.

Primary Uses and Actions

The primary action of meditation is relaxation, although often those who meditate also report that the meditation may be stimulating. Research has shown that the mental relaxation achieved through meditation can reduce stress, thereby reducing blood pressure, decreasing the heart rate, and decreasing respiration while also assisting concentration. During meditation, pain may also be reduced and depression may be eased. Thus, meditation is often suggested by physicians and psychologists as a complement to medication and other therapies.

Training

As with many complementary and alternative therapies, there are no universal standards for training in meditation. Since many meditation techniques have their origins in religion, they have often been taught by religious devotees and priests. One of the most popular meditation techniques is Transcendental Meditation (TM) which is taught by followers of Maharishi Mahesh Yogi, an Indian spiritual teacher. The TM movement offers classes in their style of mantra-based meditation throughout the United States.

Often churches, temples, and even community recreation centers offer classes in meditation. Weekend and longer meditation retreats abound. Similarly, there is a plethora of books, CDs, and DVDs that purport to teach meditation.

Sources

Bodian, Stephan. 2006. *Meditation for Dummies*. 2nd ed. Hoboken, NJ: Wiley.

Davich, Victor N. 1998. *The Best Guide to Meditation*. Los Angeles, CA: Renaissance Books.

Meditation, www.beliefnet.com/Holistic-Living/Meditation/index.aspx.

See also AYURVEDA; SPIRITUALITY, RELIGION, AND PRAYER; YOGA

Annotated Bibliography

Print Resources

- Arpaia, Joseph, and Rapgay, Lobsang. 2008. *Real Meditation in Minutes a Day: Enhancing Your Performance, Relationships, Spirituality, and Health*. Boston: Wisdom Publications. 237 pp. ISBN: 086171556X; 9780861715565.
  Meditation, when practiced regularly, can help restore memory, enhance creativity, and lead to clearer thinking. To help achieve these results, the authors have written a guide for novice meditators that will help move them toward the establishment of a regular meditation practice. Of special note are the sections that answer common questions and give advice on avoiding potential pitfalls and obstacles that may inhibit one's meditation.
- Bear, Marina. 2009. *The Little Book of Meditation: A Guide to Stress-Free Living*. Berkeley, CA: SLG Books. 96 pp. ISBN: 0943389410; 9780943389417.
  In this short book, the author presents several strategies for overcoming stress and finding relaxation through meditation. She discusses the benefits of meditation and explains several of the major meditation traditions while providing guidance on beginning a practice of meditation.
- Bodian, Stephan. 2006. *Meditation for Dummies*. 2nd ed. Hoboken, NJ: Wiley. 360 pp. ISBN: 0471777749; 9780471777748.
  Written by a long time teacher of meditation, this book provides a comprehensive overview of meditation techniques and practices. Structured similarly to other books in the Dummies series, the book can be used as a manual for those who wish to learn to meditate and as a guide for those who wish to take their meditation practice to a deeper level. Although meditation is an art that must be practiced to truly be learned, the author provides many helpful suggestions and exercises that can help the reader begin his or her journey into the world as it is revealed through meditation.
- Davich, Victor N. 1998. *The Best Guide to Meditation*. Los Angeles, CA: Renaissance Books. 350 pp. ISBN: 1580630103; 9781580630108.
  The goal of this book is to provide a guided tour of meditation and the various forms of meditation. Part 1 gives the reader a quick introduction to meditation and the establishment of a meditation practice. Part 2 examines a variety of meditation practices such as those found in Hinduism, Buddhism, Judaism, Islam, and Christianity.

The last part delves into the meditative life and gives tips on integrating meditation into all phases of live, creating a meditative home, and increasing happiness while reducing pain and stress through meditation. For readers who seek a general overview of meditation and its practice, this is an excellent choice.

➤ Didonna, Fabrizio, ed. 2009. *Clinical Handbook of Mindfulness*. New York: Springer. 523 pp. ISBN: 0387095926; 9780387095929.
This edited work contains a wealth of information on mindfulness meditation, including its history, its practice, and its clinical applications. After introductory chapters, the work includes chapters on specific illnesses that may be helped by mindfulness meditation such as anxiety disorders, obsessive-compulsive disorder, depression, addictive behavior, and post-traumatic stress disorder. Thus, it is very helpful for the therapist who wishes to integrate meditation into the treatment plans for their clients.

➤ Goldstein, Joseph. 2003, ©1993. *Insight Meditation: The Practice of Freedom*. Boston: Shambhala. 179 pp. ISBN: 1590300165; 9781590300169.
This is a guide to the practice of meditation based on Buddhist teachings. Thus, it addresses issues such as dharma, the four noble truths, and grace. Although based on Buddhism, it is also a clearly written instruction manual on the practice of meditation and offers many insights into the reaction of the human mind to meditation. Thus, for those who regularly meditate, this guide can also be a solace since it helps address many issues that they may be experiencing.

➤ Goldstein, Joseph, and Kornfield, Jack. 2001. *Seeking the Heart of Wisdom: The Path of Insight Meditation*. Boston: Shambhala. 242 pp. ISBN: 157062805X; 9781570628054.
Through exercises and clear writing, the authors introduce the reader to the teachings and practices of insight meditation. The chapters take the reader from a basic understanding of meditation to a deep understanding of life and spirituality. The first section introduces meditation in general and insight meditation in particular. In addition the authors discuss the difficulties and hindrances in developing a meditation practice. The second section seeks to help train the heart and the mind, using the life of the Buddha as an example. The third section focuses on the growth of wisdom and addresses topics such as karma, perspectives on reality, and the path of service. Although based on Buddhist teachings, this guide can be beneficial to anyone who approaches it with an open mind.

➤ Gunaratana, Henepola. 2002. *Mindfulness in Plain English*. Boston: Wisdom Publications. 208 pp. ISBN: 0861713214; 9780861713219.
Written by a teacher of meditation who became a Buddhist monk at the age of 12, this book provides an in-depth introduction to meditation. Although the author is a Buddhist, he presents meditation as a technique that transcends religions. Chapters discuss what meditation isn't, what meditation is, and what to do with your body and your mind during meditation. He provides exercises and good advice on setting up and structuring a meditation practice as well as how to deal with distractions. For anyone interesting in learning to meditate, this is a good introduction to its practice.

➤ Hoopes, Aaron. 2002. *Perfecting Ourselves: Coordinating Body, Mind and Spirit*. Hartford, CT: Turtle Press. 211 pp. ISBN: 1880336685; 9781880336687.
Through techniques such as breathing exercises, meditation, focused quietism, and conscious living, the author hopes that his readers can develop healthy habits, heal

and strengthen their bodies, reduce their tension and stress, increase the connection between their mind and body, and achieve internal balance. Reflecting these aims, the book is divided into three main sections: body, mind, and spirit. The goal of each section is to awaken our awareness of that aspect of our being so that by the end of the book we are on our way to a more perfect self.

➤ Johnston, William. 1997, ©1974. *Silent Music: The Science of Meditation*. New York: Fordham University Press. 190 pp. ISBN: 0823217752; 9780823217755.
This is not a book on how to perform meditation but a discourse on meditation presented from a variety of perspectives. The first part delves into meditation itself and examines the science of mysticism as well as brainwaves and biofeedback. Part 2 focuses on consciousness, while Part 3 looks at healing, including the healing of the mind and cosmic healing. The final part discusses intimacy, including the cosmic dimension of friendship. For those who maintain a regular contemplative or meditation practice, this book will deepen their understanding of their practice.

➤ Judy, Dwight H. 2000. *Christian Meditation and Inner Healing*. Akron, OH: OSL Publications. 130 pp. ISBN: 1878009389; 9781878009388.
Meditation is often considered an Eastern practice, but in this book the author shows how it can also be used by Christians as a means of healing and spiritual growth. Chapters discuss topics such as recovering the soul, meditating on God in creation, meditating on scripture, and the dynamics of inner healing. For Christians who wish to experience meditation but are wary of its ties to other religions, especially Buddhism, this is a very good book.

➤ Kabat-Zinn, Jon. 2005. *Wherever You Go, There You Are*. 10th anniversary ed. New York: Hyperion. 280 pp. ISBN: 1401307787; 9781401307783.
The goal of this book is to provide readers, especially those who are experiencing problems of stress, pain, or illness, with a brief and easy way to experience the essence of mindfulness meditation. For those who already practice meditation, it can help expand, deepen, and reinforce their experiences and lead to greater awareness and insight. Part 1 of the book gives the background and explores the rationale for beginning mindfulness meditation. Part 2 explains how to establish a meditation practice, while Part 3 covers a wide variety of topics and answers questions related to mindfulness.

➤ Kohn, Livia. 2008. *Meditation Works in the Daoist, Buddhist and Hindu Traditions*. Magdalena, NM: Three Pines Press. 263 pp. ISBN: 1931483086; 9781931483087.
Focusing on meditation as practiced in three traditions, the author contrasts each form of meditation, its worldview, its traditional practice, its medical adaptations, and its practice in modern settings.

➤ Kornfield, Jack. 2008. *Meditation for Beginners*. Boulder, CO: Sounds True. 93 pp. ISBN: 1591799422; 9781591799429.
Through this little book, the author teaches a simple meditation technique. After chapters that cover the ancient art of meditation, why people should meditate, and the benefits of meditation, he immediately jumps in with actual meditations that can be done in conjunction with the accompanying CD. In all, eight different meditations with different purposes are provided, such as connecting with the breath, working

with sensations in the body, working with feelings and emotions, forgiveness, and walking. The final chapter gives helpful hints on cultivating a daily meditation practice. This is an especially worthwhile book for those who wish to experience meditation without all of the added material that usually accompanies books on the topic.

➤ Koster, Frits. 2007. *Buddhist Meditation in Stress Management*. Chiang Mai, Thailand: Silkworm Books. 190 pp. ISBN: 9749511298; 9789749511299.
For many people, stress is a regular part of their lives and a cause of much illness. In this book, the author discusses the phenomenon of stress, the sources of stress, methods of stress management, and the use of meditation as a stress management tool. Although the work is based on Buddhist ideas, the concepts are universal and can be applied by most individuals, regardless of religious background. Several types of meditation are introduced, including relaxation meditation, insight meditation, and walking meditation.

➤ Langer, Ellen J. 1989. *Mindfulness*. Reading, MA: Addison-Wesley. 234 pp. ISBN: 0201095025; 9780201095029.
The simple title of this book belies the breadth of its contents. Mindfulness is a broad concept that carries with it many meanings. The author delves into this concept first by discussing its opposite, mindlessness, and the negative implications that mindlessness has in our lives. Then she introduces mindfulness and presents its nature and effect on many aspects of our lives including aging, creative uncertainty, work, decreasing prejudice, and improving our health. Her use of anecdotes from her own research enlivens the text and reinforces the ideas being presented.

➤ Mace, Chris. 2008. *Mindfulness and Mental Health: Therapy, Theory, and Science*. New York: Routledge. 188 pp. ISBN: 158391787X; 9781583917879.
The term *mindfulness* is often associated with meditation, but it is also a way of being aware. Although the concept arises out of Buddhist ideas, it has also been applied to many areas of inquiry, especially therapy. In this book, the author discusses the origins of the concept of mindfulness, the science behind it, its use in therapy, the relationship between mindfulness and mental disorder, and how mindfulness can impact mental health.

➤ Nhat Hanh, Thich. 1999, ©1987. *The Miracle of Mindfulness: An Introduction to the Practice of Meditation*. Rev. ed. Boston: Beacon Press. 140 pp. ISBN: 0807012394; 9780807012390.
The author is often considered one of the greatest proponents of mindfulness meditation in the West. In this small book, he uses anecdotes and exercises to teach the skills of mindfulness and meditation. His examples are as mundane as washing the dishes and drinking tea, but his insights are ethereal and eternal. Thus, for anyone seeking a simple yet profound practice of meditation, this book is highly recommended.

➤ Novak, John. 2008. *How to Meditate: A Step-by-Step Guide to the Art and Science of Meditation*. Rev. ed., 2nd ed. Nevada City, CA: Crystal Clarity Publishers. 199 pp. ISBN: 1565892348; 9781565892347.
This book provides a good overview of meditation Chapters discuss getting started with a meditation practice, relaxing the body, relaxing the mind, and the basic routine for meditation. In addition, the author summarizes scientific studies on meditation, the chakras, and Patanjali's eightfold path.

- Oliver, Joan Duncan, ed. 2009. *Commit to Sit: Tools for Cultivating a Meditation Practice from the Pages of Tricycle*. Carlsbad, CA: Hay House. 246 pp. ISBN: 1401921752; 9781401921750.
  Reprinting articles that originally appeared in the Buddhist magazine *Tricycle*, this book introduces the art of meditation and its ability to help individuals lead a healthy and meaningful life. The chapters define meditation, present a 28-day program for establishing a daily meditation practice, discuss issues that may arise during meditation, and demonstrate way for bringing mindfulness and compassion to daily life.
- Piver, Susan. 2008. *Quiet Mind: A Beginner's Guide to Meditation*. Boston: Shambhala. 120 pp. ISBN: 159030597, 9781590305973.
  Designed for those who wish to try meditation, this small book introduces the practice of meditation in an easy-to-understand way that can yield results quickly. The book and its accompanying CD include six different meditation practices presented by six Buddhist teachers. An additional chapter introduces six basic exercises. For those seeking a simple introduction to the art of meditation, this may be a useful resource.
- Roche, Lorin. 1998. *Meditation Made Easy*. San Francisco: HarperSanFrancisco. 198 pp. ISBN: 006251542X; 9780062515421.
  This book is designed both for those who have never meditated and those who have meditated but have trouble maintaining a meditation practice. After answering a variety of questions about meditation such as "Why should I meditate?" and "What can I do wrong?" the author introduces the reader to a simple meditation exercise. He then provides ways to go deeper into meditation and gives suggestions on fitting meditation into daily life. Since the book is easy to read and the exercises are very understandable, even the skeptical reader can begin to experience meditation quickly.
- Rodenbeck, Christina. 2008. *Meditation to Go: Learn to Relax, De-stress, Find Peace of Mind*. New York: Sterling. 142 pp. ISBN: 1856752968; 9781856752961.
  An introductory guide designed for those who are stressed, this work quickly and easily leads the reader into the world of meditation. The goal is to help establish a basic meditation practice while providing enough of the principles of meditation to help the beginner understand the actual process of meditation. The work includes photographs that help in the performance of the exercises.
- Salzberg, Sharon, and Goldstein, Joseph. 2001. *Insight Meditation: A Step-by-Step Course on How to Meditate*. Boulder, CO: Sounds True. 229 pp. ISBN: 1564559068; 9781564559067.
  This workbook, which comes with study cards and two CDs of guided meditations, is a complete introduction to the world of mindfulness meditation. It is divided into nine lessons, each of which addresses concepts such as suffering, karma, loving kindness, desire, and aversion. With these lessons, the authors take the reader step by step through the process of beginning a meditation practice. At the end of each lesson, there are exercises that reinforce the teachings and meditation experiences associated with the theme of the lesson. For those who cannot attend a meditation class but wish to learn about this healthful technique, this is a welcome alternative.

- Shear, Jonathan. 2006. *The Experience of Meditation: Experts Introduce the Major Traditions*. St. Paul, MN: Paragon House. 286 pp. ISBN: 155778857X; 9781557788573.
  Forms of meditation have arisen in a variety of places and in a variety of traditions, primarily religious. This book examines the experience of meditation from those perspectives. Individual chapters discuss meditation as perceived in Zen Buddhism, Transcendental Meditation, Taoism/qigong, yoga, Theravada Buddhism, Tibetan Buddhism, integral yoga, kriya yoga, Sufism, and Christianity. Although some meditation techniques are discussed, the focus is on the history and experience of meditation in the traditions represented. As an overview of a variety of meditation traditions, this is wonderful book.
- Shumsky, Susan G. 2002. *Exploring Meditation: Master the Ancient Art of Relaxation and Enlightenment*. Franklin Lakes, NJ: New Page Books. 254 pp. ISBN: 156414562X; 9781564145628.
  In this book, the author assists the reader in experiencing spiritual growth through meditation, simple yoga exercises, proper breathing, and the exploration of karma and past lives. It is also about healing using these techniques, about heightening spiritual insight, and about discovering enlightenment.
- Simpkins, C. Alexander, and Simpkins, Annellen M. 2009. *Meditation for Therapists and Their Clients*. New York: W. W. Norton. 324 pp. ISBN: 039370565X; 9780393705652.
  Due to its health benefits, meditation is often recommended as a way for individuals to sustain their health. This book is directed primarily toward therapists who can help their clients establish their own meditation practices. The book covers the various meditation traditions, the scientific evidence for the efficacy of meditation, and the process of establishing a meditation practice.
- Singh Khalsa, Dharma. 2002, ©2001. *Meditation as Medicine: Activate the Power of Your Natural Healing Force*. New York: Pocket Books. 352 pp. ISBN: 0743400658; 9780743400657.
  Meditation is usually thought of as a mental exercise, but in this book the author explores the health benefits of medical meditation. The first section of the book examines healing with medical meditation and explains how it works based on scientific research. The second section details the healing elements of medical meditation such as breath, posture and movement, mantra, and mental focus. The final section centers on the healing power of the chakra system, and a chapter is devoted to each of the chakras and their dysfunctions. Exercises and guided meditations are given throughout the book.
- Smith, Jonathan C. 2005. *Relaxation, Meditation, & Mindfulness: A Mental Health Practitioner's Guide to New and Traditional Approaches*. New York: Springer. 368 pp. ISBN: 0826127452; 9780826127457.
  Designed for mental health professionals, this book is a guide to a variety of approaches to relaxation. After a discussion of the basic concepts of relaxation and its use in therapy, the author presents more detailed information on yoga including stretching, progressive muscle relaxation, breathing exercises, autogenic training, imagery and relaxing self-talk, and meditation and mindfulness. Next he addresses issues of training clients to use these techniques both in general and in special situations such as with children and for pain management.

- Wallace, B. Alan. 2005. *Genuine Happiness: Meditation as the Path to Fulfillment.* Hoboken, NJ: John Wiley & Sons. 246 pp. ISBN: 047146984X; 9780471469841.
  Meditation is a technique that can transform and shape the mind, yielding greater calmness and happiness. The author strives to provide to the beginner a guide to meditation that will lead to genuine happiness. The work is based solidly in Buddhist tradition but can be used by anyone interested in learning meditation. Topics such as breathing, settling the mind, and mindfulness of the body, feelings, and mind are presented clearly. The author then discusses cultivating a good heart, compassion, and the nature of consciousness. Throughout the work, exercises are provided to introduce the reader to the experiences of the various meditations presented.
- Wallace, B. Alan. 2009. *Mind in the Balance: Meditation in Science, Buddhism, and Christianity.* New York: Columbia University Press. 244 pp. ISBN: 0231147309; 9780231147309.
  Combining theory and practice, this book examines meditation from the views of both science and spirit. The first part looks at the history of meditation and scientific studies of meditation, while Part 2 delves into the actual practice of meditation and its theoretical underpinnings. Thus, it provides a balanced view of the art of meditation and explains why meditation can be a health giving practice.
- Weiss, Gabriel S. 2008. *The Healing Power of Meditation: Your Prescription for Getting Well and Staying Well with Meditation.* Laguna Beach, CA: Basic Health Publications. 260 pp. ISBN: 1591202469; 9781591202462.
  Using evidence from medical studies, neuroscience research, clinical case histories, spiritual wisdom, and Zen philosophy, the author has produced a work that demonstrates the power of meditation. In addition to providing techniques for meditation, he also discusses how illness heals, the relationship between meditation and wellness, and ways to integrate other strategies such as using art, music, and literature to help meditation lead to healing.
- White, John. 2004. *Everything You Want to Know about TM—Including How to Do It.* New York: Paraview Special Editions. 190 pp. ISBN: 1931044856; 9781931044851.
  Transcendental Meditation (TM) is one of the most frequently practiced forms of meditation in the world. This book introduces the reader to TM, the TM movement, and to Maharishi, the main proponent and teacher of TM, while also expounding on meditation in general, on consciousness, and on enlightenment. For the beginner meditator or for those who may have an interest in TM, this is a useful resource although others will provide a better introduction to basic meditative techniques.

Internet Resources

- How to Meditate, www.how-to-meditate.org.
  Offering practical information about Buddhist meditation, this site seeks to show that Buddhist meditation can be done by anyone, even those who are busy. The directions are clear, simple, and easy to understand, and they cover the basics of breathing and posture. Several specific types of meditation are available, including introductory videos.

- Learning Meditation, www.learningmeditation.com.
  An excellent place to begin learning about meditation, this website discusses relaxation through meditation and provides a meditation room that has a variety of different spoken meditations that last from three to ten minutes each.
- Meditation, www.beliefnet.com/Holistic-Living/Meditation/index.aspx.
  The mission of Beliefnet is to help people find useful information on all topics related to spirituality, including meditation. Topics include how to start meditating, types of meditation, centering meditation, Christian meditation, and Buddhist meditation.
- The Meditation Community, www.meditationcommunity.com.
  Not affiliated with any religion, the Meditation Community is a secular group that promotes meditation and provides instruction in its practice. The website takes the beginner systematically through a simple meditation practice.
- The Meditation Infocenter, 1stholistic.com/meditation/hol_meditation.htm.
  The goal of the website is to provide in-depth information on meditation and its benefits for healing. In addition to answering basic questions on meditation, it gives good directions for beginning a meditation practice such as descriptions of postures and introduces several different types of meditation such as walking meditation, journey meditation, and vibrational meditation.
- Meditation Society of America, www.meditationsociety.com.
  The Meditation Station is useful for all those interested in meditation, whether a beginner or an expert. If provides valuable information on meditation techniques and concepts from around the world. In the beginners section it presents the basics of meditation, while other sections will appeal to the experienced meditator. Of special note is the section that discusses 108 different meditation techniques.
- The Transcendental Meditation Program, www.tm.org.
  The Transcendental Meditation technique was one of the first types of meditation to gain widespread use within the United States. This site gives an excellent introduction to TM, although it does not discuss how to do TM meditation since this must be learned in an approved class.
- The World Wide Online Meditation Center, www.meditationcenter.com.
  The goal of this site is to provide clear, easily understood instruction on how to meditate. It covers the basics of meditation, offers basic instruction on mindfulness meditation and mantra meditation, and discusses healing meditation.

Periodicals/Magazines/Journals

- *Journal of the Order of Buddhist Contemplatives*, published by the Order of Buddhist Contemplatives, 1970– . Quarterly. ISSN: 0891-1177 www.obcon.org/jobcpg.html.
  This journal includes articles focused on the practical aspects of Buddhist meditation and training written by Buddhist monks and laypersons.
- *Tricycle: The Buddhist Review*, published by the Tricycle Foundation, 1991– . Quarterly. ISSN: 1055-484X. www.tricycle.com.
  An independent magazine with a Buddhist point of view, *Tricycle* provides articles on people, art, fiction, international news, and discussions of the applications of Buddhism, including meditation, in contemporary American society.

- *The Way Fourth*, published by Tayu Meditation Center, 1979– . Irregular. No ISSN. www.tayu.org/~tayu.
  A publication of the Tayu Meditation Center, this online newsletter publishes articles on all aspects of meditation but focuses specifically on Tayu meditation, with its emphasis on self-observation and comeditation.

Chapter 15

Naturopathy and Natural Medicine

Background and History

Naturopathy is the oldest known form of medicine. From the earliest times, humankind has treated its illnesses with natural substances, including food, water, and herbs. Practicing naturopaths continue to use these substances in their practices. Sometimes called naturopathic medicine or natural medicine, naturopathy is based on the philosophy that the body has an intrinsic ability to heal and maintain itself. Over 2,400 years ago, Hippocrates formulated his concept of *vis medicatrix naturae*, or the healing power of nature, which is one of the main tenets of naturopathy. Other basic principles include treating the whole person, doing no harm by respecting the innate healing ability present in all beings, treating the cause and not the symptoms, preventing disease is the best cure, and being a teacher. Thus, naturopathy supports these ideas by relying on natural remedies instead of synthetic drugs or surgery to support the natural healing force. Naturopaths may also incorporate a wide variety of healing modalities into their practice that address the body and its ailments in different ways. Although some naturopaths eschew any application of conventional Western medicine, others regularly refer their patients to allopathic physicians, chiropractors, and other health professionals.

The use of the term *naturopathy* can be traced to 1895 in the United States when it was created by John Scheel. Benedict Lust, who studied hydrotherapy and other natural health cures in Germany, founded the first American school of naturopathy in New York. The field grew until there were naturopathic schools and naturopaths across the country. Beginning in the 1930s, naturopathy, along with other natural health professions such as homeopathy, began to decline due to the discovery of penicillin, the increased use of synthetic drugs such as antibiotics, the growth of allopathic medical education, and the increase in medical research that focused primarily on the use of drugs and surgery. Naturopathy, however, never disappeared and has witnessed resurgence in recent decades. In 1956, the National College of Naturopathic Medicine in Portland, Oregon, opened. Since then four other schools have been accredited by the Council on Naturopathic Medical Education (CNME) and two others are in candidacy status. Many other schools offer unaccredited programs in naturopathy.

Primary Uses and Actions

Naturopathy, as a medical philosophy based on the healing power of nature, uses a wide variety of techniques that facilitate the healing of the whole patient, including the body, mind, and spirit. In addition, naturopathy stresses prevention of disease or illness and education of the patient. Many techniques and therapies used in naturopathy seek to support the body in its own healing and to help patients increase their health through changes in lifestyle. In addition to prescribing herbs, a naturopath may suggest stress reduction, exercises, the use of supplements, changes to the diet, and the reduction of exposure to environmental toxins.

Before making suggestions for treatment and lifestyle changes, the naturopath will take a complete medical history that may include questions concerning family history, diet, levels of stress, sleeping habits, type of work performed, social relationships, and environment in which the patient lives and works. Since the naturopath seeks to treat the whole person, the questions may also delve into the patient's spiritual and psychological lives. A physical examination will be performed and laboratory tests may be ordered.

Treatments prescribed may include herbs and supplements, nutritional and lifestyle counseling, homeopathic medicines, detoxification, hypnosis, hydrotherapy (water therapy, which may include special baths, drinking spring water, and water exercises), acupuncture, and other techniques. Naturopaths are trained to treat a wide variety of chronic and acute disorders. In some states, they may even be allowed to perform surgery while in others they can only suggest treatments to their patients. Illnesses rising from environmental, dietary, and lifestyle factors are especially treatable by naturopathy. The goal of naturopathy, however, is not to treat the symptoms specifically but to treat the cause of the illness.

Training

Within the United States, there is no universal agreement on the training of naturopaths. The ND, or doctor of naturopathy, degree can be obtained in a variety of ways. In addition to the seven schools that are accredited or candidates for accreditation for the teaching of naturopathy, there are a wide variety of online, correspondence, and self-study programs that issue the ND degree for their graduates. Needless to say, the requirements of these various schools vary greatly. The CNME accredited schools must provide a complete, scientific education in naturopathy that includes instruction in anatomy, physiology, pathology, biochemistry, environmental/public health, and pharmacology and pharmacognosy. Most important, they must also provide supervised clinical experience. Their programs generally last for four years.

Requirements for naturopathic education and licensing vary from state to state. In at least 16 states and the District of Columbia, naturopathic doctors must complete the formal educational requirements required in an accredited school and pass the comprehensive board exams administered by the North American Board of Naturopathic Examiners (NABNE) before they can be licensed to practice naturopathy. In some states naturopaths can prescribe medicines and in others they can perform minor surgery.

The so-called "traditional naturopaths" may employ the same treatments based on the same philosophy of health offered by licensed naturopathic doctors, but they are not eligible for state licensure. Many traditional naturopaths practice in states that do not offer a license to practice naturopathy, and their education may have been secured through a source other than the CNME accredited programs. Legally, their practices are usually limited to patient education rather than the diagnosis and treatment of illness.

Many conventional physicians are now offering treatments drawn from the realm of naturopathy to their patients. The growth of integrative medicine has been phenomenal over the past two decades, and many medical colleges now offer courses on such complementary and alternative modalities.

Sources

Balch, Phyllis A. 2006. *Prescription for Nutritional Healing*. 4th ed. New York: Avery.

Pizzorno, Joseph E., Jr., and Murray, Michael T. 2006. *Textbook of Natural Medicine*. 3rd ed. 2 vols. St. Louis, MO: Churchill Livingstone Elsevier.

Thiel, Robert J. 2000. *Combining Old and New: Naturopathy for the 21st Century*. Warsaw, IN: Whitman Publications.

See also HERBS, VITAMINS, MINERALS, AND NUTRITIONAL SUPPLEMENTS

Annotated Bibliography

Print Resources

➤ Balch, James F., and Stengler, Mark. 2004. *Prescription for Natural Cures: A Self-Care Guide for Treating Health Problems with Natural Remedies, Including Diet and Nutrition, Nutritional Supplements, Bodywork, and More*. Hoboken, NJ: John Wiley & Sons. 724 pp. ISBN: 0471490881; 9780471490883.
With a focus on natural and preventative remedies, this resource is aimed at the general public and seeks to provide current, results-oriented information. The bulk of the book discusses over 90 different conditions that can benefit from natural treatment. Arranged alphabetically, the conditions range from abscesses and boils to warts and yeast infections. For each condition, the entry includes general symptoms, root causes, testing techniques, treatment that may include a wide variety of different healing modalities, and different types of herbal remedies that can help treat the condition. In a separate section, the authors provide general information on a variety of treatment methods, including diet and nutrition, fasting, nutritional supplements, herbal medicine, homeopathy, Bach flower remedies, aromatherapy, and others. This is a very helpful book that will be of great benefit to many readers.

➤ Balch, James F., Stengler, Mark, and Young-Balch, Robin. 2008. *Prescription for Drug Alternatives: All-Natural Options for Better Health without the Side Effects*. Hoboken, NJ: John Wiley & Sons. 496 pp. ISBN: 0470183993; 9780470183991.
The authors argue for using natural medicines to achieve good health. The chapters, each of which focuses on a specific health issue, compare pharmaceutical drugs and natural remedies that have similar effects. Ailments covered include, among others, allergies, anxiety, atherosclerosis, common cold, diabetes, headache, obesity, and prostate enlargement.

➤ Balch, Phyllis A. 2006. *Prescription for Nutritional Healing*. 4th ed. New York: Avery. 869 pp. ISBN: 1583332367; 9781583332368.
The goal of this work is to provide a resource both for individuals and their health care providers that discusses a more natural approach to healing. It is divided into three parts. Part 1 introduces the elements of health and provides basic information on nutrition, vitamins, minerals, amino acids, antioxidants, herbs, and supplements. Part 2 lists common disorders, from acne to yeast infections, provides a description

of the disorder, suggests nutrients and herbs that can be helpful in treating the disorder, and makes recommendations for other actions that can also be helpful in dealing with the problem. The third part includes descriptions of a wide variety of techniques that can be used to treat health problems. Many of these treatments can be used in conjunction with traditional methods.

- Bowden, Jonny. 2008. *The Most Effective Natural Cures on Earth: The Surprising Unbiased Truth about What Treatments Work and Why*. Beverly, MA: Fair Winds Press. 358 pp. ISBN: 1592332919; 9781592332915.
  Written for a general audience, this book explores over 75 common ailments, from allergies and cancer to menopause and stress. For each condition, the author provides natural cures that can aid in healing.
- Chaitow, Leon. 2008. *Naturopathic Physical Medicine: Theory and Practice for Manual Therapists and Naturopaths*. New York: Churchill Livingstone Elsevier. 577 pp. ISBN: 0443103909; 9780443103902.
  This text covers the breadth of naturopathic physical medicine, which is primarily concerned with the treatment and rehabilitation of musculoskeletal dysfunction but can also be used in the treatment of a variety of health problems. In addition to introducing the concept of naturopathic physical medicine, the book includes chapters on assessment and palpation, treatment protocols, rehabilitation, general health enhancement, hydrotherapy, and electrotherapy. This work is not for the general reader but will be helpful for those health professionals seeking to broaden their knowledge of other techniques and modalities that may be useful in treating their patients and clients.
- Gottlieb, Bill. 2008, ©2000. *Alternative Cures: More Than 1,000 of the Most Effective Natural Home Remedies*. New York: Ballantine Books. 796 pp. ISBN: 0345505395; 9780345505392.
  In this guide, the author has compiled over 1,000 safe and effective alternative home remedies for over 150 ailments as suggested by 300 doctors and natural healers. Part 1 lists the health concerns, from acne to wrinkles. The suggested remedies include foods, herbs, supplements, and the use of therapies such as homeopathy, massage, acupressure, meditation, relaxation, and hydrotherapy. Part 2 discusses 22 different types of alternative healing methods such as acupressure, affirmations, movement education, and yoga therapy. The final part lists useful resources, including a guide to acupressure points, guidelines for the safe use of the natural remedies included in the book, and sources for many of the products suggested. Due to its breadth of coverage, this is a useful, inexpensive book.
- Hoffer, Abram, and Prousky, Jonathan. 2006. *Naturopathic Nutrition: A Guide to Nutrient-Rich Food & Nutritional Supplements for Optimum Health*. Toronto: CCNM Press. 350 pp. ISBN: 1897025157; 9781897025154.
  This is a guide to the therapeutic use of nutrient-rich foods and nutritional supplements both to improve overall health and to prevent disease. After an enlightening discussion of the health costs of the modern high-tech diet, the authors present the benefits of a naturopathic diet based on what they term the optimum diet, which permits optimal absorption of needed nutrients. They also present a compelling argument for the use of nutritional supplements including vitamins, minerals, amino

acids, and essential fatty acids. The work concludes with several nutritional therapy case studies and a listing of the nutrient content of many common foods.

- Hudson, Tori. 2008. *Women's Encyclopedia of Natural Medicine: Alternative Therapies and Integrative Medicine for Total Health and Wellness*. Rev. and updated ed. New York: McGraw-Hill. 500 pp. ISBN: 0071464735; 9780071464734.
  Written for women by a naturopathic physician, this book provides information on complementary and alternative therapies that can help women achieve good health. The author discusses topics such as bio-identical hormones, vitamin supplementation, herbs, diet, and exercise that can be used to treat a wide array of female health issues such as menopause, heart conditions, and yeast infections.
- Lloyd, Iva. 2009. *The Energetics of Health: A Naturopathic Assessment*. New York: Churchill Livingstone. 250 pp. ISBN: 0443069557; 9780443069550.
  Students and medical clinicians will find this guide helpful due to its examination of naturopathic assessment. Chapters cover the underlying theories of both traditional and complementary systems of medicine and focus specifically on naturopathic medicine. Other chapters discuss the human energy system, symptom patterns, causes of symptoms and diseases, the therapeutic encounter, physical assessment, disease patterns, and treatment strategies.
- Meletis, Chris D., Zabriskie, Nieske L., and Rountree, Bob. 2008. *Clinical Natural Medicine Handbook*. New Rochelle, NY: Mary Ann Liebert. 465 pp. ISBN: 0913113441; 9780913113448.
  Designed for practicing clinicians, this book provides guidelines, protocols, and literature reviews for the clinical use of nutrition, nutraceuticals, and botanicals based on recent medical and scientific research. The handbook focuses on common diseases and conditions that health care providers regularly see in their practices. For each condition, the authors provide diagnostic information including prevalence, pathophysiology, risk factors, symptoms, and associated conditions as well as treatment guidelines and protocols that incorporate conventional approaches (medical and surgical) in addition to nutraceuticals, botanicals, lifestyle modifications, and other naturopathic approaches.
- Mindell, Earl, and Hopkins, Virginia. 2009. *Prescription Alternatives: Hundreds of Safe, Natural, Prescription-Free Remedies to Restore and Maintain Your Health*. 4th ed. New York: McGraw-Hill. 440 pp. ISBN: 0071600310 9780071600316.
  Now in its fourth edition, this work gives valuable information on an array of alternative treatments and dietary supplements in addition to information on prescription drugs. Topics covered include heart disease, digestive diseases, infections, sleep disorders, depression, osteoporosis, asthma, obesity, attention deficit disorder, and hormone replacement.
- Murray, Michael T., and Pizzorno, Joseph. 1998. *Encyclopedia of Natural Medicine*. Rev. 2nd ed. Rocklin, CA: Prima Publishing. 946 pp. ISBN: 0761511571; 9780761511571.
  Written for the general reader, this book provides an excellent introduction to natural health. The authors first focus on what they call the four cornerstones of good health: a positive mental attitude, a healthy lifestyle, a health-promoting diet, and supplementary measures. They then examine ways to enhance the systems of the body, including detoxification, immune support, and stress management. The final section of the

book lists over 70 different health problems and gives background information on the problem, therapeutic considerations, and a summary of ways to treat the problem. Thus, this is a very helpful resource that will be of great assistance to many readers.

➤ Pizzorno, Joseph E., Jr., and Murray, Michael T. 2006. *Textbook of Natural Medicine.* 3rd ed., 2 vols. St. Louis, MO: Churchill Livingstone Elsevier. 1620 pp. ISBN: 0443073007 (set); 9780443073007 (set).

Although designed as a textbook on natural medicine, this is also a wonderful and useful reference book for anyone seeking information on a wide variety of health-related topics. The two volumes are divided into six sections. The first section focuses on the philosophy of natural medicine, while section 2 examines a wide variety of diagnostic procedures that are not commonly used in allopathic medicine such as cell signaling analysis, heavy metal assessment, and the urine indican test. A variety of therapeutic modalities are discussed in the third section, including acupuncture, ayurveda, homeopathy, exercise, faith, glandular therapy, and fasting. Section 4 includes chapters on several syndromes and special topics such as chronic candidiasis, chronic fatigue syndrome, food allergies, and sports nutrition. Of special interest are the final two sections. Section 5 covers the pharmacology of natural medicines and presents detailed information on over 60 different substances from allium sativum (garlic) to carnatine and echinacea to zingiber officinale (ginger). The last section, specific health problems, has its own volume and provides information on 70 ailments. For each ailment, the entry gives a diagnostic summary, general considerations, therapeutic considerations, including the use of botanical medicines, and various therapeutic approaches to treating the ailment. The entire work is solidly based on the scientific literature and includes over 10,000 citations to peer-reviewed research reports and articles.

➤ Pizzorno, Joseph E., Murray, Michael T., and Joiner-Bey, Herb. 2008. *The Clinician's Handbook of Natural Medicine.* St. Louis, MO: Churchill Livingstone. 818 pp. ISBN: 0443067236; 9780443067235.

Over 80 common conditions are covered by the authors, from acne and affective disorders to vaginitis and varicose veins. Based on scientific studies, the entries give diagnostic procedures, general considerations, therapeutic considerations, and therapeutic approaches for each condition as well as flowcharts to help clinicians decide on the proper treatment.

➤ Rost, Amy. 2009. *Natural Healing Wisdom & Know-How: Useful Practices, Recipes, and Formulas for a Lifetime of Health.* New York: Black Dog & Leventhal Publishers. 496 pp. ISBN: 1579128009; 9781579128005.

Loaded with charts, lists, tips, instructions, diagrams, and illustrations, this work covers a variety of natural healing techniques including herbal healing, naturopathy, homeopathy, Eastern medicine, energy healing, mind–body healing, and healing with foods.

➤ Sierpina, Victor, ed. 2007. *1000 Cures for 200 Ailments: Integrated Alternative and Conventional Treatments for the Most Common Illnesses.* New York: Collins. 1000 pp. ISBN: 006112029; 9780061120299.

Covering a wide array of common illnesses and ailments, this book provides treatment options drawn from conventional medicine as well as alternative practices. The illnesses are arranged into nine categories: skin and hair; eyes and mouth; ears, nose, and throat; digestive system and urinary tract; respiratory system and circulation; aches and pains; personal complaints, such as hot flashes and impotence; mind and spirit; and first aid. The entry for each illness follows a set format and gives methods of diagnosis, symptoms, and treatment goals followed by suggested treatments from conventional medicine, traditional Chinese medicine, naturopathy, homeopathy, and herbalism. Additional tips are provided that often suggest other types of therapy. This is a very useful resource to have in the home due to the breadth of ailments and the variety of treatments suggested, including allopathic medicine.

- Thiel, Robert J. 2000. *Combining Old and New: Naturopathy for the 21st Century*. Warsaw, IN: Whitman Publications. 296 pp. ISBN: 1885653085; 9781885653086.
  This book is intended both for licensed health professionals and for general readers who have an interest in natural health practices. It covers the philosophy of naturopathy and many of the treatments utilized by naturopaths. It presents the history of naturopathy, naturopathic philosophy, toxemia as a cause of disease, the laws of cure, simple ways to ensure health, and naturopathic assessment using reflexes, pulse analysis, and iridology. Treatments discussed include light and color, sound and music, rest and sleep, exercise, manipulation such as massage and reflexology, water and hydrotherapy, foods and diet, vitamins, glandulars and enzymes, herbology, and homeopathy.
- Vasey, Christopher. 2009. *The Naturopathic Way: How to Detox, Find Quality Nutrition, and Restore Your Acid-Alkaline Balance*. Rochester, VT: Healing Arts Press. 133 pp. ISBN: 1594772606; 9781594772603.
  This book seeks to help readers restore their good health through detoxification, proper nutrition, and achieving a proper acid–alkaline balance within the body. According to the author, disease results from toxicity in the body due to the internal cellular environment being clogged with waste products. By eliminating these wastes and using the proper natural supplements, health can be restored.
- Wilen, Joan, and Wilen, Lydia. 2008. *Healing Remedies: More Than 1,000 Natural Ways to Relieve Common Ailments, from Arthritis and Allergies to Diabetes, Osteoporosis, and Many Others!* New York: Ballantine Books. 336 pp. ISBN: 034550335X; 9780345503350.
  Using home remedies, the authors give recipes and suggestions to help control health issues such as high blood pressure, cholesterol, headaches, digestive problems, and obesity. Often, the suggestions are as simple as eating apples to help lower blood pressure or inhaling boiling apple cider vinegar to eliminate a headache.

Internet Resources

- American Association of Naturopathic Physicians, www.naturopathic.org.
  The American Association of Naturopathic Physicians represents licensed or licensable naturopathic physicians in North America who graduated from one of the four-year, accredited schools of naturopathic medicine. The website provides good information on naturopathic medicine and on maintaining one's health using a preventive, natural, and holistic perspective.
- American Naturopathic Medical Association, www.anma.com.
  Maintained by the nation's oldest and largest association of naturopathic physicians, this website contains information on legislation affecting the practice of naturopathy

as well as news stories. The site also includes archived contents from the *Journal of the American Naturopathic Medical Association* starting in 2000.

- The Coalition for Natural Health, www.naturalhealth.org.
  The Coalition for Natural health seeks to promote everyone's right to choose natural healing techniques. The website features updates on legislation, reports from each state on the status of alternative therapies, articles on a variety of alternative treatment methods, and even a section on using alternative treatments for animals.
- An Introduction to Naturopathy, nccam.nih.gov/health/naturopathy.
  Produced by the National Center for Complementary and Alternative Medicine, this is an excellent introduction to naturopathy and its key principles.
- NaturoDoc, www.naturodoc.com.
  Produced by Dr. Thomas S. Lee, a naturopathic physician, NaturoDoc offers a wide variety of information on a variety of complementary and alternative medical treatments. The library includes hundreds of articles on natural health, herbal remedies, alternative treatments, and naturopathy.
- Naturopathic Medicine Network, www.pandamedicine.com/index.html.
  The Naturopathic Medicine Network seeks to promote naturopathic medicine and natural health care, to provide information and resources on naturopathic medicine, and to support communication and information sharing between naturopathic physicians and other health care providers. The website also provides a directory of naturopaths.
- Naturopathy Online, naturopathyonline.com.
  This is a good source of general information on naturopathy. It covers medical conditions, treatments that can be done at home, recipes for healthy meals, and background information on medical treatment including naturopathic medicine, homeopathy, herbology, and hydrotherapy.

Periodicals/Magazines/Journals

- *The International Journal of Naturopathic Medicine*, published by ND News & Review, 2008– . Irregular. ISSN: 1938-0046. www.intjnm.org.
  IntJNM publishes articles and research of interest to the practice of naturopathic medicine. The goal of the journal is to develop a greater understanding of health and disease in ways that help naturopaths prevent, identify, and treat illness while also helping patients achieve optimum health.
- *Natural Health*, published by American Media Inc., 1971– . Ten times a year. ISSN: 1067-9588. www.naturalhealthmag.com.
  A magazine aimed at the consumer, *Natural Health* examines all aspects of living a healthy life, with an emphasis on lifestyle, eating healthy foods, maintaining fitness, and using supplements and other nutrients to enhance health.
- *Naturopathy Digest*, published by MPA Media, 2006– . Monthly. ISSN: 1559-0399. www.naturopathydigest.com.
  A trade magazine for those interested in naturopathy, *Naturopathy Digest* provides current information on the naturopathic profession, including the philosophy of naturopathy and technical and clinical information for the practice of naturopathic medicine.

Chapter 16

Neuro-Linguistic Programming

Background and History

Developed in the 1970s by psychotherapists John Grinder and Richard Bandler, neuro-linguistic programming (NLP) is based on the theory that life experiences, beginning at birth, determine how you see and approach the world. By examining how you created your own world and how you learned to think and feel, an NLP practitioner can help you change your actions by restructuring how you derive meaning from the world.

NLP grew out of the study of communication. Grinder and Bandler studied the works and psychotherapy sessions of Fritz Perls, Virginia Satir, and Milton Erickson. Grinder and Bandler determined that excellence in communication as demonstrated by Perls, Satir, and Erickson resulted in their greater success in treating patients. They also found that top executives and top salespeople also modeled these excellent communication skills. As a result, Grinder and Bandler aimed to create a model of such successful communication that others could learn and use in their own therapy sessions. In addition, individuals can learn these models and apply them to their own intrapersonal and interpersonal communication.

NLP makes the basic assumption that internal mental processes, especially problem solving, memory, and language all consist of visual, auditory, kinesthetic and sometimes olfactory and gustatory representations that are activated when you think about or engage in problems or activities. These representations are constantly being formed and accessed and thereby they impact behavior and performance. NLP, as a therapy, aims to change behavior by modifying these internal representations.

Primary Uses and Actions

The focus of NLP therapy is change, and the first question often asked by the therapist is, "What do you want?" One model that is often used in therapy is the logical levels model, which addresses the client's identity, beliefs and values, capability, behavior, and environment. These levels help structure our experience, yet they also help identify the level of the problem that is being addressed. By addressing the problem on its appropriate level, the other levels will also be affected.

Although it is primarily a form of psychotherapy, NLP is effective in helping with stress reduction, problem solving, and relationship and communication issues. It has also been used in helping clients deal with a range of other health challenges, such as migraines, pain, phobias, trauma, and allergies. Since NLP addresses the belief system of the individual, exposing those beliefs can lead to change that can then lead to better health.

One of the major uses of NLP has been in the realm of business. Many people have used NLP therapy or training to become better salespeople, better negotiators, or better communicators.

Training

There are many books, workshops, and seminars on NLP, however, the Society of Neuro-Linguistic Programming is the only organization that offers certification for NLP practitioners. The Society of NLP offers certification at two levels: practitioner and master practitioner. Workshops and seminars are offered worldwide that are approved by the Society of NLP. There are no official licensing requirements by state governments, although some offer the title "Licensed Practitioner of Neuro-Linguistic Programming" to those who complete their training.

Sources

Bandler, Richard, and Grinder, John. 1979. *Frogs into Princes: Neuro Linguistic Programming*. Moab, UT: Real People Press.

Bavister, Steve, and Vickers, Amanda. 2008. *NLP*. Blacklick, OH: McGraw Hill.

Linden, Anné, and Perutz, Kathrin. 2008. *Mindworks: An Introduction to NLP*. Bethel, CT: Crown House Publishing.

See also EYE MOVEMENT DESENSITIZATION AND REPROCESSING

Annotated Bibliography

Print Resources

➤ Bandler, Richard. 2008. *Get the Life You Want*. Deerfield Beach, FL: Health Communications. 229 pp. ISBN: 0757307760, 9780757307768.

Written by one of the founders of neuro-linguistic programming, this book distills his ideas into a highly readable format that is accessible to any reader. The goal of NLP is help individuals overcome their problems and develop the kinds of life they want. In this book, Bandler presents the major techniques of NLP in a way that can be quickly applied without the help of a psychotherapist. The stories and examples provide extra guidance to the reader and give an understanding of the brain and its working. Part 2 provides techniques to deal with resolving fears and phobias, bad memories, grief, bad relationships, and bad decisions. Part 3 suggests ways to get through habits, big events, tests, and other obligations. The final part helps the reader learn to have fun and love, to meet people, to exercise, to become more organized, to make more money, and to make big decisions. Thus, the book can help in most aspects of life.

➤ Bandler, Richard, and Fitzpatrick, Owen. 2009. *Conversations with Richard Bandler: Two NLP Masters Reveal the Secrets to Successful Living*. Deerfield Beach, FL: Health Communications. 354 pp. ISBN: 0757313817; 9780757313813.

In this book, a practitioner of NLP talks with one of the founders of the technique, and both give their own personal and professional insights into the life-changing processes that NLP can facilitate. The book includes many exercises to help readers change their lives and become happier, more confident, and more successful.

➤ Bavister, Steve, and Vickers, Amanda. 2008. *NLP*. Blacklick, OH: McGraw Hill. 256 pp. ISBN: 0071602593; 9780071602594.

If you are looking for a good source of information on NLP or if you wish to be a better communicator, this book will fulfill such needs. The authors cover all aspects of NLP in an understandable manner. Individual chapters discuss the main concepts of NLP including representational systems, submodalities, meta programs, values and beliefs, well-formed outcomes, states and emotions, anchoring, sensory acuity and calibration, rapport, modeling, and others. In addition, helpful exercises which reinforce the concept are given at the end of each chapter.

- Bradbury, Andrew. 2006. *Develop Your NLP Skills*. 3rd ed. Philadelphia: Kogan Page. 151 pp. ISBN: 0749445580.
  This is a short, easy-to-read summary of NLP with the overall goal of being a practical guide to increasing business excellence. The special focus of the author is providing an understanding of what happens when people communicate and then using that knowledge to increase the effectiveness of interpersonal transactions, including building better relationships, replacing conflict, managing one's own mental activities, and setting effective organizational goals.

- Cameron-Bandler, Leslie. 1985. *Solutions: Practical and Effective Antidotes for Sexual and Relationship Problems*. San Rafael, CA: FuturePace. 259 pp. ISBN: 0932573010; 9780932573018.
  Using anecdotes and examples from therapy sessions, including transcript excerpts, the author uses techniques derived from NLP to provide direction on how to live a happier and more fulfilling life. Although most of the material in the book focuses on the relationships of couples and on sexuality, the principles can be applied in all areas of life. The ideas book can be useful both to the therapist but also to the reader seeking to change his or her life.

- Linden, Anné, and Perutz, Kathrin. 2008. *Mindworks: An Introduction to NLP*. Bethel, CT: Crown House Publishing. 270 pp. ISBN: 1845900863; 9781845900861.
  This book presents Neuro-Linguistic Programming in a form that can be used by anyone. The goal is to provide simple techniques that can unlock the potential that resides in everyone. Organized by the seven major principles of NLP, the book offers a systematic way to restructure your thoughts so that your desires and potential can be realized. Easy to read with abundant examples, this is an excellent introduction to NLP that can be of help to all readers.

- McDermott, Ian, and Jago, Wendy. 2001. *Brief NLP Therapy*. Thousand Oaks, CA: Sage Publications. 181 pp. ISBN: 0761959653; 9780761959656.
  This book is a practical introduction to NLP and its basic principles. Although useful for therapists, it is also a helpful resource for clients and for anyone interested in learning more about NLP, its theoretical foundations, and its goals.

- Molden, David. 2007. *NLP Business Masterclass: Driving Peak Performance with NLP*. 2nd ed. Harlow: Financial Times Prentice Hall. 342 pp. ISBN: 0273707906; 9780273707905.
  Focusing specifically on business, this book presents techniques drawn from NLP to help the reader in being successful and creating change. The book is divided into four sections. The first section discusses the principles of NLP, while the second explains the core patterns of behavior and thinking that underlie the skills necessary to succeed. The third section gives a variety of tools, techniques, and skills that can create change. Finally, section 4 gives models of excellence so that the principles and techniques are reinforced.

- Ready, Romilla, and Burton, Kate. 2004. *Neuro-Linguistic Programming for Dummies.* Hoboken, NJ: John Wiley & Sons. 331 pp. ISBN: 0764570285; 9780764570285.
  This book seeks to capture the essentials of NLP and to encourage readers to take the action needed to shape their own lives by providing practical ideas on using NLP to help resolve issues or to make changes in their lives. It is arranged so that it can be read straight through or so that individual chapters can be dipped into for specific information. Both the basic assumptions and the detailed techniques of NLP are addressed, providing an excellent introduction to using NLP for change. Exercises and examples are given throughout to help the reader apply the techniques quickly and effectively.
- Ready, Romilla, and Burton, Kate. 2008. *Neuro-Linguistic Programming Workbook for Dummies.* Hoboken, NJ: Wiley. 282 pp. ISBN: 0470519738; 9780470519738.
  Organized like other books in the Dummies series, this is an excellent overview of NLP for the general reader. The authors take readers through the basic principles of NLP and give exercises on how to apply these principles to their own lives. The goal of the book is to help readers assess their own thought patterns, communicate confidently and effectively, build rapport, manage their emotions, break bad habits, and set goals and achieve success. All this is done using the humor that the series is known for.
- Thomson, Garner, and Khan, Khalid. 2008. *Magic in Practice: Introducing Medical NLP: The Art and Science of Language in Healing and Health.* London: Hammersmith Press. 302 pp. ISBN: 1905140193; 9781905140190.
  Focusing specifically on the medical use of NLP, this book gives medical and health care professionals the tools they need to begin using techniques and principles from NLP with their clients and patients. The authors use real-life case studies as well as research and clinical experience to demonstrate how NLP can be used as an intervention to help treat an array of problems, such as chronic fatigue syndrome, thyroid health, infertility, menopause, and diabetes.
- Tosey, Paul, and Mathison, Jane. 2009. *Neuro-Linguistic Programming: A Critical Appreciation for Managers and Developers.* New York: Palgrave Macmillan. 233 pp. ISBN: 0230516033; 9780230516038.
  NLP has often been used most successfully in businesses, especially to facilitate personnel training. In this book, the authors explore the theory and the research that bolster NLP. In addition, they trace the development of the technique and examine the ethics and values of the practice of NLP.

Internet Resources

- Anchor Point Institute, www.nlpanchorpoint.com/index.html.
  Anchor Point Institute provides training in NLP and publishes the *Anchor Point Magazine*. Their website also provides links to introductory information on NLP as well as resources from around the world. In addition, Anchor Point publishes books, videos, and audiotapes on NLP.
- Neuro-Linguistic Programming Articles, www.intonlp.com/about.
  This is an excellent source of well-written articles on Neuro-Linguistic Programming. The articles are arranged into categories such as anchoring, chunking, positive

thinking, and submodalities. The website also provides links to a variety of other useful sites and resources.

- Neurolinguisticprogramming.com, www.neurolinguisticprogramming.com.
  This is one of the major sites for information on Neuro-Linguistic Programming. Of special note are the frequently asked questions (FAQs), which provide answers about various aspects of NLP and links to other helpful websites. Another helpful feature is the glossary of NLP terms.
- NLP Institutes, www.nlpinstitutes.com.
  This is the best site for those seeking a listing of licensed trainers of NLP from around the world. Links to other resources such as the NLP Store and other top NLP sites are provided.
- NLPInfo.com, www.nlpinfo.com.
  The purpose of this website is to introduce Neuro-Linguistic Programming to a wider audience. It provides links to a variety of resources such as other NLP websites, periodicals that discuss NLP, training for NLP therapists, and NLP organizations. The site also includes an excellent, brief introduction to NLP, exercises based on NLP, and a listing of events.

Periodicals/Magazines/Journals

- *Anchor Point Magazine: The Practical Journal of NLP*, published by Anchor Point Institute, 1987– . Monthly. ISSN: 0895-366X. www.nlpanchorpoint.com/magmainnew.html.
  Anchor Point Magazine covers all aspects of NLP. The website for the magazine includes a searchable index to articles in the print version of the magazine as well as selected scanned articles.
- *John's HOT NLP Tips Newsletter*, published by NLP-Newsletter.com, 2005– . Monthly. No ISSN. www.nlp-newsletter.com.
  Available freely through electronic delivery to registered users, this newsletter is composed of tips for the practicing NLP therapist.

Chapter 17

Reflexology

Background and History

Reflexology, at its simplest, is foot massage, and has probably been performed for as long as the human species has walked upright. As it is currently practiced, the thumbs and fingers are used to stimulate reflex points on the feet and hands. This action, in turn, through the reflexive action of the body, treats the area of the body associated with the foot or hand reflex point. According to reflexology, every part of the foot and hand, as well as other body parts such as the ear, corresponds to a specific part or organ of the body.

As a therapeutic technique, a form of massage that incorporated reflexology was probably practiced in China over 5,000 years ago, based on the pressure points known from acupuncture. An Egyptian tomb painting from the Physician's Tomb in Saqqara dating from over 4,000 years ago seems to show some sort of foot massage or manipulation. In the later sixteenth century, several books were written related to reflexology. In the United States, various Native American tribes used foot reflexology as part of their healing practices.

The modern use of reflexology traces its origins to 1913 when Dr. William H. Fitzgerald began his research into a method of healing that later became known as "zone therapy." Dr. Fitzgerald, an American ear, nose and throat specialist, probably became interested in zone therapy while working in Vienna, Austria. When he returned to the United States, he began to use this therapy in his practice. According to zone therapy, the body is divided into ten zones, five on each side of the body. Within each zone, there is an energy link between all the parts of the body that are located within that zone. By applying pressure in one area of the zone, pain could be reduced in other areas located within that zone. Dr. Fitzgerald applied pressure primarily to the finders and hands, sometimes using clothespins on the fingertips or rubber bands wrapped around the fingers. He also found that pressure applied to other areas of the body, such as the toes, ankles, wrists, and even the ears, had a similar healing result.

A colleague and student of Fitzgerald, Dr. Edwin F. Bowers, is generally credited with actually coining the term "zone therapy." Others, including Dr. Joe Shelby Riley, built on the work of Fitzgerald and Bowers. Dr. Riley produced detailed diagrams and drawings showing the reflex points of the feet and also included the ear in his work. Eunice D. Ingham, a student of Dr. Riley, is considered the founder of modern reflexology. Her work focused primarily on the feet, using pressure on the soles and tops of the feet and also on the toes. She mainly used her fingers and thumb to apply pressure, avoiding the gadgets that most zone therapists used. Through her work on patients, she discovered and codified the relationships between areas of the feet and parts of the body. She published three influential books, *Stories the Feet Can Tell*, *Zone Therapy and Gland Reflexes*, and *Stories the Feet Have Told*, that helped spur on the spread of reflexology around the world.

Primary Uses and Actions

Currently, reflexology is regularly used in a variety of medical settings, most often to help treat chronic pain and pain arising from cancer and its treatment, yet it can be used as a treatment for any illness, usually as a complement to other medical therapies. Reflexology can also be used to help maintain good health and to prevent illness. Skilled reflexologists can even detect disease or illness early in their course through massaging of the reflex areas. Early treatment can help prevent the disease or illness from developing. Relaxation is probably the most cited benefit of reflexology since it is an easy way to reduce stress, which itself can lead to health problems.

The action of reflexology has not been proven scientifically. The theory espoused by many reflexologists is that the technique works on several levels including the physical, the mental, and the spiritual. Others say that it works through the energetic system that resides within the human body. By stimulating specific points on the foot, hand, or ear, a reflexive action results within the nervous system or the energetic system, thereby creating a situation that can relieve stress and lead to healing. Some reflexologists argue that this reflexive action is mitigated through the body's glandular system. Still others maintain that reflexology works through the meridian system as explained by traditional Chinese medicine.

Training

As with many complementary and alternative healing techniques, there is no mandated course of training to be a reflexologist. Many who practice reflexology may have simply read a book about the technique, while others may have attended a workshop. Yet, there are ongoing attempts to standardize and strengthen training in reflexology. The American Commission for Accreditation of Reflexology Education and Training is a voluntary, nongovernmental accrediting organization that sets educational standards for reflexology in America. Similarly, the American Reflexology Certification Board has as its mission the voluntary certification of reflexologists in the United States. The board provides testing which, when passed, provides national certification to the reflexologist. It also maintains a listing of those who have become nationally certified as well as a listing of schools that offer courses that are prerequisites for taking the certification exam. Most states do not have any licensing requirements for the practice of reflexology. Several states, and some cities, require licensing as a massage therapist.

Sources

Brown, Denise Whichello. 2006. *Reflexology*. New York: Sterling Publishing.

Kunz, Barbara, and Kunz, Kevin. 2003. *Reflexology: Health at Your Fingertips*. New York: DK Publishing.

Mackereth, Peter A., and Tiran, Denise, eds. 2002. *Clinical Reflexology: A Guide for Health Professionals*. New York: Churchill Livingstone.

Wolfe, Frankie Avalon. 2006. *The Complete Idiot's Guide to Reflexology*. New York: Alpha.

See also THERAPEUTIC MASSAGE AND BODYWORK; TRADITIONAL CHINESE MEDICINE, ACUPUNCTURE, AND ACUPRESSURE

Annotated Bibliography

Print Resources

- Andrews, Synthia, and Dempsey, Bobbi. 2007. *Acupressure & Reflexology for Dummies*. Hoboken, NJ: Wiley Publishing. 340 pp. ISBN: 0470139420; 9780470139424.
This book provides an introduction to both reflexology and acupressure. It is aimed at the novice with an interest in learning more about these two related healing modalities and how to use them on oneself or a loved one. The introductory section discusses the essentials of acupressure and reflexology, touching on the history of both modalities, the healing session, basic anatomy, and proper technique. The second section focuses on promoting emotional and physical wellness, while the third section discusses common ailments and pains such as backaches, headaches, and digestive problems. Specific needs and concerns, such as treatments for children, women, or the elderly, are addressed in the fourth section. The final section examines myths and misconceptions about acupressure and reflexology and ways that these techniques can enrich one's life. The illustrations, primarily line drawings, are clear yet not as abundant as in other introductory works.

- Brown, Denise Whichello. 2001. *Reflexology Basics*. New York: Sterling Publishing. 128 pp. ISBN: 0806978457; 9780806978451.
Wonderfully illustrated with crisp color images, this is an excellent general introduction to reflexology. After a short chapter on the benefits and theory of reflexology, the author delves directly into treating the body through reflexology. She instructs on how to prepare the client to receive a treatment and how to warm up the foot so that it is more receptive to treatment. The chapter on reflexology treatment techniques is clear and easy to follow. Next comes a detailed step-by-step guide to using reflexology that addresses all areas of the foot. The chapter on the systems of the body provides additional details on treating the circulatory, digestive, endocrine, lymphatic, musculoskeletal, reproductive, respiratory, and urinary systems.

- Brown, Denise Whichello. 2003. *Teach Yourself Hand Reflexology*. Chicago: Contemporary Books. 150 pp. ISBN: 0071429794; 9780071429795.
After a brief explanation of hand reflexology, its history, and its principles, the author presents the structure of the hands, preparation for hand reflexology, reflexology techniques, a step-by-step sequence to use in performing hand reflexology, using essential oils on the hands, and using hand reflexology to treat common ailments. Although this is a small book, it does a good job in covering using hand reflexology on oneself as well as treating others. The line drawings show the basic reflex points clearly.

- Brown, Denise Whichello. 2006. *Reflexology*. New York: Sterling Publishing. 256 pp. ISBN: 1402735626; 9781402735622.
Wonderfully illustrated, this book provides a complete introduction to both foot and hand reflexology. The detailed color photographs and clear text lead the reader through complete treatment sessions on the feet and the hands. The color charts of the feet and hands are extremely helpful. This is one of the best, clearest introductions to reflexology.

- Dougans, Inge. 2006. *The New Reflexology: A Unique Blend of Traditional Chinese Medicine and Western Reflexology Practice for Better Health and Healing.* New York: Marlowe & Company. 324 pp. ISBN: 1569242895; 9781569242896.
  In this book, the author combines reflexology, as it is practiced in the Western world, with concepts drawn from traditional Chinese medicine, especially the principles of the 12 meridians and the 5 elements. She discusses the foundations of modern reflexology, the principles of Chinese medicine, the application of the meridians to reflexology, mapping the feet, and the anatomy, structure, and conditions of the feet. Building on these theoretical foundations, she then applies them to the treatment sequence.
- Faure-Alderson, Martine. 2008. *Total Reflexology: The Reflex Points for Physical, Emotional, and Psychological Healing.* Rochester, VT: Healing Arts Press. 165 pp. ISBN: 1594772479; 9781594772474.
  Incorporating reflexology with acupuncture, naturopathy, homeopathy, and the chakra system, this book provides a new method of mapping the entire foot to fine-tune the pressure points while also explaining how to work with the emotional reactions that may be released when physical conditions are treated using these pressure points. The work includes 25 color diagrams of the foot to help the user determine the precise pressure points with which to work. Thus, it is useful for both the professional reflexologist as well as the layman.
- Forem, Jack. 1999. *Healing with Pressure Point Therapy: Simple, Effective Techniques for Massaging Away More Than 100 Common Ailments.* Paramus, NJ: Prentice Hall Press. 389 pp. ISBN: 0735200068; 9780735200067.
  Divided into three parts, this book guides the reader through the use of pressure points to provide healing or symptom reduction for a wide variety of ailments. The first part discusses the fundamentals of pressure point therapy, including how pressure point therapy works and the benefits one can derive from it. Part 2 focuses on specific types of pressure point therapy, including acupressure, shiatsu, and reflexology. Part 3 guides the reader through applying these therapies to common problems from acne and allergies to toothache and weight control. Various diagrams depict the proper pressure points to use for healing purposes.
- Gillanders, Ann. 2002. *The Busy Person's Guide to Reflexology: Simple Routines for Home, Work, & Travel.* Hauppauge, NY: Barron's. 143 pp. ISBN: 0764119672; 9780764119675.
  In addition to being an introductory book on reflexology, this book is also a manual for a healthy lifestyle. Thus, instead of chapters devoted to reflexology techniques, the chapters focus on lifestyle, including preparing for the day, traveling in balance, staying on top at work, relaxation and recreation, and prevention and cure. Within each chapter, helpful tips on maintaining one's health is interspersed with specific reflexology treatments that are relevant to the topic. Since it may be difficult to perform reflexology on one's own feet, the author also gives detailed instruction on hand reflexology. The illustrations, all of which are color photographs, provide clear assistance in performing the techniques discussed. This is an excellent book for doing reflexology on oneself or on a partner.
- Hall, Nicola M. 2000. *Reflexology—A Way to Better Health: Foot and Hand Massage for Relaxation and Treating Many Ailments.* Dublin: Newleaf. 192 pp. ISBN: 0717130959; 9780717130955.

Providing an excellent introduction to reflexology, this book covers the theory of reflexology, gives good descriptions and illustrations of the reflex areas on the hands and feet, and discusses how to give a reflexology treatment. The author also covers the treatment of a variety of disorders. The line drawings used for illustrating principles are helpful, but other works that have color photographs provide a better visualization of the reflex points.

- Jones, Sonia. 2009. *Simply Reflexology*. New York: Sterling/Zambezi. 134 pp. ISBN: 1402754558; 9781402754555.
  In this short book, the author presents the basics of reflexology, including its history and techniques. The detailed instructions take the reader step by step through giving a treatment.

- Keet, Louise. 2009. *The Reflexology Bible: The Definitive Guide to Pressure Point Healing*. New York: Sterling. 400 pp. ISBN: 1402766211; 9781402766213.
  Designed for anyone interested in learning about reflexology, this is a good guide to finding the pressure points that can help boost immunity, fight stress, and stimulate the healing processes of the body. It is well illustrated and gives step-by-step instructions on how to perform reflexology on others, including the special needs of children and the elderly.

- Keet, Louise, and Keet, Michael. 2007. *Hand Reflexology: Stimulate Your Body's Healing System*. London: Hamlyn. 128 pp. ISBN: 0600615936; 9780600615934.
  Extremely well-illustrated, this book gives an excellent introduction to hand reflexology. After short chapters on the history, use, and theories of reflexology, the authors proceed to detailing how to perform a hand reflexology session including preparation, opening moves, closing moves, and basic techniques. They then present 10 minute treatment sessions for treating common conditions and balancing the systems of the body. The final chapter discusses specialized uses of hand reflexology, such as its use during pregnancy, with babies and young children, for terminal illness, and for emotional well-being.

- Kolster, Bernard C., and Waskowiak, Astrid. 2005. *The Reflexology Atlas*. Rochester, VT: Healing Arts Press. 255 pp. ISBN: 1594770662; 9781594770661.
  Wonderfully illustrated with excellent color photographs and drawings, this book covers the basics of reflexology massage on the foot, hand, ear, and head. In addition, Shiatsu massage is covered. The final section covers specific ailments that can be treated with reflexology massage, including allergies, back pain, digestive problems, headache, knee pain, and sleep problems. Other books provide more depth on hand and foot reflexology.

- Kunz, Barbara, and Kunz, Kevin. 2003. *Reflexology: Health at Your Fingertips*. New York: DK Publishing. 160 pp. ISBN: 0789493535; 9780789493538.
  Providing step-by-step directions using excellent color photographs, this book takes the reader through providing treatment sessions on both the hands and the feet to others as well as to oneself. The authors briefly introduce the history and theory of reflexology and provide excellent maps of the reflex areas of the feet and hands. Their chapter on taking care of the hands and feet discusses the anatomy of the hands and feet, self-help tools, and relaxation exercises. The bulk of the book provides a

detailed sequence for giving a reflexology session, while the final chapter addresses specific health concerns.

- Kunz, Barbara, and Kunz, Kevin. 2006. *Hand Reflexology: Simple Routines for Health and Relaxation*. 1st American ed. New York: DK Publishing. 160 pp. ISBN: 0756620602; 9780756620608.
  After chapters on the principles and benefits of reflexology in general, the authors present chapters on taking care of the hands, the hand reflexology session, and using reflexology to target specific health concerns. The chapter on the hand reflexology session is especially useful and presents both performing a session on another and also on oneself. Specific health concerns addressed include stress, headaches, backache, neck pain, carpal tunnel syndrome, and arthritis.
- Kunz, Barbara, and Kunz, Kevin. 2009. *Complete Reflexology for Life*. New York: DK Publishing. 352 pp. ISBN: 0756655803; 9780756655808.
  This may be the best single book on reflexology. The authors take the reader through the principles of reflexology, proper techniques, using minisessions for specific problems, employing reflexology through the life span, addressing specific health concerns, and using reflexology for rejuvenation. The work abounds with color photographs and illustrations that are enhanced with directional arrows to help the beginner know how to apply pressure properly. Charts of the feet and hands are given to assist in locating specific reflex points. Often, illustrations are given to assist in self-treatment. If only one book on reflexology can be purchased for a collection, this should be it.
- Kunz, Kevin, and Kunz, Barbara. 2005. *The Complete Guide to Foot Reflexology*. 3rd ed. Albuquerque, NM: RRP. 230 pp. ISBN: 0960607013; 9780960607013.
  This is one of the best books that introduces the theory and techniques of foot reflexology. The text takes the reader from being a complete novice to being able to provide a reflexology treatment. The authors do an admirable job in summarizing the theory of reflexology and in providing enough information to make the reader able to begin to use reflexology immediately. The chapter on technique is especially noteworthy in that it teaches the correct techniques in a straightforward way. The authors provide detailed instructions on how to work with the foot and how to use the reflexology "desserts." They give good tips on how to read the foot to determine stresses, how to manage a treatment session, and how to set up a reflexology practice. The chapter on anatomy and physiology is helpful in providing a basic background that can be quickly applied. The table of disorders provides a chart that gives the disorder, the reflex areas on the foot, a schematic drawing of the foot locations, and a description and emphasis section that discusses the disorder and where to place special emphasis during a treatment session.
- Mackereth, Peter A., and Tiran, Denise, eds. 2002. *Clinical Reflexology: A Guide for Health Professionals*. New York: Churchill Livingstone. 200 pp. ISBN: 0443071209; 9780443071201.
  Designed for professionals in health care, this book explores a variety of topics related to reflexology, such as theories and origins, ethical and legal principles, research, and practicing refloxology safely and effectively. It also discusses applications of reflexology in specialized clinical settings such as maternity, neonatal care, and palliative care. Reflexology techniques themselves are not directly discussed.

- McLaughlin, Chris, and Hall, Nicola. 2000. *Secrets of Reflexology*. New York: DK Publishing. 224 pp. ISBN: 078946778X; 9780789467782.
  This little book provides a great amount of useful information on reflexology. It is divided into six sections: principles of reflexology, reflexology basics, a basic foot reflexology session, a basic hand reflexology session, reflexology for healing, and reflexology for special cases. Clear color illustrations, including many photographs of the feet and hands, assist the reader in actually performing the reflexology moves discussed. The section on reflexology for healing is especially helpful. It gives directions for treating conditions such as respiratory disorders, digestive disorders, urinary disorders, headaches, and sleeping difficulties. Using reflexology on children, during pregnancy, and on older people is presented in the section on special cases.
- Schaefer, Monika. 2008. *Reflexology Massage*. New York: Sterling. 95 pp. ISBN: 1402747632; 9781402747632.
  Over 100 color photographs and diagrams give the reader excellent instructions on how to perform reflexology on others or on oneself. The author discusses how to do reflexology by examining the proper grips and holds to use, the pinching techniques, and the manipulation of the critical zones on both the hands and the feet.
- Seager, Adrian. 2005. *Reflexology and Associated Aspects of Health: A Practitioner's Guide*. Berkeley, CA: North Atlantic Books. 168 pp. ISBN: 1556435673; 9781556435676.
  Aimed at the reflexology practitioner, the book provides additional information to help both reflexologists and their patients understand the broader concept of health. Topics include techniques for loosening the foot and ankle in preparation for treatment, an introduction to dermatology with a special focus on the foot, nutrition, energy as related to the body including a discussion of the chakras and the meridians, research on reflexology, and treating stroke patients.
- Vennells, David F. 2001. *Reflexology for Beginners: Healing through Foot Massage of Pressure Points*. St. Paul, MN: Llewellyn Publications. 238 pp. ISBN: 0738700983; 9780738700984.
  A good, general introduction to reflexology, this book provides enough background and discussion of techniques to permit one to begin practicing reflexology immediately. Although well illustrated, other books provide greater detail in their illustrations. The chapters on practical advice and case studies are especially instructive. The author also includes a discussion of the use of meditation to help produce a state of relaxation in the body.
- Vennells, David F. 2005. *Healing Hands: Simple and Practical Reflexology Techniques for Developing Good Health and Inner Peace*. New York: O Books. 182 pp. ISBN: 1905047126; 9781905047123.
  Although focusing on the hands alone, this is a good introduction to reflexology in general. In addition to providing excellent instruction on how to perform reflexology on the hands, the author discusses traditional Chinese medicine and managing a reflexology practice. The appendixes include information on meditation, essential oils that can be combined with hand reflexology, Reiki, and Bach flower remedies.
- Voner, Valerie. 2003. *The Everything Reflexology Book: Manipulate Zones in the Hands and Feet to Relieve Stress, Improve Circulation, and Promote Good Health*. Avon, MA: Adams Media. 289 pp. ISBN: 1580629636; 9781580629638.

The goal of this book is to provide the reader with everything that he or she needs to know to be able to give a reflexology treatment. This goal is accomplished through a logical progression from the history and theory that underlie reflexology to working through each of the body's systems. Although the text is clearly written, the lack of sufficient illustrations reduces the usefulness of the book. Used in conjunction with other books that provide more detailed illustrations, this book will be a good resource.

- Watson, Susan A., and Voner, Valerie. 2009. *Practical Reflexology: Interpretation and Techniques*. Boston: McGraw Hill. 405 pp. ISBN: 0073510955; 9780073510958.
  This is a good, thorough introduction to reflexology. Chapters cover the principles of reflexology, anatomy and pathologies of the foot, mapping of the feet, relaxation techniques for the foot, proper technique, and ethics for the practicing reflexologist. One chapter discusses the business aspects of developing a practice, while others cover each of the body systems.
- Wolfe, Frankie Avalon. 2006. *The Complete Idiot's Guide to Reflexology*. New York: Alpha. 264 pp. ISBN: 1592575293; 9781592575299.
  Written in a lighthearted, easy-to-read style, this book nevertheless provides a good introduction to reflexology, including its history, foot anatomy, and use in maintaining a healthy lifestyle. The new edition focuses more on how to use reflexology on yourself and others to improve overall health. The use of reflexology to maintain the health of the body's various systems is presented using plenty of illustrations. The author also discusses other healing techniques such as aromatherapy to enhance health.
- Wright, Janet. 2003. *Reflexology and Acupressure: Pressure Points for Healing*. Summertown, TN: CRCS Wellness Books. 128 pp. ISBN: 1570671494; 9781570671494.
  Wonderfully illustrated, this book gives basic instruction in using foot reflexology and acupressure to treat common problems such as pain, digestive disorders, premenstrual syndrome, and prostate problems. The illustrations assist in performing both reflexology and acupressure either on oneself or on others.

Internet Resources

- American Commission for Accreditation of Reflexology Education and Training, www.acaret.org.
  ACARET seeks to promote and advance the profession of reflexology in America by establishing uniform national standards for reflexology. Such accreditation is voluntary yet demonstrates that the accredited educator meets professional standards and possesses the competency to teach reflexology. The website lists accredited reflexology educators who uphold educational standards as promoted by ACARET.
- American Reflexology Certification Board, www.arcb.net.
  An independent testing agency, the American Reflexology Certification Board offers a voluntary national certification program. The goal of the certification program is to ensure that those reflexologists qualifying for certification practice the profession in accord with national standards. The board does not accredit teachers or a specific curriculum. The website does provide a list of reflexology schools as well as certified reflexologists.

- International Council of Reflexologists, www.icr-reflexology.org.
  The International Council of Reflexologists seeks to provide a forum for the exchange of ideas and information among reflexologists by hosting a biennial international conference and by promoting World Reflexology Week. The site includes a variety of resources, including links to reflexology associations from around the world.
- Reflexology Association of America, www.reflexology-usa.org.
  The Reflexology Association of America is composed of professional reflexologists, reflexology schools, and reflexology students from around the United States. Its goals include the endorsement of professional standards and ethics, excellence in education in reflexology, and providing reliable information to the general public about reflexology. The site provides links to reflexology schools, reflexologists who are members of the RAA, business members, and reflexology laws by state.
- Reflexology Research Project, www.reflexology-research.com.
  Created and hosted by Kevin and Barbara Kunz, authors of many books on reflexology, this site covers all aspects of reflexology, including both feet and hands. Of special note are the articles that report on the efficacy of reflexology.

Periodicals/Magazines/Journals

- *Reflexions: The Journal of Reflexology Research Project*, published by the Reflexology Research Project, 1980– . Quarterly. No ISSN. www.reflexology-research.com.
  Published only in an online format, this newsletter includes articles that vary from research on the efficacy of reflexology to new techniques and how-to information.
- *Reflexology World*, published by Reflexology World, 1996– . Quarterly. ISSN: 1327-2047. www.reflexologyworld.com.
  An independent reflexology magazine published in Australia that is available only through subscription, *Reflexology World* includes articles on reflexology business practices and management, on current trends, case studies, foot conditions, product reviews, conference reports, new reflexology techniques, interviews with reflexologists, and other related news and events.

Chapter 18

Reiki

Background and History

Reiki is a gentle, hands-on healing technique that originated in Japan and has spread worldwide. The term *Reiki* is usually translated as "universal life energy" and is composed of two Japanese characters: *Rei*, meaning universal, spirit, mysterious power, gift, or essence, and *Ki*, meaning energy or vital life force (similar to the Chinese term *chi* or *qi*).

According to the traditional story of its founding, Reiki was "rediscovered" by Mikaomi Usui at the end of the nineteenth century. Although much about his life is a mystery, the inscription on his tomb at the Saihoji temple in the Toyotama district of Tokyo reveals that Usui was born on August 14, 1864. In the early twentieth century, probably after 1914, as the result of a 21-day retreat on Mount Kurama during which he fasted and meditated, he felt the Reiki energy at the top of his head. This experience led to the development of the Reiki healing system. Usui also formulated five guiding principles related to Reiki: don't get angry today, don't worry today, be grateful today, work hard today, and be kind to others today.

Dr. Usui taught Reiki to over 2,000 people and established both a clinic for the use of Reiki as a healing technique and the Usui Reiki Ryoho Gakkai (Usui Reiki Healing Method Society). He died in 1926. Some stories claim that Usui was a Christian and served as the principal of Doshisha University in Kyoto and later studied at the University of Chicago, seeking to discover how Jesus could heal the sick. These stories, however, seem apocryphal, since no evidence has surfaced to verify them. Although Reiki was popular in Japan before World War II, its use declined over time.

Among others who were initiated into Reiki by Dr. Usui was Chujiro Hayashi, a retired naval officer who was still on reserve status. Hayashi also trained Reiki practitioners and opened a clinic in Tokyo where patients could live while they were in treatment. Into this clinic came Hawayo Kawamuru Takata in 1935. Takata was born on December 24, 1900, on the island of Kauai, Hawaii. In 1917, she married Saichi Takata, who died in 1930. Always frail and sickly and having two small children to raise alone, she suffered from exhaustion and other diseases. In 1935, Takata journeyed to Tokyo to visit her parents and to inform them that her sister had died. During this time she was admitted to a hospital for rest and surgery, but she heard a voice telling her that an operation was not necessary. She asked her doctor if there was another way to be healed, and he told her about Hayashi's clinic. After living at the clinic for four months, she was completely healed. She received her preliminary training in Reiki, levels one and two, and returned to Hawaii in 1937. Back home in Hawaii she set up a Reiki clinic. When Hayashi visited her in Hawaii in 1938, she received her Reiki III training and was informed that she would be his successor. Hayashi died in 1941, and with the coming of World War II most Reiki in Japan ceased. Thus, Takata became the conduit of Reiki to the Western world.

Over her lifetime, Takata maintained her healing clinic and also taught Reiki, initiating 22 Reiki masters. From these individuals, Reiki has spread around the world with thousands of individuals now offering Reiki healings.

Primary Uses

Reiki can be used to treat any illness or disease, whether physical, mental, emotional, or spiritual. It can be used alone or in combination with other therapies such as allopathic medicine, chiropractic, or herbal remedies. Reiki works on the energetic level of the human body, thereby affecting all other levels. Since Reiki is a manifestation of universal energy, it possesses its own intelligence and will work where it is needed. Thus, the Reiki practitioner is a conduit for the healing, not the healer per se. In general terms, Reiki can be thought of as bringing balance into an individual, and this balance will help affect the healing. Sometimes results will be immediate, but in most cases the healing will take place over time.

In a treatment session, the Reiki practitioner, often referred to as the healer, will use a variety of hand positions. The individual receiving the treatment remains clothed at all times and will generally be lying down, often on a massage table. Usually the healer's hands are placed directly on the body, but some practitioners will keep the hands suspended above the individual. Although the hand positions can vary slightly, in general there are four positions on the head, five on the front of the body, five on the back, and often one to three on the legs and feet. Each position can be held for up to five minutes. During a treatment session, clients and healers are free to talk, especially if any specific issues surface. Since Reiki often leads to an experience of deep relaxation, the treatment is usually done in silence.

In addition to treating others, Reiki practitioners can also treat themselves, using modified hand positions.

Training

Although Reiki, by definition, is a channeling of universal energy and can be learned by anyone, training and attunements are necessary to become a healer or practitioner. There are three levels of training, called degrees, which must be taught by a Reiki master/teacher. Each degree is accompanied by a ceremony referred to as an attunement in which the energetic channels are cleansed and opened so that the student can be a channel for the energy associated with Reiki. In the first degree, the student learns the basics of Reiki, its history, and treatment protocol. After receiving the first degree attunements, students practice giving treatments to themselves and others. At this stage, the students are considered to be Reiki healers.

The second degree involves receiving not only additional training and attunements but also receiving three symbols for use in healing sessions. Two of the symbols assist in healing both physical and emotional issues, while the third assists in performing healings at a distance, either in time or space.

The third degree training and attunements confer on the student the title of Reiki master/teacher. After this training, the individual is then permitted to teach others about Reiki and to pass on the attunements and symbols. Usually an individual who wishes to receive the third degree must have been practicing Reiki for at least a year.

There are no national associations that certify or license Reiki practitioners and no states regulate its use.

Sources

Brown, Fran. 1992. *Living Reiki: Takata's Teachings*. Mendocino, CA: LifeRhythm.

Lübeck, Walter, Petter, Frank Arjava, and Rand, William Lee. 2004, ©2001. *The Spirit of Reiki: The Complete Handbook of the Reiki System: From Tradition to the Present: Fundamental, Lines of Transmission, Original Writings, Mastery, Symbols, Treatments, Reiki as a Spiritual Path in Life, and Much More*. Twin Lakes, WI: Lotus Press.

Stein, Diane. 1995. *Essential Reiki: A Complete Guide to an Ancient Healing Art*. Freedom, CA: The Crossing Press.

See also ENERGY MEDICINE AND ENERGY HEALING; SPIRITUALITY, RELIGION, AND PRAYER

Annotated Bibliography

Print Resources

➤ Beckett, Don. 2009. *Reiki: The True Story: An Exploration of Usui Reiki*. Berkeley, CA: North Atlantic Books. 229 pp. ISBN: 158394267X; 9781583942673.
The traditional story of Reiki traces its founding back to Makao Usui. In this book, the author presents an in-depth history of Reiki in Japan through the testimony of some of Usui's students. In addition, he provides a manual for the practice of Reiki, discusses the nature of Reiki energy, and examines the chakra system, yin and yang, and the Five Transformations. He then concludes with a discussion of the future of Reiki.

➤ Bevell, Brett. 2009. *Reiki for Spiritual Healing*. Berkeley, CA: Crossing Press. 167 pp. ISBN: 1580911943; 9781580911948.
This is a general guide for Reiki practitioners and for the interested laypersons to learn to use Reiki as a way to awaken their spirit. The author presents new Reiki symbols and techniques and explores the use of Reiki as a means to provide healing treatments across lifetimes and to clear karmic and spiritual blocks that hinder their connection with the divine nature of the world.

➤ Brown, Fran. 1992. *Living Reiki: Takata's Teachings*. Mendocino, CA: LifeRhythm. 97 pp. ISBN: 0940795108; 9780940795105.
Written by one of the 22 individuals who were made Reiki master/teachers by Hawayo Takata, this slim volume is a must-read for anyone interested in Reiki as it is practiced in the West. Hawayo Takata, as the student of Chujiro Hayashi, became the conduit who brought Reiki out of Japan prior to the outbreak of World War II. Thus, she helped keep the Usui System of Natural Healing alive. Since Reiki is generally taught orally by a master who imparts the knowledge to his or her students, the words and stories of Takata are of special importance and are wonderful sources for illustrating the story of Reiki and the art of using it as a healing technique.

➤ Burack, Marsha. 1995. *Reiki: Healing Yourself & Others: A Photo-Instructional Art Book*. Encinitas, CA: Lo Ro Productions. 145 pp. ISBN: 188044139X; 9781880441398.
For the individual who is just learning Reiki, the wonderful illustrations in this book will be a godsend. The author provides a good, though brief, explanation of the

chakras, the endocrine glands, and the use of Reiki in healing oneself as well as others. The photographs of the hand positions, along with their captions, will guide the novice Reiki practitioner through the steps of performing a healing.

- Jones, Philip. 2009. *Simply Reiki.* New York: Sterling/Zambezi. 128 pp. ISBN: 1402744927; 9781402744921.
  In this short book, the author introduces Reiki and its healing techniques. The book does a good job of explaining Reiki and how it can be used for healing oneself and others.
- Lübeck, Walter, and Petter, Frank Arjava. 2003. *Reiki Best Practices: Wonderful Tools of Healing for the First, Second, and Third Reiki Degree.* Twin Lakes, WI: Lotus Press. 292 pp. ISBN: 0914955748; 9780914955740.
  This book provides a wide range of healing techniques that incorporate Reiki into them. The techniques are as varied as treating animals with Reiki, treating comatose patients with Reiki, charging food and drinks with Reiki, finding lost objects with Reiki, and sex with Reiki. This book is most useful to those who have already been attuned to Reiki and wish to use it in broader ways.
- Lübeck, Walter, Petter, Frank Arjava, and Rand, William Lee. 2004, ©2001. *The Spirit of Reiki: The Complete Handbook of the Reiki System: From Tradition to the Present: Fundamental, Lines of Transmission, Original Writings, Mastery, Symbols, Treatments, Reiki as a Spiritual Path in Life, and Much More.* Twin Lakes, WI: Lotus Press. 304 pp. ISBN: 0914955675; 9780914955672.
  For those who seek additional information on the history and development of Reiki, this is an excellent book. The authors provide an in-depth history of Reiki, discuss the basics of Reiki energy, present Reiki as it is practiced in the Western world and in Japan, and examine the future of Reiki.
- McKenzie, Eleanor. 2009. *The Reiki Bible: The Definitive Guide to Healing with Energy.* New York: Sterling. 400 pp. ISBN: 1402770030; 9781402770036.
  Designed to be a comprehensive guide to Reiki, this book covers the origins and development of Reiki, the anatomy of the human energy system, and the three levels of Reiki attunement. The author uses photographs to demonstrate all of the hand positions, and she offers advice for offering Reiki treatments to friends and family and for helping heal common ailments.
- Miles, Pamela. 2006. *Reiki: A Comprehensive Guide.* New York: Jeremy P. Tarcher/Penguin. 265 pp. ISBN: 1585424749; 9781585424740.
  Miles provides a good general introduction to Reiki and its practice. She describes the levels of Reiki and offers sound advice on finding and choosing a Reiki practitioner for personal healing or for Reiki training. She also discusses the relationship between Reiki, science, medical research, and integrative medicine.
- Morris, Joyce J., and Morris, William R. 1999. *Reiki: Hands That Heal.* York Beach, ME: Weiser Books. 174 pp. ISBN: 1578631181; 9781578631186.
  This is a useful book that delves more into the practical sides of operating a Reiki practice. Chapters such as "Treatment Guidelines" and "Professional Ethics" will assist both those who are just beginning the Reiki journey and those that have been practicing for years. The chapter on hand positions is excellent, with good illustrations and

charts of the physical, mental/emotional, and spiritual attributes, signs, and systems for each location.

- Paul, Nina L. 2006. *Reiki for Dummies.* Hoboken, NJ: Wiley Publishing. 334 pp. ISBN: 0764599070; 9780764599071.
  Written for the complete novice, this book provides a basic introduction to the history of Reiki while exploring more deeply the experience of receiving and giving Reiki treatments. Of special note is the section titled "Becoming Well-Versed in Reiki," which gives helpful hints on seeking Reiki training, using the Reiki symbols, healing others with proper hand positions, healing yourself, and using crystals with Reiki. The author also discusses the use of Reiki with other health practices. She includes ways to use Reiki in everyday situations and for personal growth. She concludes the book by discussing common myths about Reiki.

- Petter, Frank Arjava. 1997. *Reiki Fire: New Information about the Origins of the Reiki Power: A Complete Manual.* Twin Lakes, WI: Lotus Light Publications. 126 pp. ISBN: 0914955500; 9780914955504.
  Examining the Japanese origins of Reiki, Petter provides the best single story of Dr. Usui's development of Reiki. Petter also discusses the training necessary to become a Reiki practitioner, the hand positions used in healing, and topics such as the heart, the body, the mind, and the esoteric background of Reiki. Thus, the book is a good introduction to Reiki as a healing modality.

- Petter, Frank Arjava, Yamaguchi, Tadao, and Hayashi, Chujiro. 2003. *The Hayashi Reiki Manual.* Twin Lakes, WI: Lotus Press. 109 pp. ISBN: 0914955756; 9780914955757.
  This is an excellent book that explains, in great detail, the Hayashi Reiki system as taught by Dr. Chujiro Hayashi, one of the early pioneers of Reiki in Japan. First, the authors discuss Dr. Hayashi and his contributions to Reiki. Then one of the authors recounts the story of his mother and her training in Reiki under Dr. Hayashi. Wonderfully illustrated, each hand position used in the "blood circulation technique" created by Dr. Hayashi is explained. The final chapter discusses diseases of specific organ systems and the best hand positions to use.

- Rand, William Lee. 2000, ©1991. *Reiki: The Healing Touch: First and Second Degree Manual.* Southfield, MI: Vision Publications. Various pp. ISBN: 1886785058; 9781886785052.
  Probably the best single resource for the beginning student of Reiki, this book provides excellent background on Reiki, including its history and use. Designed for classes that teach the first two levels of Reiki, clear explanations of performing a Reiki healing are given. Of special note is the section on developing a Reiki practice that provides helpful tips on setting up and managing one's own healing practice.

- Rowland, Amy Zaffarano. 2008. *Reiki for the Heart and Soul: The Reiki Principles as Spiritual Pathwork.* Rochester, VT: Healing Arts Press. 243 pp. ISBN: 1594772525; 9781594772528.
  Instead of focusing on Reiki as a healing technique, this is a meditation on the five Reiki principles. Thus, the exercises and teachings can be used as a guide for spiritual growth, both for Reiki practitioners and for anyone interested in Reiki.

- Stein, Diane. 1995. *Essential Reiki: A Complete Guide to an Ancient Healing Art.* Freedom, CA: The Crossing Press. 156 pp. ISBN: 0895947366; 9780895947369.

Covering all aspects of Reiki from the novice to the expert, this is the single best book that is available on Reiki. As a Reiki master/teacher, Stein is amply qualified to produce such a work. The book is arranged by the degrees of Reiki. Thus, the section of the first degree discusses the story of Reiki and a typical healing session. The Reiki symbols, distance healing, and opening the kundalini are discussed under the second degree section. Finally, the section of the third degree, that of Reiki master/teacher, provides information on the third degree symbols, on performing attunements, on teaching Reiki, and on the use of Reiki as a step on the path to enlightenment. The work is well illustrated, providing drawings of all the symbols, hand positions for healing, and anatomy as related to energetic healing.

➤ Stein, Diane. 2007. *Essential Reiki Teaching Manual: A Companion Guide for Reiki Healers.* Berkeley, CA: Crossing Press. 147 pp. ISBN: 1580911811; 9781580911818.
Designed for the Reiki master/teacher, this book is a guide to teaching others about Reiki. Topics covered include preparing oneself to teach Reiki, preparing the teaching space, passing the Reiki attunements, and teaching Reiki. The author includes useful handouts for all three levels of Reiki instruction.

➤ Stiene, Bronwen, and Stiene, Frans. 2003. *The Reiki Sourcebook.* New York: O Books. 366 pp. ISBN: 1903816556; 9781903816554.
The goal of this book is to collect together a vast array of information on Reiki. Thus, it is not a book for reading but for reference. The authors provide detailed discussions of the word *Reiki*, the treatment session, training courses, the history of Reiki beginning with Mikao Usui and continuing in the Western world, characteristics of Reiki branches, scientific studies of Reiki, Japanese Reiki techniques, Western Reiki techniques, and various directors to schools, associations, and Internet resources. The glossary is very helpful in defining words that the reader or Reiki student may encounter.

➤ Stinnett, Gay. 2009. *A Measure of Joy: Opening to the Energy of Reiki.* Albuquerque, NM: Fresco Fine Art Publications. 95 pp. ISBN: 1934491136; 9781934491133.
Using both text and photography, this is a simple introduction to Reiki. The author gives many examples from her own life and how the gift of Reiki changed her forever.

➤ Usui, Mikao, and Petter, Frank Arjava. 1999. *The Original Reiki Handbook of Dr. Mikao Usui.* Translated by C. M. Grimm. Twin Lakes, WI: Lotus Press. 79 pp. ISBN: 0914955578; 9780914955573.
In this little book, the author presents the results of his quest to find the roots of Reiki at its source: the handbook of Dr. Mikao Usui, the founder of Reiki healing in Japan. This is the first English translation of the section of Dr. Usui's handbook that gives detailed descriptions of the hand positions that he taught for the treatment of specific illnesses. In addition to giving good translations of the original Japanese, excellent color photographs and drawings enhance the text and provide visual representation of the written text. Also included are the hand positions to use for disorders of specific body systems, childhood diseases, women's health, and contagious diseases.

➤ Vennells, David F. 1999. *Reiki for Beginners: Mastering Natural Healing Techniques.* St. Paul, MN: Llewellyn Publications. 336 pp. ISBN: 1567187676; 9781567187670.
Providing a good introduction to Reiki, the author writes in an easy to understand style. Line drawings provide visual representations of the major hand positions used

in Reiki. Also included are brief stories written by Reiki practitioners about what Reiki has meant to them.

Internet Resources

- The International Association of Reiki Professionals, iarp.org.
  The International Association of Reiki Professionals is a professional association of the global Reiki community. Its goals include promoting the use of the healing effects of Reiki throughout the world and providing members with the tools to enhance and expand their practices.
- The International Center for Reiki Training, www.reiki.org.
  This is one of the most comprehensive websites devoted to Reiki. The International Center for Reiki Training offers classes, publishes the *Reiki News Magazine*, and sells a variety of Reiki-related products. The director of the center, William Lee Rand, is known around the world for his teaching of Reiki.
- James Deacon's Reiki Pages, www.aetw.org.
  This site provides a wealth of information on Reiki including the Reiki symbols, the Reiki principles, early Reiki documents, terminology, various Japanese Reiki styles, and the history of Reiki.
- The Reiki Alliance, www.reikialliance.com.
  The Reiki Alliance traces its lineage back directly to Hawayo Takata and the masters that she initiated. The site provides useful information on Reiki and also gives a listing of Reiki teachers affiliated with the Reiki Alliance.
- The Reiki Page, reiki.7gen.com.
  Produced by David Herron, The Reiki Page is loaded with useful information on Reiki for both practitioners and clients, its history, and its practice.

Periodicals/Magazines/Journals

- *Radiance Technique Journal*, published by the Radiance Technique International Association Inc., 1980– . Semi-annual. ISSN: 1040-5836. www.trtia.org.
  Received with membership, this publication features news from members of their use of the Radiance Technique and information on peace projects in the U.S. and abroad.
- *Reiki News Magazine*, published by the International Center for Reiki Training, 2002– . Quarterly. ISSN: 1539-6533. www.reikinm.com.
  Probably the single best source of current information on Reiki, *Reiki News Magazine* provides a variety of articles about Reiki written by experienced Reiki practitioners.
- *The Reiki Times*, published by IARP: International Association of Reiki Professionals, 1995– . Monthly. ISSN: 1081-8529. www.iarpreiki.org/The_Reiki_Times_Magazine.
  Covering the global Reiki community, articles in this magazine provide useful information on the practice of Reiki.

Chapter 19

Rolfing and Structural Bodywork

Background and History

Rolfing, also known as structural integration, was developed by Dr. Ida Rolf and is a technique for relieving pain and stress. Dr. Rolf, a biochemist who received her degree in 1920 from the College of Physicians and Surgeons of Columbia University, explored many forms of alternative healing including homeopathy, osteopathy, chiropractic, and yoga in a search to treat her own physical ailments. She was fascinated by the idea of manipulation to achieve proper alignment and functioning of the body. Through this research she developed her idea that the body should be aligned with gravity. Misalignment causes stress on the soft tissues of the body, especially the muscles, fascia, tendons, and ligaments. Such misalignment can be caused by physical or emotional stress, which causes the fascia to tense or harden. Over time, Rolf established techniques to release these stresses or tensions, resulting in a healthier individual, both physically and emotionally.

In 1971, Rolf founded the Rolf Institute for Structural Integration in Boulder, Colorado, to train practitioners of her technique. Dr. Rolf died in 1979, but her institute continues to instruct students on her methods.

Primary Uses and Actions

Although Rolfing is primarily a technique that manipulates the structure of the body, it can also be considered a holistic healing technique because changes in structure can impact the physical, emotional, and energetic aspects of the individual. At the beginning of a Rolfing session, the Rolfer will evaluate the client's movement and posture, which help determine the specific goals of the session. Most clients will begin with what is called the Ten-Series because the treatment consists of ten one-hour sessions in which the whole body is systematically balanced so that the structure and the function of the entire body improve. Each session focuses on a specific region of the body, although the whole body is also considered in designing the treatment.

During the session, the Rolfer will use his or her elbows, fingers, hands, and knuckles to apply firm, sometimes uncomfortable, pressure to stretch and manipulate the fascia so that holdings can be released and misalignments corrected. In contrast to massage, which can also relax tight muscles, Rolfing seeks not only to relax muscles but also to reshape and realign the body so that it is balanced in gravity.

Rolfing is not recommended for those with cancer, rheumatoid arthritis, or other inflammatory conditions.

Training

The Rolf Institute of Structural Integration is the only source through which one can receive the training to become a certified Rolfer. The basic certification process can take between 18 and 24 months. Students must have a good understanding of human anatomy, physiology, and kinesiology in addition to the techniques of Rolfing. The training also includes a clinical component in which the student works under the supervision of instructors. After successful completion of the entire course sequence, the student becomes a certified Rolfer. There are currently over 1,500 certified Rolfers in 26 countries.

Sources

Rolf, Ida P. 1989. *Rolfing: Reestablishing the Natural Alignment and Structural Integration of the Human Body for Vitality and Well-Being.* Rochester, VT: Healing Arts Press.

Rolf, Ida P., edited by Feitis, Rosemary. 1990, ©1978. *Rolfing and Physical Reality.* Rochester, VT: Healing Arts Press.

The Rolf Institute of Structural Integration, www.rolf.org.

See also THE ALEXANDER TECHNIQUE; FELDENKRAIS METHOD; THERAPEUTIC MASSAGE AND BODYWORK

Annotated Bibliography

Print Resources

➤ Bond, Mary. 1996, ©1993. *Balancing Your Body: A Self-Help Approach to Rolfing Movement.* Rochester, VT: Healing Arts Press. 214 pp. ISBN: 0892816422; 9780892816422.
This book gives a basic introduction to the concepts and teachings of Ida Rolf and provides exercises that let the reader experience these principles firsthand. Each chapter presents a specific concept—for example, breath—and then it gives a set of scripts that guide the reader through exercises that explore the concept physically. The scripts can either be read aloud by a partner or recorded for personal use. The exercises can yield both physical and emotional changes.

➤ Bond, Mary. 2007. *The New Rules of Posture: How to Sit, Stand, and Move in the Modern World.* Rochester, VT: Healing Arts Press. 225 pp. ISBN: 1594771243; 9781594771248.
Based largely on the ideas and teachings of Ida Rolf, this book is a manual that teaches proper posture. Although such posture will vary by individual, the basic principles are the same. The author takes the reader through the process of becoming conscious of the body, establishing healthy breathing patterns, and establishing proper alignment of the pelvic floor, the shoulders, the feet, and the head. She also introduces the concept of healthy walking. This is an excellent book that can help relieve pain caused by incorrect posture in walking, sitting, and standing.

➤ Karrasch, Noah. 2009. *Meet Your Body: CORE Bodywork and Rolfing Tools to Release Bodymindcore.* Philadelphia: Singing Dragon. 184 pp. ISBN: 1848190166; 9781848190160.
Using techniques drawn from Rolfing, the author seeks to show how to release the old fears, traumas, and stresses that many of us hold onto. Once they are released, we can begin to regain health and feel better. In this book, the author discusses his concept of the bodymindcore, the inherent connection between our minds and our

bodies and how the connective tissue can be manipulated to permit free movement that results in better overall health, well-being, and happiness.

- Rolf, Ida P. 1989. *Rolfing: Reestablishing the Natural Alignment and Structural Integration of the Human Body for Vitality and Well-Being*. Rochester, VT: Healing Arts Press. Original ed., *Rolfing: The Integration of Human Structures*, 1977. 304 pp. ISBN: 0892813350; 9780892813353.
  In this book, Rolf provides the anatomical background and structural principles of her technique. She discusses the structure of the body and focuses especially on the muscles responsible for maintaining the body in gravity. The book provides excellent discussions of the fascia, feet, the psoas muscle, pelvis, joints, spine, and movement. Almost 1,000 photographs and drawings amply illustrate almost every point made in the text. This book must be included in any collection on CAM techniques.
- Rolf, Ida P., edited by Feitis, Rosemary. 1990, ©1978. *Rolfing and Physical Reality*. Rochester, VT: Healing Arts Press. Original ed., *Ida Rolf Talks about Rolfing and Physical Reality*. 215 pp. ISBN: 0892813806; 9780892813803.
  After an introduction to the history of the development of the Rolfing technique, the editor provides quotations from Ida Rolf in which she tells about her life, about the human body, and about Rolfing. Of special interest is the way Rolf talks about how she works with clients and how psychological issues often surface as a result of her work.
- Schultz, R. Louis, and Feitis, Rosemary. 1996. *The Endless Web: Fascial Anatomy and Physical Reality*. Berkeley, CA: North Atlantic Books. 126 pp. ISBN: 1556432283; 9781556432286.
  This is a very good introduction to the anatomy of the fascia, or connective tissue, which is manipulated during Rolfing treatment. Using clear illustrations and photographs, this book helps both those who are giving and those who are receiving Rolfing and other techniques such as myofascial release understand how the myofascial system works, its role in supporting the body, and how its manipulation can be therapeutic.
- Sise, Betsy. 2005. *The Rolfing Experience: Integration in the Gravity Field*. Prescott, AZ: Hohm Press. 295 pp. ISBN: 1890772526; 9781890772529.
  This is an excellent book that introduces the reader to the basics of Rolfing and the experience of receiving Rolfing treatments. For those interested in receiving Rolfing, Part 3 addresses what happens during a treatment session and also discusses the issue of pain that may be experienced during the treatment. Interspersed throughout the book are stories and before and after photographs of individuals who have received Rolfing.
- Smith, John. 2005. *Structural Bodywork: An Introduction for Students and Practitioners*. New York: Elsevier Churchill Livingstone. 232 pp. ISBN: 0443100101; 9780443100109.
  Building on the ideas of Ida Rolf, the author takes an eclectic approach to discussing the concept of structural bodywork that is built on three primary ideas: the human body has a structure that can be reorganized, the connective tissue network is important in this structure, and the dynamics of posture vary between individuals and must be taken into account. Aimed at a wide range of health professionals, from massage therapists, to psychologists, to nurses, this book provides both an introduction to the

background and history of structural bodywork and to the somatic organization of the body. In addition, the bulk of the book presents a practical manual of working with the body's structure from the sagittal, frontal, and transverse planes with the shoulder girdle and the leg. Clear directions and illustrations assist in applying the information presented throughout the book.

Internet Resources

- The Rolf Institute of Structural Integration, www.rolf.org.
  Founded by Ida P. Rolf in 1971, The Rolf Institute of Structural Integration is the only organization that can certify practitioners as Rolfers and Rolf Movement Practitioners. The institute also provides continuing education for practitioners of the Rolf Method of Personal Structural Integration and educates the public on both the principles of structural integration and the health benefits of the Rolf method. For those seeking information on Rolfing, this is the single best source.

Periodicals/Magazines/Journals

None found.

Chapter 20

Spirituality, Religion, and Prayer

Background and History

No one knows when religion began, but one of its primary purposes was probably the health of the worshipers. People used ritual and prayer in the hopes of preserving their health or for healing. This use of religion and ritual is attested by the offerings often left at sanctuaries. For example, at the sanctuary of Asclepius near Epidaurus in Greece, many small offerings in the shape of body parts have been found. The same ritualistic use of such votive offerings is still seen at Lourdes in France and at other sites renowned for their healing powers. Most religions use intercessory prayer with their deity or deities to seek help for those who are ill. Even today, prayer circles can be found in most Christian churches and on the Internet that have as their expressed purpose the requesting of healing.

According to research supported by the National Center for Complementary and Alternative Medicine, prayer is the most frequently used form of alternative therapy. The center reports that 45 percent of the respondents had used prayer for health reasons. Of these, 43 percent had prayed for their own health, almost 25 percent had had others pray for them, and almost 10 percent had participated in a prayer group for their own health.

Although prayer is the most used form of alternative therapy, other CAM modalities also have a religious or spiritual basis or origin. These include meditation, yoga, tai chi, qigong, and many energy healing techniques such as Reiki.

Primary Uses and Actions

Prayer, spirituality, and other religious practices can be used for any illness, whether physical, psychological, or spiritual. Although much research has been conducted on the effect of prayer on healing, the healing mechanism itself cannot be specifically determined.

Training

No training is needed to use spirituality, prayer, or religion for healing purposes. Many religions, however, do include rituals for the healing of the sick, and these rituals must often be performed by trained priests. For example, in many parts of the world, shamans must be trained by other shamans before they can perform the sacred rituals of healing. In the United States, seminaries, including those serving protestant and Catholic churches and Jewish synagogues and temples, often include coursework on counseling and working with those who are sick. Some offer the master's degree in pastoral counseling, which permits the recipient to work in hospitals, nursing homes, and other health care facilities offering their services, one of which is prayer with patients and their families.

Sources

Chamberlain, Theodore J., and Hall, Christopher A. 2001, ©2000. *Realized Religion: Research on the Relationship between Religion and Health*. Philadelphia, PA: Templeton Foundation Press.

Dossey, Larry. 1996. *Prayer Is Good Medicine: How to Reap the Healing Benefits of Prayer*. San Francisco, CA: HarperSanFrancisco.

Dossey, Larry. 1997, ©1993. *Healing Words: The Power of Prayer and the Practice of Medicine*. New York: HarperPaperbacks.

See also ENERGY MEDICINE AND ENERGY HEALING; MEDITATION

Annotated Bibliography

Print Resources

- Chamberlain, Theodore J., and Hall, Christopher A. 2001, ©2000. *Realized Religion: Research on the Relationship between Religion and Health*. Philadelphia, PA: Templeton Foundation Press. 239 pp. ISBN: 189015153X; 9781890151539.
  Based on over 300 research reports, the authors examine the relationship between religion and health. Each chapter focuses on a specific topic and includes a detailed bibliography. The first two chapters discuss the role of prayer in healing and health and the effects of faith healing. The next group of chapters explores the relationship of religion and well-being with specific attention given to mental health, life satisfaction, mental disorders, marital satisfaction, suicide, and alcohol use and abuse. The final chapters stress the need for future empirical research and posit Christianity as a model for religion's relationship to health.
- Csordas, Thomas J. 2002. *Body/Meaning/Healing*. New York: Palgrave Macmillan. 321 pp. ISBN: 0312293925; 9780312293925.
  Drawn from the research experiences of the author, this book seeks to set forth two agendas, one empirical and the other theoretical. The empirical agenda presents an analysis of religious healing from which an understanding of the therapeutic process can be generalized. The second agenda seeks to explore the notion of embodiment as a way through which to understand human experience in culture. Examples used in the book are drawn from research on Catholic charismatics, from cancer studies of Navajos, and from North American psychotherapy, among others. For those readers with a philosophical bent, this work will be of interest.
- Dale, Cyndi. 2009. *The Subtle Body: An Encyclopedia of Your Energetic Anatomy*. Boulder, CO: Sounds True. 487 pp. ISBN: 1591796717; 9781591796718.
  This work is intended to cover the full scope of human energetic anatomy. Part 1 explores energy and energy healing, while Part 2 examines human anatomy and has a chapter devoted to each of the bodily systems as well as the cells, DNA, metabolism, and the senses. The third section is devoted to energy fields and includes chapters on topics as diverse as natural energy fields, magnetism, and sacred geometry. The

fourth part focuses on the channels of energy and the channels of light such as the meridians and the acupuncture points. The fifth part includes chapters on energy bodies, the kundalini, the chakra system, and Jewish kabbalah. Finally, Part 6 examines a variety of energy practices.

- Dossey, Larry. 1996. *Prayer Is Good Medicine: How to Reap the Healing Benefits of Prayer*. San Francisco, CA: HarperSanFrancisco. 249 pp. ISBN: 0062514245; 9780062514240.
  Approached from a nonsectarian viewpoint, this book examines the role of prayer in healing. The author summarizes the evidence for the efficacy of prayer, discusses the controversy of including prayer in medical treatment, examines the concept of prayer, and presents examples of how to pray.
- Dossey, Larry. 1997, ©1993. *Healing Words: The Power of Prayer and the Practice of Medicine*. New York: HarperPaperbacks. 405 pp. ISBN: 0061043834; 9780061043833.
  Using personal anecdotes from his own medical practice, the author explores the place of prayer in healing and health. In the first part of the book, prayer and healing are discussed in general, while in Part 2 the factors that influence the efficacy or prayer are addressed. In the final section, he presents the scientific evidence that the beliefs of the patient and the doctor can affect the outcome of treatment and uses discoveries of modern physics to explain these effects.
- Dossey, Larry. 1999. *Reinventing Medicine: Beyond Mind–Body to a New Era of Healing*. San Francisco: HarperSanFrancisco. 271 pp. ISBN: 0062516442; 9780062516442.
  Using medical research to support his ideas, the author examines the spiritual dimension of healing and argues that conventional medicine needs to be reinvented to incorporate the ideas of mind–body medicine into the treatment of the whole person. To reinvent medicine, he argues that prayer and intentions be used to promote healing, that nonverbal communication between physician and the patient be recognized for its importance, and that the intuition of health care providers be further developed. Although of interest to the general reader, physicians should read this book and try to incorporate the author's ideas into their practices.
- Ellens, J. Harold. 2010. *The Healing Power of Spirituality: How Faith Helps Humans Thrive*. 3 vols. Santa Barbara, CA: Praeger/ABC-CLIO. 989 pp. ISBN: 0313366454; 9780313366451.
  This three volume series strives to provide a scientific exploration of faith and well-being. Volume one examines the healing power of personal spiritualities such as I Ching and Transcendentalism. Volume two focuses on healing in the context of Christianity, Judaism, and other major world faiths. Finally, Volume 3 is much broader in scope and explores the psychodynamics of the connection between healing and spirituality, including topics such as the role of biochemical and chemical reactions in heightening psychospiritual perception.
- Graham, Helen. 1993. *Magic Shop: Healing with the Imagination*. York Beach, ME: Samuel Weiser. 228 pp. ISBN: 0877287708; 9780877287704.
  The exercises in this book aid you in delving into your own subconscious to help bring about healing. Using such techniques of the imagination can also help you relax, improve your health, and increase your awareness of your personal physical, emotional, and spiritual needs.

- Hollins, Susan. 2009. *Religions, Culture and Healthcare: A Practical Handbook for Use in Healthcare Environments.* New York: Radcliffe Publishing. 143 pp. ISBN: 1846192609; 9781846192609.

  Health care professionals, including doctors, nurses, therapists, and even chaplains, will find this a useful resource that offers practical information on each of the major world faiths and their cultural manifestations. The relationship of each faith to health care is examined, providing needed information for those working with individuals from these various faith communities.

- Koenig, Harold George. 2001. *The Healing Power of Faith: How Belief and Prayer Can Help You Triumph Over Disease.* New York: Simon & Schuster. 331 pp. ISBN: 0684852977; 9780684852973.

  Combining anecdotal stories and scientific research, this book examines the relationship between faith and health, especially living a healthier life and healing from disease. The author addresses topics such as faith and life satisfaction, marriage and family, depression, stress, cardiovascular disease, and the immune system. The strength of this work is its strong foundation based on the research literature drawn from a variety of medical disciplines.

- Koenig, Harold George. 2008. *Medicine, Religion, and Health: Where Science and Spirituality Meet.* West Conshohocken, PA: Templeton Foundation Press. 234 pp. ISBN: 1599471418; 9781599471419.

  Building on the most current literature, this is one of the newest books to address the convergence of medicine and religion. Although many research studies are cited, the author has written this book for nonspecialists and the general reader. After first arguing for clear definitions of religion and spirituality to facilitate precisely defined objectives for research, he presents the psychological and social factors that influence the physical body. Over the span of several chapters, he then provides his thesis that religion has a potential to influence both mental and physical health. The last two chapters summarize the studies of religious involvement and longevity and discuss the potential applications of research on the spiritual and religious effects on health. Thus, the author takes this controversial issue and presents a clear articulation of the relationship between health and religion and spirituality.

- Koenig, Harold George, McCullough, Michael E., and Larson, David B. 2001. *Handbook of Religion and Health.* New York: Oxford University Press. 712 pp. ISBN: 0195118669; 9780195118667.

  This book is a reaction to the increasing interest of researchers and clinical practitioners in the relationship between religious faith and medicine. It summarizes the results of over 1,200 research studies and 400 research reviews. Chapters focus on a wide variety of topics drawn from both mental health and physical disorders. Thus, the effect of religion on depression, suicide, alcohol and drug use, marital instability, and personality are addressed in the section on mental health while illnesses such as heart disease, cancer, disability, and health behaviors are included in the physical disorders. Other topics presented include the use of health services, clinical applications, and priorities for future research. At its time, this was an excellent summary of the knowledge then available, and it still retains historic significance, although other works have summarized more recent research.

- Kunz, Dora, comp. 1995. *Spiritual Healing*. Wheaton, IL: Quest Books. 333 pp. ISBN: 0835607143; 9780835607148.
  A compilation of a variety of works by many authors including noted writers on CAM, this book is unified by its theme of the relationship between spirituality and healing. Part 1 examines healing as a worldview and how that worldview is changing in response to the growing use of CAM therapies. Part 2 looks into the unseen sources of healing, especially the spirit. In Part 3, the authors discuss new dimensions in healing, especially the concept of holistic medicine. The psyche and its effects are the focus of Part 4, while the human energy system underlies Part 5. Thus, taken together, the authors both question the way conventional medicine heals and postulate a new paradigm for understanding the art of healing
- Levin, Jeffrey S. 2001. *God, Faith, and Health: Exploring the Spirituality–Healing Connection*. New York: John Wiley. 256 pp. ISBN: 0471355038; 9780471355038.
  In this interesting book, the author explores the scientific literature and concludes that there is compelling evidence that a relationship exists between health and spiritual belief and practices such as prayer, attending worship services, meditation, and faith in God or a higher power. Examples are drawn from diverse practices such as Christianity, Judaism, and yoga. The work is divided into three parts. The first discusses the health effects of public religion, such as attending religious services. The second focuses on the health effects of private spirituality, such as the emotional impact of worship, religious beliefs, and faith. The last part examines energy, consciousness, healing, and the future of medicine. The author argues that mind–body medicine should be expanded to include the spirit, thereby forming body-mind-spirit medicine.
- Matthews, Dale A., and Clark, Connie I. 1999, ©1998. *The Faith Factor: Proof of the Healing Power of Prayer*. New York: Penguin Books. 322 pp. ISBN: 0140275754; 9780140275759.
  Starting from the premise that "faith is good medicine," the authors present their view of "whole-person medicine," which focuses on caring for the whole person, not just their organs and tissues. To support their views, they present the science of prayer and faith as drawn from the scientific, clinical literature, especially as related to healing the body, mind, and addictions. They also discuss spirituality and provide guidance on developing a spiritual program, prayer, reading the Bible, and living in a spiritual community. The final chapter attempts to synthesize spirituality and healing and lays out a plan for twenty-first century medicine.
- Sha, Zhi Gang. 2006. *Soul Mind Body Medicine: Techniques for Optimum Health and Vitality*. Novato, CA: New World Library. 362 pp. ISBN: 1577315286; 9781577315285.
  The basic premise of this work is that if the soul is healed first, then the healing of the mind and body will naturally follow. To facilitate the healing of the soul, the author demonstrates that love and forgiveness are the key to healing the soul. From this simple theory, he then presents techniques, such as universal meditation and the four power techniques, which can be used by anyone to hasten healing. The core of the book is a set of instructions on using his techniques to heal common ailments, including conditions of the head, ears, heart, abdomen, joints, and skin.

- Sorajjakool, Siroj, Carr, Mark F., and Nam, Julius J. 2010. *World Religions for Healthcare Professionals*. New York: Routledge. 179 pp. ISBN: 0789038137; 9780789038135.
  This short work discusses American Indian religions, Hinduism, Buddhism, Chinese religions, Sikhism, Islam, Judaism, and Christianity. Designed for health care workers, the entries discuss the health-related beliefs and practices of the major world religions. Its greatest strength is being a guide to health care etiquette for those working with individuals of different faiths.
- Stavish, Mark. 2007. *Kabbalah for Health & Wellness*. Woodbury, MN: Llewellyn Publications. 216 pp. ISBN: 0738709778; 9780738709772.
  This is an introductory text on kabbalah for those who have an interest in the healing arts, specifically in energy healing. The work contains many exercises that reinforce the concepts being taught. Chapters address issues of energy healing, prayer, meditation, ritual, the etheric body, and the practice of kabbalah and its major ideas.
- Turner, Edith. 2006. *Among the Healers: Stories of Spiritual and Ritual Healing around the World*. Westport, CT: Praeger. 183 pp. ISBN: 0275987299; 9780275987299.
  Written by an anthropologist, this work examines spiritual healing traditions from around the world. Through examples drawn from anthropological fieldwork in Ireland, Africa, Mexico, Russia, Israel, Brazil, Europe, and the United States, the author examines such topics as energy healing, the experience of power, the presence of spirits, the idea of communitas, and patterns of healing. Thus, she broadens the topic of complementary and alternative healing into the realm of the spiritual and approaches it from a variety of angles.
- Woods, Richard. 2008. *Wellness: Life, Health and Spirituality*. Chester Springs, PA: Dufour Editions. 271 pp. ISBN: 1847300928; 9781847300928.
  In his book, Woods argues that a healthy spiritual life helps people live longer and happier lives, contribute to society, and also suffer from less discontent. He attributes this to a positive link between physical, emotional, and mental health and spirituality. He also argues that those who have a healthy spiritual life also contribute more to society, thereby helping to create a better world.

Internet Resources

- Beliefnet.com, www.beliefnet.com.
  The mission of Beliefnet is to provide people with information on a wide variety of spiritual paths so that they can discover comfort, hope, clarity, strength, and happiness. This includes health and holistic living. The site gives excellent background on topics as diverse as healthy living, emotional health, yoga, meditation, personal growth, and astrology, in addition to guides to most of the world's major religious traditions.
- Center for Spirituality and Healing, www.csh.umn.edu.
  The Center for Spirituality and Healing of the University of Minnesota seeks to enhance the health and well-being of patients through research, clinical care, and other programs that integrate health, healing, and spirituality. Programs are available for health care professionals and for consumers.
- Center for Spirituality and Health, www.ufspiritualityandhealth.org.
  In addition to offering classes at the undergraduate, graduate, and professional levels, the Center for Spirituality and Health of the University of Florida also sponsors

seminars and conducts research on the relationship between religious traditions, spirituality, biomedical science, and health.

- The Center for Spirituality, Theology and Health, www.spiritualityandhealth.duke.edu.
  Based in the Center for Aging at Duke University, the Center for Spirituality, Theology and Health conducts interdisciplinary research on the relationship between spirituality, theology, and health with an emphasis on older adults.
- The George Washington Institute for Spirituality and Health, www.gwish.org.
  Known as GWish, this institute performs research and offers educational programs for physicians and other health care providers, including clergy and chaplains, on the clinical issues related to spirituality and health.
- Institute for Spirituality and Health, www.religionandhealth.org.
  With its home at the Texas Medical Center, the Institute for Spirituality and Health offers programs and information on wellness, compassionate health care, and research on the intersection of health, healing, and spirituality.

Periodicals/Magazines/Journals

- *Body + Soul: Whole Living*, published by Martha Stewart Living Omnimedia LLC, 1974– . Bimonthly. ISSN: 1539-0004. www.wholeliving.com.
  Covering topics as diverse as alternative and holistic medicine, natural foods, self-help exercises, and spirituality, this magazine seeks to provide articles that address all aspects of a healthy lifestyle.
- *Breath of God*, published by Lee Publishing, 2006– . Bimonthly. ISSN: 1930-5923. www.breathofgodmag.com.
  Focused on the modern Christian woman, *Breath of God* tackles topics such as marriage, parenting, living as a single woman, faith in the workplace and home, fitness, recipes, spirituality from a Christian perspective, and medical news.
- *Christian Counseling Today*, published by American Association of Christian Counselors, 1993– . Quarterly. ISSN: 1076-9668. www.aacc.net/resources/publications/#.
  Featuring articles of interest to Christian counselors, this quarterly magazine includes topics such as marriage and family counseling, spirituality, abuse, pastoral care, sexual conflicts, and the church as a healing community.
- *The Christian Science Journal*, published by the Christian Science Publishing Society, 1883– . Monthly. ISSN: 0009-5613. www.spirituality.com/journal/index.jhtml.
  One of the oldest continuously published journals on spirituality, *The Christian Science Journal* publishes articles on Christian healing as understood by practitioners of Christian Science. Its goal is to help readers understand the practice of Christian Science in their daily lives and to report instances of healings within the Christian Science community.
- *Christian Science Sentinel*, published by the Christian Science Publishing Society, 1898– . Weekly. ISSN: 0009-563X. www.spirituality.com/sentinel/index.jhtml.
  A sister publication to *The Christian Science Journal*, *Christian Science Sentinel* is a weekly newsletter that explores current world events from a Christian Science perspective. It also includes articles on how Christian Science can be effective in bringing healing to any situation.

- *Creations Magazine: Inspiring the Soul*, published by Path of Peace Inc., 1987– . Bimonthly. No ISSN. www.creationsmagazine.com.
  Containing articles, poems, and photography on spirituality, this magazine also examines alternative health, the environment, and spiritual growth with the goal of increasing the reader's physical, emotional, and spiritual health.
- *EnlightenNext: The Magazine for Evolutionaries*, published by EnlightenNext, 1991– . Quarterly. ISSN: 1080-3432. www.enlightennext.org/magazine.
  Written for contemporary spiritual seekers, *EnlightenNext* offers a new way of approaching life. The goal of the magazine is to help create a better future for all through an examination of core questions such as who are we and why are we here.
- *Explore: The Journal of Science & Healing*, published by Elsevier Inc., 2005– . Bimonthly. ISSN: 1550-8307. www.elsevier.com/locate/explore.
  A scholarly journal, *Explore* seeks to examine the healing arts, consciousness, and spirituality using scientific principles. It examines both conventional and alternative medicine.
- *Healing Ministry*, published by Weston Medical Publishing, LLC, 1995– . Quarterly. ISSN: 1087-1586. www.healingministryjournal.com.
  A peer-reviewed, quarterly journal, *Healing Ministry* publishes articles, research studies, and human interest studies of the power of faith, prayer, and spirituality, especially as they relate to death, bereavement, and counseling for those who are drug or alcohol dependent. The journal also includes spiritual healing techniques, profiles of those in the healing ministry, and book reviews.
- *The International Journal for the Psychology of Religion*, published by Routledge, 1991– . Quarterly. ISSN: 1050-8619. www.informaworld.com/smpp/title~content=t775653664.
  An academic journal, this publication reports on research in the psychology of religion, especially on the methods, theories, and applications of psychological research as related to the scholarly study of religion.
- *International Journal of Children's Spirituality*, published by Routledge, 1966– . Three times a year. ISSN: 1364-436X. www.tandf.co.uk/journals/titles/1364436X.asp.
  International and multicultural in scope, the articles in this journal present research on the expression of spirituality in children around the world. Articles also discuss the philosophical and practical foundations for morality as well the development of spirituality of both children and young people.
- *The International Journal of Transpersonal Studies*, published by International Journal of Transpersonal Studies, 1982– . Semi-annual. ISSN: 1321-0122. www.transpersonalstudies.org.
  One of the major academic journals in transpersonal studies, *ITJS* explores issues related to the concept of higher consciousness, expanded self/identity, spirituality, and human potential. The journal includes articles on the theory, research, and practice of transpersonal studies. Each issue consists of three sections that include original peer-reviewed articles, special topics dedicated to specific themes, and comments from readers.

- *The Journal of Christian Healing*, published by the Association of Christian Therapists, 1979– . Semi-annual. ISSN: 0738-2944. actheals.org/Publications/Additional_Sources.html.
  This journal of an association of health care professionals with strong Roman Catholic and Christian roots publishes articles on topics such as the healing of trauma, research on the science of healing and spirituality, and living the life of a committed Christian health care practitioner.
- *Journal of Health & Healing*, published by Wildwood Lifestyle Center & Hospital, 1975– . Quarterly. ISSN: 1044-2790. www.wildwoodhealth.org/index.php/resources/thejournalofhealthandhealing.
  The Journal of Health & Healing seeks to emphasize living a healthful lifestyle. It includes articles on herbs, nutrition, medicine, gardening, diseases and their treatments, emotional health, and cooking using vegan recipes
- *Journal of Psychology and Christianity*, published by Christian Association for Psychological Studies Inc., 1982– . Quarterly. ISSN: 0733-4273. www.caps.net/index.php?option=com_content&view=article&id=201&Itemid=237.
  This peer-reviewed, scholarly journal includes theoretical, clinical, and research-based articles on the relationship between Christianity and the psychological and pastoral professions.
- *Journal of Psychology and Theology: An Evangelical Forum for the Integration of Psychology and Theology*, published by Biola University, Rosemead School of Psychology, 1973– . Quarterly. ISSN: 0091-6471. www.biola.edu/jpt.
  Based on an evangelical understanding of Christianity, the *Journal of Psychology and Theology* presents articles and research on the relationship between theology and psychology and how these concepts affect individuals in the professional, clinical setting.
- *Journal of Religion and Health*, published by Springer New York LLC, 1961– . Quarterly. ISSN: 0022-4197. springerlink.metapress.com/content/104938.
  This scholarly journal seeks to understand the relationship between various religious traditions and research on medicine and health. Papers that are both theoretical and practical in scope are included.
- *Journal of Religion & Spirituality in Social Work: Social Thought*, published by Taylor & Francis, 1993– . Quarterly. ISSN: 1542-6432. www.tandf.co.uk/journals/WRSP.
  Dedicated to exploring the relationship between social justice and religion, the *Journal of Religion & Spirituality in Social Work: Social Thought* provides a forum for scholars, researchers, and practitioners to debate issues of policy development and the delivery of social services. It includes articles on spirituality and ethics, justice and peace, the role of religion in the social services, and the philosophy of social work.
- *Journal of Religion, Disability & Health: Bridging Clinical Practice and Spiritual Supports*, published by Taylor & Francis, 199[illegible]– . Quarterly. ISSN: 1522-8967. www.tandf.co.uk/journals/WRDH.
  Aimed at those with disabilities and their families, this journal provides an interfaith, interdisciplinary forum on issues of spirituality and religion in health and human services such as the ethical, moral, and spiritual issues raised by individuals

with disabilities in health care and rehabilitation services. Articles address issues of research, policies, and practices with the goal of supporting inclusive communities.

- *Journal of Religion, Spirituality & Aging: The Interdisciplinary Journal of Practice, Theory & Applied Research*, published by Taylor & Francis, 1985– . Quarterly. ISSN: 1552-8030. www.tandf.co.uk/journals/WRSA.
  Focusing on the needs and resources of the elderly, this journal provides an interdisciplinary exploration of issues such as ethics, death, long-term care, retirement, and other subjects focusing on the elderly. The goal of the journal is to provide scholarly information on aging and spirituality to professionals such as physicians, therapists, social workers, nurses, and counselors.
- *Journal of Spirituality in Mental Health*, published by Taylor & Francis, 1952– . Quarterly. ISSN: 1934-9637. www.tandf.co.uk/journals/WSPI.
  A professional, peer-reviewed journal devoted to the scholarly study of spirituality, this publication can serve as a resource both for those in the counseling and psychotherapeutic disciplines and for those interested in research on the relationship between spirituality and mental health.
- *The Journal of the American Society for Psychical Research*, published by the American Society for Psychical Research, 1907– . Quarterly. ISSN: 0003-1070. www.aspr.com/jaspr.htm.
  This journal is devoted to publishing scholarly, research-based articles on parapsychology and psychic phenomena, such as clairvoyance, extrasensory perception, precognition, psychokinesis, and psychic healing.
- *Journal of Transpersonal Psychology*, published by Association for Transpersonal Psychology, 1969– . Semi-annual. ISSN: 0022-524X. www.atpweb.org/journal.asp.
  A major journal in the field of transpersonal psychology, the articles in the *Journal of Transpersonal Psychology* examine clinical methods as well as personal, social, and spiritual understanding of modern life and psychology. Topics include the relationship between psychology and spiritual states, experiences, practices, and concepts.
- *Light of Consciousness: Journal of Spiritual Awakening*, published by Truth Consciousness at Desert Ashram, 1988– . Three times a year. ISSN: 1040-7448. light-of-consciousness.org.
  Light of Consciousness is dedicated to those who are seeking to awaken consciousness in their lives. The ultimate goal of the journal and the truth consciousness ashrams is personal and global transformation based on the teachings of Swami Amar Jyoti.
- *Miracles Magazine*, published by Institute for Personal Religion, 1983– . Bimonthly. ISSN: 1061-3927. www.miraclesmagazine.org.
  Based on *A Course in Miracles*, this bimonthly magazine seeks to supplement the course by providing daily meditations, quotations, jokes, parables, prayers, poems, and seasonal perspectives.
- *Psychic Reader*, published by Deja Vu Publishing, 1975– . Monthly. No ISSN. www.dejavupublishing.com/psychic-reader-magazine.
  In addition to publishing interviews of spiritual leaders and articles on spiritual topics, the magazine also discusses topics such as parapsychology, alternative healing, religion and theology.

- *SageWoman: Celebrating the Goddess in Every Woman*, published by BBI Media Inc., 1983– . Quarterly. ISSN: 1068-1698. www.sagewoman.com.
  Dedicated to celebrating the Goddess, articles focus on the spirituality of women and include artworks created by women and the wisdom inherent in women and the Goddess.
- *Self-Realization Magazine*, published by Self-Realization Fellowship Inc., 1925– . Quarterly. ISSN: 0037-1564. bookstore.yogananda-srf.org/Self-Realization-Magazine-c28.html.
  Founded by Yogi Paramahansa Yogananda, this is the official magazine of the Self-Realization Fellowship. Features include spiritual principles related to life, death, reincarnation, a personal relationship with God, and healing of the body, mind, and soul through the application of spiritual principles taught by the Fellowship.
- *Shaman's Drum: A Journal of Experiential Shamanism and Spiritual Healing*, published by Cross-Cultural Shamanism Network, 1985– . Quarterly. ISSN: 0887-8897. shamansdrum.org.
  Shaman's Drum explores the concept of shamanism across cultures. Articles discuss topics such as Native American healing, ethnic spirituality, and shamanic methodologies.
- *Shift: At the Frontiers of Consciousness*, published by Institute of Noetic Sciences, 1986– . Quarterly. ISSN: 1556-3359. www.noetic.org/publications/magazine.cfm.
  Containing articles, interviews, research summaries, and essays on the people and ideas of consciousness research, this magazine seeks to explore how we think about knowing. The goal of the magazine is to expand our views of consciousness and help us transform our beliefs, values, and actions.
- *Spirituality & Health: The Soul/Body Connection*, published by Spirituality & Health Media, 1998– . Bimonthly. ISSN: 1520-5444. www.spirituality-health.com/spirit.
  This general interest magazine publishes articles on all aspects of personal growth such as spirituality and beliefs, music, and the arts. It provides practical resources that can be used for personal exploration and practice such as self-tests, guides to spiritual practice, and interviews with and insights from spiritual teachers, researchers, and practitioners.
- *Spirituality and Health International*, published by John Wiley & Sons, 2004– . Quarterly. ISSN: 1743-1867. www3.interscience.wiley.com/journal/112094329/home/Product Information.html.
  The aim of this peer-reviewed journal is to publish high-quality, scholarly articles that discuss spirituality and its relationship with health. Thus, it is of interest to those involved in health care. Topics include all facets of spirituality, prayer, meditation, sacred architecture in healing, the health of the environment, "new age" spirituality, and psychotherapy.
- *Strength for the Day: God's Words of Hope and Healing*, published by Concordia Publishing House, 1962– . Monthly. No ISSN. www.cph.org/t-magazines-strength.aspx.
  Each issue focuses on a specific topic that helps the reader deal with the issues and emotions that arise in daily life such as stress, illness, loss, and anxiety through prayers, Bible verses, hymns, humor, and short articles.

- *Suffering: The Stauros Notebook*, published by Stauros U.S.A., 1982– . Quarterly. ISSN: 1557-9751. www.stauros.org/notebooks.
  The Stauros Center reaches out to those who suffer, whether physically or spiritually. In this newsletter, the center provides articles and stories that present perspectives on suffering drawn from various religious traditions and addresses issues arising from those coping with disabilities, illness, grief, isolation, injustice, or death.
- *Synchronicity: The Magazine*, published by Synchronicity Publishing Ltd., 1993– . Bimonthly. ISSN: 1198-760X. www.synchronicitymagazine.ca.
  Designed for those with an interest in holistic living, healthier relationships, complementary and alternative medical therapies, alternative spirituality and personal healing, this magazine offers articles on balancing the mind, body, and spirit to achieve greater harmony and health.
- *Tathaastu: So Be It*, published by Planet Archives LLC, 2007– . Bimonthly. ISSN: 1937-4917. tathaastumag.com.
  With its focus on holistic healing, spirituality, and a healthy lifestyle, this general interest magazine seeks to nurture the mind, body, and soul through practices such as meditation, yoga, ayurveda, and feng shui.
- *Weavings: A Journal of the Christian Spiritual Life*, published by the Upper Room Publications, 1986– . Bimonthly. ISSN: 0890-6491. www.upperroom.org/weavings.
  Each article in *Weavings* explores a single theme dealing with a contemporary issue through articles, meditations, poetry, and fiction. The magazine promotes a healthy and faithful lifestyle rooted in a Christian heritage.

Chapter 21

Tai Chi and Qigong

Background and History

Tai chi, often written "t'ai chi" and sometimes called tai chi chuan or taiji, is a martial art that originated in China. Although its ultimate origins are difficult to trace with accuracy, the first teacher of tai chi is considered to be Chang San-feng (Zhang Sanfeng), who, according to legend, lived from 1279 to 1368. He introduced a style of martial art that involved 13 postures based on the movements of five animals: tiger, dragon, leopard, snake, and crane; many of the postures or movements still used today in tai chi derive their names from these animals. Others trace the development of tai chi much earlier to the ancient teachers of Taoism.

The exercises in tai chi involve slow, relaxed, and gentle movements accompanied by deep breathing and meditation. The purpose of the exercises is to help the flow of qi, or vital energy, throughout the body. Qi regulates a person's spiritual, emotional, mental, and physical health. Thus, tai chi is often practiced for its health benefits in addition to its use as a form of exercise. Tai chi exercises are composed of prescribed movements, with the simplest using 13 postures while the more complex styles may have dozens. There are five major styles of tai chi, each of which is named after the Chinese family that developed it: Chen style, Yang style, Wu or Wu/Hao style of Wu Yu-hsiang, Wu style of Wu Ch'uan-yü and Wu Chien-ch'uan, and Sun style. Each style is represented by its own specific types of movement and postures and may vary on the speed at which the postures or poses are performed. Currently, there are dozens of new and hybrid styles that have branched from these five main styles.

Qigong, or ch'i kung, refers to a wide variety of exercises that involve methods of accumulating, circulating, and working with qi or energy within the body. Qigong can be practiced to maintain health, for therapy, and for spiritual growth. The roots of qigong can be traced back millennia, and it is currently practiced wherever ethnic Chinese have settled. In many parks in China, you can see the old and young, men and women, rich and poor, the educated and the uneducated all practicing qigong together.

Primary Uses and Actions

Since they provide a low-impact aerobic workout, tai chi and qigong are taught in a variety of settings including hospitals, medical clinics, community recreation centers, and even senior centers. The physical benefits of strengthening, stretching, and conditioning have made them very popular, especially with baby boomers and seniors. In addition, their practice relieves stress, increases coordination and flexibility, improves balance, and reduces pain and stiffness. Widely practiced in China and in other countries with substantial Chinese populations, both are growing in popularity in the United States and other Western nations.

Training

In the United States, there are no regulations, standards, or certifications for the training of tai chi or qigong teachers. As a result, it is important to ask potential instructors about their qualifications and training. Many schools of acupuncture include instruction in qigong and tai chi for their students, and some acupuncturists teach their clients these techniques.

Sources

Douglas, Bill. 2005 *Complete Idiot's Guide to T'ai Chi and QiGong*. 3rd ed. Indianapolis: Alpha Books.

Frantzis, Bruce Kumar. 2006. *Tai Chi: Health for Life: How and Why It Works for Health, Stress Relief and Longevity*. Berkeley, CA: Blue Snake Books.

Tai Chi: An Introduction, http://nccam.nih.gov/health/taichi.

See also TRADITIONAL CHINESE MEDICINE, ACUPUNCTURE, AND ACUPRESSURE

Annotated Bibliography

Print Resources

- Dang, Tri Thong. 1994. *Beginning T'ai Chi*. Rutland, VT: C. E. Tuttle. 67 pp. ISBN: 0804820015; 9780804820011.
  Using simple drawings of the body with arrows depicting movement, this is a short introduction to a simplified t'ai chi exercise composed of 24 specific movements. For the beginner, this will provide a sample of the practice of tai chi.
- Douglas, Bill. 2005. *Complete Idiot's Guide to T'ai Chi and QiGong*. 3rd ed. Indianapolis: Alpha Books. 322 pp. ISBN: 1592574203; 9781592574209.
  Written in a very accessible style, this book is a well-illustrated guide to learning the basics of both tai chi and qigong. The chapters introduce the reader systematically into the practice of tai chi first and then to qigong. The first part gives the background to the practice of tai chi and discusses its health benefits, while the second prepares the reader for taking a class or using the book to begin to practice the tai chi exercises. Part 3 teaches the basics of qigong, which prepares the reader for the actual practice of qigong. Thus, for those who wish a simple, yet complete, introduction to tai chi and qigong, this is a useful resource that can also be used as a supplement for a formal class.
- Frantzis, Bruce Kumar. 2006. *Tai Chi: Health for Life: How and Why It Works for Health, Stress Relief and Longevity*. Berkeley, CA: Blue Snake Books. 320 pp. ISBN: 1583941444; 9781583941447.
  This is not a how-to book on tai chi but one that examines the health benefits of its practice. The author introduces the origins of tai chi, its various forms, and how it can be used for specific health benefits. He also discusses the way tai chi can help reduce and manage stress and its effect on longevity. Other topics include using tai chi for physical and emotional self-defense, tai chi and spirituality, and choosing the appropriate tai chi style and teacher. Although it does not teach any tai chi forms,

this is a wonderful book that will answer many questions on the use of tai chi for a better life.

- Hong, Youlian, ed. 2008. *Tai Chi Chuan: State of the Art in International Research.* New York: Karger. 244 pp. ISBN: 380558489X; 9783805584890.
  Widely used in China as a health exercise, tai chi chuan provides many benefits to its practitioners. This book collects a variety of scientific studies on the efficacy of tai chi from around the world. The first group of chapters addresses the biomechanical and physiological characteristics of tai chi, such as muscle strength and endurance in older practitioners of tai chi and the improvement of cardiorespiratory capacity as a result of tai chi exercise. The second set of chapters examines balance control and the prevention of falls as a result of tai chi. The third group focuses on the mental health and social aspects of tai chi, while the final section looks at the clinical applications of tai chi. Taken together, these various chapters give a good scientific overview of some of the health benefits that regular exercise using tai chi may give to its practitioners.
- Iknoian, Therese, and Fuentes, Manny. 2001. *T'ai Chi for Dummies.* New York: Wiley Publishing. 332 pp. ISBN: 0764553518; 9780764553516.
  The authors introduce tai chi in this fun to read and easy to use book. The clear drawings and good directions will have the reader performing the tai chi and qigong moves quickly. The chapters systematically take the reader through the principles of tai chi, the specific moves of the Yang style short form, and establishing a regular practice.
- Kauz, Herman. 2009. *Tai Chi Handbook: Exercise, Meditation and Self-Defense.* New York: Overlook Press. 174 pp. ISBN: 1590201795; 9781590201794.
  The author does a good job of explaining the Chinese art of tai chi and its benefits of improved health. In addition, the uses of tai chi as a form of both meditation and self-defense are covered. Ample photographs accompany the text and provide good descriptions of the basic postures.
- Kobayashi, Petra, and Kobayashi, Toyo. 2008. *Tai Chi Chuan: Becoming One with the Tao.* Tokyo; North Clarendon, VT: Tuttle Pub. 192 pp. ISBN: 0804837643; 9780804837644.
  Suited for both beginners and advanced practitioners, this is a good, complete presentation of tai chi chuan.
- Liao, Waysun. 2009. *Chi: Discovering Your Life Energy.* 1st Shambhala ed., rev. ed. Boston: Shambhala. 156 pp. ISBN: 1590306953; 9781590306956.
  For those wishing to learn more about the concept of chi, this is a good introduction. The author, a tai chi and Taoist master, offers an understandable explanation of chi and its relationship to good health and vitality. Thus, those who practice tai chi or qigong and those who work with energy healing techniques such as acupuncture or shiatsu and their clients will gain a greater understanding of chi and energy by reading this book and practicing the breathing techniques and exercises.
- Robinson, Ronnie. 2009. *Total Tai Chi: The Step-by-Step Guide to Tai Chi at Home for Everybody.* Rev. ed. New York: Sterling. 144 pp. ISBN: 1844837238; 9781844837236.
  This is a good book for those who wish to learn basic tai chi. After an introduction to tai chi and its history and philosophy, the author takes you step by stop through several

beginning positions using both photos and grids of the movements. By the end of the book the novice can perform the short Yang form.

- Yang, Yang, Grubisich, Scott A., and Feng, Zhiqiang. 2008, ©2005. *Taijiquan: The Art of Nurturing, The Science of Power*. Champaign, IL: Zhenwu Publications. 253 pp. ISBN: 0974099015; 9780974099019.
  This is a good general introduction to taijiquan. Chapters cover the foundations of the practice including the mental, physical, and spiritual aspects of the art, finding a teacher, doing Wuji meditation, and the practice of taiji itself. An appendix gives a brief history of taijiquan and the modern Chen style of practice.
- Zhang, Fuxing. 1996. *Handbook of T'ai Chi Ch'uan Exercises*. Boston: Samuel Weiser. 198 pp. ISBN: 0877288917; 9780877288916.
  Using over 600 illustrations, the author presents three forms of tai chi exercises. The forms include a short form, a long form, and push hands. Each form is presented in detail so that the reader can begin to perform the movements immediately. For those who have already learned a style of tai chi, this will be a handy reference to many of the moves used in the various forms.

Internet Resources

- Everyday Tai Chi, www.everyday-taichi.com/index.html.
  Covering all aspects of both tai chi and qigong, this site provides information on styles, forms, exercises, training, and accessories. It even includes an examination of human anatomy as related to tai chi.
- National Qigong Association, www.nqa.org.
  Supporting all forms and styles of qigong, the website of the National Qigong Association offers information and articles on qigong and on the work of the association. Of special note are the links for finding qigong teachers, a questionnaire for assessing your energy, and information on the annual conference of the association.
- Qigong Association of America, www.qi.org.
  This website of one of the major associations for qigong in the United States offers pages on qigong forms, articles about qigong, a teacher registry, a list of recommended books, a message board, and other services.
- Qigong Institute, www.qigonginstitute.org/main_page/main_page.php.
  The Qigong Institute offers excellent information on qigong including a directory of qigong teachers and therapists, dissertations, scientific papers, classes and workshops, and materials to help in the study of qigong.
- Tai Chi: An Introduction, nccam.nih.gov/health/taichi.
  Produced by the National Center for Complementary and Alternative Medicine, this is an excellent introduction to tai chi. The site includes an overview of tai chi, its use in the United States, the status of tai chi research, side effects and risks, and training, licensing, and certification.
- T'ai Chi Chih, www.taichichih.org.
  This site provides a good introduction to the Tai Chi Chih form of tai chi developed by Justin Stone. It consists of 19 stand-alone movements and one specific pose. Although based on tai chi, Tai Chi Chih is not considered a martial art and is completely

nonviolent. It can be learned by anyone regardless of level of physical fitness, coordination, or age and can be modified for those with physical limitations

- Tai Chi Health, www.taichihealth.com/health.html.
  Based on the Yang style of tai chi, this website discusses the fundamentals of the exercise, introduces Yang style, and provides information on the origins of tai chi, the health benefits of its practice, guidelines for establishing a practice, and the mind/body principles of tai chi.

Periodicals/Magazines/Journals

- *The Empty Vessel: A Journal of Contemporary Taoism*, published by Abode of the Eternal Tao, 1993– . Quarterly. ISSN: 1073-7480. www.abodetao.com.
  With a goal of exploring and disseminating a nonreligious Taoist philosophy and practice, this journal includes articles, interviews, and stories that touch on all aspects of Taoist thought including tai chi, traditional Chinese medicine, and qigong. The journal also includes art, poetry, and book and video reviews.
- *Qi: The Journal of Traditional Eastern Health & Fitness*, published by Insight Graphics, 1991– . Quarterly. ISSN: 1056-4004. qi-journal.com.
  Qi: The Journal of Traditional Eastern Health & Fitness and its companion website, Qi-Journal.com, provide coverage of topics related to "qi" such as traditional Chinese medicine, tai chi, qigong, feng shui, herbology, and acupuncture. It also presents general articles on Chinese culture, philosophy, meditation, Taoism, Buddhism, and calligraphy.
- *Tai Chi & Alternative Health*, published by John Ding, 1994– . Quarterly. ISSN: 1355-8307. www.taichiwl.demon.co.uk/tcah.html.
  A British magazine, *Tai Chi & Alternative Health* publishes articles on all aspects of tai chi chuan including history, theory, applications of tai chi as a martial art. Other articles provide interviews with tai chi masters and cover such alternative health topics as acupuncture, reflexology, and aromatherapy.
- *T'ai Chi: The International Magazine of T'ai Chi Ch'uan*, published by Wayfarer Publications, 1977– . Bimonthly. ISSN: 0730-1049. www.tai-chi.com.
  Focusing on the various styles of tai chi chuan, qigong, Chinese philosophy, and traditional Chinese medicine, this magazine is intended for the general reader. It is filled with interesting articles and photographs.
- *Taijiquan Journal*, published by Taijiquan Journal, 2000– . Quarterly. ISSN: 1528-6290. www.taijiquanjournal.com.
  Covering all aspects of tai chi, *Taijiquan Journal* presents articles on the history, philosophy, study, and teaching of tai chi as well as information for practitioners and instructors.

Chapter 22

Therapeutic Massage and Bodywork

Background and History

The origins of massage and bodywork are clouded by time. Almost all cultures have practiced some form of massage, as evidenced by the widespread use of massage and bodywork in traditional medical practices. Cave paintings from 15,000 BCE may depict massage or healing touch therapy. Cultures as varied as Rome, Greece, Egypt, China, India, Persia, and Japan all had some form of massage. In Rome, massage was a standard adjunct to a visit to the baths. In traditional Chinese medicine a form of massage called *tui na*, which includes acupressure, kneading, and percussive stimulation, is often used in treatments. Similarly, in Japan, shiatsu massage, which also incorporates acupressure, is used. In ayurveda, massage is traditionally used to help balance the doshas.

Although the use of massage never disappeared from the healing arts, its use as a recognized therapeutic technique surged again beginning in the 1970s. Some experts estimate that over 20 million Americans receive a therapeutic massage each year, although the total number receiving some form of bodywork is undoubtedly much higher. It is estimated that there are over 1,500 massage therapy schools, college programs, and training programs throughout the United States. Although Swedish massage and deep tissue massage are the most taught modalities, over 250 different types of massage and bodywork can currently be identified. Other types of massage and bodywork include lymphatic massage, sports massage, neuromuscular massage, structural bodywork such as Rolfing, Hellerwork, myofascial release, craniosacral therapy, trigger point therapy, therapeutic touch, the Alexander Technique, the Feldenkrais Method, Reiki, the Rosen Method, and the Trager Approach, some of which are represented by their own chapters.

Primary Uses and Actions

Massage and bodywork can be used as therapeutic approaches to help treat a wide variety of ailments, especially when combined with conventional medical care. Research on massage has shown that it has many effects on the body. Of special note is its use in treating muscle pain and spasms, pain that arises from injury, headaches, temporomandibular joint syndrome, and conditions related to stress. Massage and bodywork are especially useful in helping the client relax, in relieving anxiety, and in increasing flexibility. Often, massage and bodywork can be rejuvenating and help relieve sinus and lung congestion. Some research has shown that massage benefits the cardiovascular system, the immune system, the nervous system, and the endocrine system.

Training

In 2006, there were an estimated 118,000 massage therapists actively employed or self-employed. Many others may practice massage therapy part time. As of 2007, 38 states and the District of Columbia had passed laws regulating massage therapy in some way, with most requiring that massage therapists complete a formal education program approved by the state or accredited by an independent accrediting agency and pass a national certification examination or a state exam.

Formal education in massage therapy usually takes place in a massage therapy school, a college, or a specialized training program. These programs usually require instruction in anatomy, physiology, kinesiology, business practices, professional ethics, first aid, and clinical practice of massage techniques. The various training programs may provide instruction in a variety of massage modalities and may also include instruction in topics such as myofascial release, reflexology, and aromatherapy.

Once the massage training program has been completed, massage therapists may choose to take the National Certification Examination for Therapeutic Massage and Bodywork (NCETMB), which is administered by the National Certification Board for Therapeutic Massage and Bodywork. Many states require that all massage therapists pass this test before they can legally practice massage therapy. Once the NCETMB is passed, the therapist may use the designation that he or she is Nationally Certified in Therapeutic Massage and Bodywork (NCTMB). Many states also recognize the examinations and licensing offered through the Federation of State Massage Therapy Boards.

Other types of bodywork require different types of education. Some, such as myofacial release and craniosacral therapy, require only weekend courses to become a certified practitioner, although more advanced courses are also available. Others, such as Rolfing and the Alexander Technique, require attendance at courses spread over months and sometimes years before certification is granted.

Sources

Ashley, Martin. 2005. *Massage: A Career at Your Fingertips: The Complete Guide to Becoming a Bodywork Professional.* 5th ed. Somers, NY: Enterprise.

Loving, Jean E. 1999. *Massage Therapy: Theory and Practice.* Stamford, CT: Appleton & Lange.

Massagetherapy.com, www.massagetherapy.com.

See also The Alexander Technique; Ayurveda; Feldenkrais Method; Rolfing and Structural Bodywork; Traditional Chinese Medicine, Acupuncture, and Acupressure

Annotated Bibliography

Print Resources

➤ Anderson, Sandra K. 2008. *The Practice of Shiatsu.* St. Louis, MO: Mosby Elsevier. 240 pp. ISBN: 0323045804; 9780323045803.

Shiatsu combines elements of traditional Chinese medicine and various forms of Japanese massage. This is an excellent introductory guide for students of massage and Shiatsu as well as for practitioners of other forms of massage. The history and theories of Shiatsu are presented in an understandable manner, and the basic shiatsu massage session is presented clearly with ample illustrations.

- Andrade, Carla-Krystin, and Clifford, Paul. 2008. *Outcome-Based Massage: From Evidence to Practice*. 2nd ed. Philadelphia: Wolters Kluwer Health/Lippincott Williams & Wilkins. 497 pp. ISBN: 0781767601; 9780781767606.
  Aimed at health care professionals, the authors seek to provide a text that focuses on integrating massage techniques based on clinical decision making and psychomotor skills into the therapy of patients for either the promotion of wellness or the remediation of the impairments, limitations, or disabilities of the patient. Part 1 details client examination and treatment planning while Part 2 presents specific treatment techniques and discharge planning. The treatments include superficial reflex techniques, superficial fluid techniques, neuromuscular techniques, connective tissue techniques, passive movement techniques, and percussive techniques.
- Ashley, Martin. 2005. *Massage: A Career at Your Fingertips: The Complete Guide to Becoming a Bodywork Professional*. 5th ed. Somers, NY: Enterprise. 300 pp. ISBN: 0964466252; 9780964466258.
  For anyone interested in pursuing a career in massage therapy and for massage students, this book should be consulted. The author provides a good overview of the profession, discusses the variety of career options available as well as the tasks of opening a massage office and marketing massage services, delves into the difficult topics of sex and gender as related to massage, and presents detailed and practical information on running a massage business, including business basics, insurance, income taxes, and keeping client and financial records. Also included are sources of equipment and other information on massage, a listing of bodywork organizations and training opportunities, and a state-by-state directory of massage schools.
- Aslani, Marilyn. 1997. *Massage for Beginners*. New York: HarperPerennial. 79 pp. ISBN: 0062733982; 9780062733986.
  Written for the individual who wishes to learn massage for personal use, not to practice massage professionally, this is a very good, well-illustrated manual that provides the basic techniques of massage. The format is also helpful in that the book has been designed with a folding base that permits it to stand upright so that it can be referred to throughout a massage session, whether on a partner or on oneself.
- Benjamin, Patricia J. 2009. *Professional Foundations for Massage Therapists*. Upper Saddle River, NJ: Pearson Prentice Hall. 372 pp. ISBN: 0131717367; 9780131717367.
  The goal of this book is to prepare massage therapists to run their own businesses. Chapters cover topics such as personal development and professionalism, social and communication skills, goal-oriented planning, documentation and SOAP (subjective, objective, assessment, and plan) notes, business and professional ethics, and managing finances.
- Benjamin, Patricia J., and Tappan, Frances M. 2010. *Tappan's Handbook of Healing Massage Techniques*. 5th ed. Boston: Pearson. Various pp. ISBN: 0135142237; 9780135142233.
  Providing students with massage techniques and approaches from around the world, this is a textbook for the beginning massage therapy student. In addition to providing a solid, if brief, foundation of massage theory and Western massage, the authors also cover contemporary massage and bodywork, such as myofascial massage, lymphatic drainage massage, foot reflexology, and polarity therapy. Asian bodywork is covered

in its own chapter. Special applications, such as sports and fitness, mother and child, terminally ill and dying, and healthy aging are also addressed. This edition includes "Practice Sequences," which provide step-by-step directions for using the techniques included in the text.

- Braun, Mary Beth, and Simonson, Stephanie. 2008. *Introduction to Massage Therapy.* 2nd ed. Philadelphia: Lippincott, Williams & Wilkins. 625 pp. ISBN: 0781773741; 9780781773744.
  As a textbook for the entry-level massage student, this work covers all the basics of massage therapy. It provides a good background on the history of massage, professional ethics, medical terminology, anatomy and physiology, massage equipment, client positioning and draping, massage strokes and flow, and therapeutic applications. In addition, using massage on special populations such as athletes, pregnant women, and chronically ill patients is included. The authors also briefly address other therapies such as acupressure, reflexology, and hydrotherapy. The last chapter focuses on the business side of a massage therapy practice. Excellent color illustrations enhance the text.
- Caldwell, Eddie. 2001. *Remedial Massage Therapy.* Champaign, IL: Corpus Publishing. 224 pp. ISBN: 1903333024; 9781903333020.
  The author provides a comprehensive guide to remedial massage, which can be used to treat a variety of conditions, but is especially useful for injuries arising from sports and other activities. All aspects of massage are addressed, including the history of massage, different massage techniques, muscles and joints, assessing and treating the client, treating specific areas of the body, and managing a massage practice.
- Cassar, Mario-Paul. 2004. *Handbook of Clinical Massage: A Complete Guide for Students and Professionals.* 2nd ed. New York: Churchill Livingstone. 351 pp. ISBN: 044307349X; 9780443073496.
  This work, which is written for students and practitioners, explores the application of massage to the treatment of disease, dysfunctions, and musculoskeletal imbalances. In addition to introducing basic massage techniques and discussing the effects of massage, the author focuses on the clinical application of massage, arranged by the various bodily systems. Separate chapters focus on massage for the back, the lower limbs, the abdomen, the chest, the upper limb, and the face, head, and neck.
- Clay, James H., and Pounds, David M. 2008. *Basic Clinical Massage Therapy: Integrating Anatomy and Treatment.* 2nd ed. Philadelphia: Lippincott Williams and Wilkins. 443 pp. ISBN: 0781756774; 9780781756778.
  Primarily a textbook for advanced massage therapy students, this work integrates instruction in clinical massage therapy with instruction in human anatomy. Clinical massage therapy seeks to relieve complaints of pain and dysfunction through the manipulation of soft tissues. Thus, this book is a guide to performing such massage by providing detailed directions and clear color illustrations that show the anatomy and the therapeutic techniques simultaneously, greatly aiding the learning of these techniques.
- Cohen, Don. 1995. *An Introduction to Craniosacral Therapy: Anatomy, Function, and Treatment.* Berkeley, CA: North Atlantic Books. 115 pp. ISBN: 155643183X; 9781556431838.
  This is an excellent introduction to craniosacral therapy. The author covers all aspects of the craniosacral system including the craniosacral fluid, the anatomy and function

of the craniosacral system within the body, palpation to determine the rhythm or pulse of the craniosacral system, the fundamental principles of performing craniosacral therapy, unwinding, the dural tube, and cranial adjusting. Good examples, exercises, and illustrations help to clarify the material covered.

- Davies, Clair. 2004. *The Trigger Point Therapy Workbook: Your Self-Treatment Guide for Pain Relief.* 2nd ed. Oakland, CA: New Harbinger Publications. 323 pp. ISBN: 1572243759; 9781572243750.
  Designed as a guide for self-treatment, this workbook teaches how to assess trigger points and how to manipulate them to relieve pain. The first three chapters discuss trigger points in general and provide guidelines for massaging them to treat pain. The remaining chapters focus on specific areas of the body such as the head and neck, the elbow and forearm, and the hip and knee. The illustrations provide useful graphic depictions of the location of the major trigger points. A separate chapter addresses the use of trigger point therapy in massage and provides detailed directions for massage therapists to incorporate this therapy into their massage routines.
- DeLaune, Valerie. 2008. *Trigger Point Therapy for Headaches & Migraines: Your Self-Treatment Workbook for Pain Relief.* Oakland, CA: New Harbinger Publications. 165 pp. ISBN: 1572245255; 9781572245259.
  Focusing specifically on headaches and migraines, this book seeks to provide individuals the tools they need to use trigger point therapy to relieve their pain. The author provides background information on trigger points, on the causes of headaches and migraines, on temporomandibular joint dysfunction, and on self-help techniques using trigger point therapy. She then focuses specifically on the muscles of the face, scalp, and neck and their trigger points. Photographs are used to demonstrate the location and manipulation of the relevant trigger points. For those who suffer from headaches, migraines, and temporomandibular joint disorder, this book will be a great help.
- Finando, Donna. 2005. *Trigger Point Self-Care Manual for Pain-Free Movement.* Rochester, VT: Healing Arts Press. 200 pp. ISBN: 1594770808; 9781594770807.
  Using self-massage, stretching, and wet heat and/or ice, this guide is designed for use in working on one's own trigger points to assist in the relief of pain and in the healing of muscular injuries. The book is arranged by major area of the musculoskeletal system: head and face; neck and upper back; shoulder; elbow, arm, and hand; torso; low back, buttock, hip, and thigh; groin and inner thigh; thigh and knee; and lower leg, ankle, and foot. Under each section, she discusses the major muscles and their trigger points. She also gives stretches that can help alleviate pain and facilitate healing. The line drawings of stretches, muscles, and trigger points work seamlessly with the directions for applying trigger point massage as needed.
- Finando, Donna, and Finando, Steven J. 2005. *Trigger Point Therapy for Myofascial Pain: The Practice of Informed Touch.* Rochester VT: Healing Arts Press. 244 pp. ISBN: 1594770549; 9781594770548.
  Designed for health care professionals, this book examines the use of trigger point therapy to treat myofascial pain. The introductory chapters present the nature of muscles and trigger points, the relationship between qi, movement, and health, the use of informed touch as a healing modality, and the diagnosis and treatment of

myofascial pain. The rest of the book presents the major muscles and their trigger points arranged by the major sections of the musculoskeletal system. For each muscle, the entry gives the proximal attachment, the distal attachment, action, palpation, pain pattern, causative or perpetuating factors, satellite trigger points, affected organ systems, associated zones, meridians, and points, stretching exercises, and strengthening exercises.

- Fritz, Sandy. 2009. *Mosby's Fundamentals of Therapeutic Massage.* 4th ed. St. Louis, MO: Mosby/Elsevier. 799 pp. ISBN: 0323048617; 9780323048613.
  This is a complete introduction to massage therapy, including its history, professional and legal issues, medical terminology, indications and contraindications for massage, and hygiene, sanitation, and safety. The author also addresses body mechanics and provides good discussions of the basic massage manipulation techniques. In a section that is not found in many other introductory texts on massage, she discusses wellness education focusing on stress, body, mind, and spirit.
- Fritz, Sandy, Chaitow, Leon, and Hymel, Glenn M. 2008. *Clinical Massage in the Healthcare Setting.* St. Louis, MO: Mosby/Elsevier. 827 pp. ISBN: 0323039960; 9780323039963.
  Designed for those who work in clinical settings such as hospitals, hospice care, and long-term care, this text covers the essentials of clinical massage, indications and contraindications for therapy, massage methods, range of motion testing, SOAP note documentation, and a general protocol for offering massage therapy. Case studies and a palliative protocol give additional support for those working in such settings.
- Fritz, Sandy, Grosenbach, M. James. 2009. *Mosby's Essential Sciences for Therapeutic Massage: Anatomy, Physiology, Biomechanics and Pathology*. 3rd ed. St. Louis, MO: Mosby/Elsevier. 698 pp. ISBN: 0323048692 9780323048699.
  This is a complete textbook for learning massage therapy. Loaded with more than 700 color illustrations, it provides overviews of anatomy and disease, detailed directions for doing massage, and information on biomechanics and pathology concepts.
- Gilchrist, Roger. 2006. *Craniosacral Therapy and the Energetic Body: An Overview of Craniosacral Biodynamics.* Berkeley, CA: North Atlantic Books. 211 pp. ISBN: 1556435800; 9781556435805.
  The goal of this book is to provide the therapeutic principles of biodynamic craniosacral therapy. The initial chapters present the history of craniosacral therapy, key principles and the basic dynamics of the breath of life, one of the core concepts of craniosacral therapy. Following this introduction, the author focuses more on the therapeutic aspect of craniosacral therapy. Thus, in addition to being of interest to the general reader who wishes to learn more about in craniosacral therapy, the author's approach will also engage the craniosacral therapist.
- Heller, Joseph, and Henkin, Bill. 2004. *Bodywise: An Introduction to Hellerwork for Regaining Flexibility and Well-Being*. Berkeley, CA: North Atlantic Books. 260 pp. ISBN: 155643524X; 9781556435249.
  The purpose of this book is to explain the functioning of the human body so that you can feel more alive in your own body, to increase pleasure and decrease problems with it, and to explore the interconnections of you, your body, and the greater universe. Thus, examining the way you perceive and think about your own body will

facilitate more efficient and graceful movement, leading to greater ease and balance in other aspects of life by reducing pain, stress, tension, and discomfort. Part 1 examines the body, its use in everyday life, its role in our consciousness and its plasticity, and bodywork. Part 2 delves into Hellerwork and how it can affect our body and our lives.

➤ Hollis, Margaret, and Jones, Elisabeth. 2009. *Massage for Therapists: A Guide to Soft Tissue Therapy*. 3rd ed. Ames, IA: Wiley-Blackwell. 206 pp. ISBN: 1405159162; 9781405159166.
This is a logically arranged general guide to massage therapy. After an overview of human anatomy and physiology, the authors address topics such as contra-indications for massage, examination and assessment, preparation for massage, massage manipulations, and massage of specific body regions. Additional chapters address aromatherapy, shiatsu, and myofascial release.

➤ Hover-Kramer, Dorothea, and Mentgen, Janet. 2002. *Healing Touch: A Guide Book for Practitioners*. 2nd ed. Albany: Delmar Thomson Learning. 254 pp. ISBN: 0766825191; 9780766825192.
Intended as a basic textbook on the concepts and techniques of healing touch, this book can be used in a class or by anyone who is interested in touch therapies. The author and her colleagues discuss the history of healing touch, research related to the effectiveness of touch therapy, the human energy system including the chakras, and the techniques used in healing touch. She also presents how to integrate healing touch with other healing modalities and how the practitioner should approach self-care.

➤ Kern, Michael. 2005. *Wisdom in the Body: The Craniosacral Approach to Essential Health*. Rev. ed. Berkeley, CA: North Atlantic Books. 338 pp. ISBN: 1556435592; 9781556435591.
One of the fastest growing natural therapies, craniosacral therapy is used for the treatment of a wide array of conditions. In this book, Kern discusses the history of craniosacral work and its core concepts. Of special note are the chapters on the primary respiratory mechanism, the intelligent body, and the patterns of experience and their effects on health and disease. He then presents methods of diagnosis and the essentials of treatment. Additional chapters focus on a holistic view of healing, on stress and trauma, and on pregnancy, birth, and children. The book is written in an understandable manner that makes it accessible to any reader who wishes to learn more about craniosacral therapy.

➤ Krieger, Dolores. 1993. *Accepting Your Power to Heal. The Personal Practice of Therapeutic Touch*. Santa Fe, NM: Bear & Co. 197 pp. ISBN: 1879181045; 9781879181045.
This is one of the classics of bodywork written by one of the founders of therapeutic touch. Although Krieger recognizes that therapeutic touch does not provide a "miracle cure," it is helpful in the treating a variety of conditions from PMS, headaches, asthma, reproductive problems, and cancer. In this straightforward book, she demonstrates how anyone can master this healing technique.

➤ Krieger, Dolores. 1997. *Therapeutic Touch Inner Workbook*. Santa Fe, NM: Bear & Co. 205 pp. ISBN: 1879181398; 9781879181397.
Building on her work in developing therapeutic touch, the author presents an exploration of the healing act. Thus, the book discusses healing, energy, the setting

of healing, consciousness, and relationships. Within many chapters are exercises to expand the therapists understanding of healing. For example, in the chapter on emotional states the exercise centers on using a journal to explore your own moods. For therapists who use therapeutic touch or another energy healing technique, this workbook will deepen their understanding of the work that they are doing.

- Krieger, Dolores. 2002. *Therapeutic Touch as Transpersonal Healing.* New York: Lantern Books. 291 pp. ISBN: 1590560108; 9781590560105.
  Written by one of the founders of therapeutic touch, this book was designed for therapeutic touch therapists and others who want to take the healing process to a deeper level of consciousness. It examines three frames of reference: conceptual, experiential, and teaching/learning. The conceptual frame of reference explores healing as a concept and then progresses through the universal healing field, the human energy field, the nature of consciousness, and the chakra system. In the section on the experiential frame of reference, the author explores the power of compassion and the energetic forces that are active during the therapeutic touch process. The final part, the teaching/learning frame of reference, focuses on the healer and the teacher as well as on learning styles.

- Kunz, Dora. 2004. *The Spiritual Dimension of Therapeutic Touch.* Rochester, VT: Bear & Co. 262 pp. ISBN: 1591430259; 9781591430254.
  Building on the healing power of therapeutic touch, this book deepens the examination of the efficacy of therapeutic touch by exploring the interrelationship between the healer and the patient. During a therapeutic touch session, the healer and the patient often experience an expanded level of consciousness that partakes of the spiritual dimension. In this book, the author explores this dimension of healing as she discusses consciousness and healing, the context of therapeutic touch, the nature of therapeutic touch, the chakras and the therapeutic touch process, and clinical applications of therapeutic touch.

- Loving, Jean E. 1999. *Massage Therapy: Theory and Practice.* Stamford, CT: Appleton & Lange. 300 pp. ISBN: 0838561616; 9780838561614.
  This is a carefully written, complete introduction to massage therapy. Starting with the philosophy and history of massage, the author progresses through topics such as professional practice, law, and ethics; the effects and benefits of massage; and sanitation, safety, and personal hygiene. She then introduces the science and art of massage, preparing for and consulting with the client, and the major massage strokes used in a session. Other massage approaches such as cranialsacral therapy, myofascial techniques, and seated massage are introduced and a chapter is devoted to assessing the client so that the proper massage session can be designed. The final chapters are devoted to self-care and wellness for both the therapist and the client and to applying therapeutic massage to the specific needs of the client.

- Macrae, Janet. 1988. *Therapeutic Touch: A Practical Guide.* New York: Knopf. 91 pp. ISBN: 039475588X; 9780394755885.
  This short book is a good, basic introduction to therapeutic touch as a healing technique. After a short chapter that introduces therapeutic touch and its guiding principles, the rest of the book is devoted to giving a treatment, using therapeutic touch in daily practice, and self-transformation through therapeutic touch.

- Mairi, Audrey. 2006. *Trager for Self-Healing: A Practical Guide for Living in the Present Moment.* Tiburon, CA: H. J. Kramer; Novato, CA: New World Library. 222 pp. ISBN: 1932073191; 9781932073195.
  While discussing the Trager Approach, the author also teaches how to receive enlightenment through the physical body using exercises grounded in ordinary physical movements. The goal of the book is to increase one's awareness of the present moment through the exercises presented in the book based on the work of Milton Trager. The Trager Approach uses both touch and physical movement to open oneself to experience a feeling of lightness and bliss. The author takes the reader through the basics of the Trager Approach, adds techniques and tools to facilitate changes in the body/mind, and concludes with several stories of how the approach works.
- Manheim, Carol. 2008. *The Myofascial Release Manual.* 4th ed. Thorofare, NJ: Slack. 285 pp. ISBN: 1556428359; 9781556428357.
  After a brief discussion of the history of myofascial release, the anatomy of the fascia, and protocols for using the technique, the author presents both basic and advanced myofascial release techniques. Ample illustrations and directions guide the therapist through using the techniques. Of special note are the advanced techniques, which include topics such as pelvic floor release, skin and scar mobility, and trigger point releases. Separate sections are devoted to the initial assessment of the client and for posture evaluation.
- Mumford, Susan. 2009. *The Massage Bible: The Definitive Guide to Soothing Aches and Pains.* New York: Sterling. 400 pp. ISBN: 1402770014; 9781402770012.
  Covering a wide array of massage techniques, this guide helps introduce the novice massage therapist to different techniques that they can use in their practice of massage therapy. The work gives advice on how to perform massage to relieve common ailments and offers lifestyle tips.
- Premkumar, Kalyani. 2004. *The Massage Connection: Anatomy and Physiology.* 2nd ed. Baltimore, MD: Lippincott Williams & Wilkins. 677 pp. ISBN: 0781734762; 9780781734769.
  Providing a highly detailed introduction to anatomy and physiology, this book is intended to meet the specific needs of massage therapy students and professionals. Separate chapters are devoted to each body system. Ample color illustrations, review questions, and coloring exercises all enhance the learning experience. Information boxes, pathology boxes, and special consideration boxes related to massage provide additional useful information. Although designed for massage therapy students, anyone with an interest in learning about human anatomy and physiology will benefit from reading this book.
- Rosen, Marion. 2003. *Rosen Method Bodywork: Accessing the Unconscious through Touch.* Berkeley, CA: North Atlantic Books. 133 pp. ISBN: 1556434189; 9781556434181.
  In this book, Rosen shares her own experiences in working with people and their bodies while also providing an excellent introduction to her method of bodywork. In addition, she expands beyond using the work on individuals and shows how an individual's growth as a result of treatment can have a ripple effect on the world. The Rosen Method is a way that a person can access his or her feelings and experiences through the muscle tensions of the body. Through this manual, Rosen provides the

reader with the tools and techniques to aid people in releasing these tensions which can, in turn, lead to physical and psychological healing. The chapters cover the major components of the Rosen Method and its practice.

- Rosen, Marion, and Brenner, Sue. 1991. *The Rosen Method Movement.* Berkeley, CA: North Atlantic Books. 97 pp. ISBN: 1556431171; 9781556431173.
The Rosen Method of bodywork involves the use of range of motion and stretching exercises to lubricate the joints, expand the chest, and loosen the diaphragm. Doing so creates relaxation and reduces holding patterns in the body so that the body can be reshaped without hurting it. It also increases awareness of how the body is put together and is interconnected. The result of Rosen exercises is often a feeling of joy and an increase in the sense of balance and rhythm. In addition, function and mobility as well as health can be maintained, even in older age. In this book, the authors present the background theory of Rosen Work, discuss what happens in a class, and demonstrate the exercises and exercise sequences that are used. Although the exercises work best when in a class with an experienced teacher, the book does provide good illustrations and directions so that they can be done at home.

- Saeger, Jan L., and Kyle-Brown, Donna. 2008. *New Foundations in Therapeutic Massage and Bodywork.* Dubuque, IA: McGraw Hill. 597 pp. ISBN: 0073025828; 9780073025827.
In addition to providing the fundamental principles and practical applications of massage, this work also examine topics such as massage for hospice patients and survivors of abuse and massage routines for common ailments such as carpal tunnel syndrome, thoracic outlet syndrome, and fibromyalgia. The ultimate goal of the book is to prepare the student therapist to succeed in passing the National Certification Exam.

- Salvo, Susan G. 2007. *Massage Therapy: Principles and Practice.* 3rd ed. St. Louis, MO: Saunders Elsevier. 904 pp. ISBN: 1416036520; 9781416036524.
For those seeking a comprehensive textbook on massage therapy, this is one of the best sources. The author does a marvelous job covering just about every topic that the massage therapist will need to know. The first section gives a historical perspective on massage, discusses the therapeutic relationship, and examines the tools needed for a massage practice, such as the massage table, the massage media (cream, butters, oils and gels, lotion, powder, and liniments), and even the furniture and fixtures needed in the massage room. The second section introduces topics such as infection control and hygiene, massage physiology and contraindications, body and table mechanics, Swedish massage, assessment and planning, pregnancy and infant massage, and adaptive massage. Anatomy and physiology are the focus of the third section, which comprises almost half the book. Each system is discussed in detail. The fourth section gives instruction in other therapies such as hydrotherapy, foot reflexology, sports massage, seated massage, and Eastern massage therapies. Business practices comprise the fifth section.

- Sayre-Adams, Jean, and Wright, Stephen G. 2001. *The Theory and Practice of Therapeutic Touch.* 2nd ed. New York: Churchill Livingstone. 158 pp. ISBN: 0443070822; 9780443070822.
This short book is a complete introduction to therapeutic touch. Chapters cover the background of therapeutic touch, review the literature and research on its effectiveness,

provide a conceptual framework for its practice, present the essentials of the practice, and discuss the development of a therapeutic touch practice.

- Scheumann, Donald W. 2007. *The Balanced Body: A Guide to Deep Tissue and Neuromuscular Therapy*. 3rd ed. Philadelphia: Lippincott Williams & Wilkins. 248 pp. ISBN: 0781763088; 9780781763080.
  This book provides a comprehensive approach to deep tissue massage and neuromuscular therapy that seek to provide tension release in the muscles of the body. Lessons in the book include discussions of the connective tissue, breath and support in the body, aligning the upper extremity, establishing a firm foundation, stabilizing the core, and balancing the neck and head. Clear illustrations and text direct the therapist through each technique. Case studies provide contextual information on applying the techniques given in the book.

- Sharkey, John. 2008. *The Concise Book of Neuromuscular Therapy: A Trigger Point Manual*. Berkeley, CA: North Atlantic Books. 236 pp. ISBN: 1556436734; 9781556436734.
  Since neuromuscular therapy treats soft tissue pain and injury, a detailed knowledge of the anatomy of the muscular system and the related trigger points is required of the therapist. This book provides such information. The author gives an overview of the functional anatomy, discusses the muscles, fascia, and the kinetic chain, and then discusses the trigger points and patient assessment. In addition, the book provides an excellent review of the major skeletal muscles. For each muscle, the entry gives a drawing of where it is located, the muscle name, origin, insertion, action, kinetic chain comment, trigger point comment, and the nerve that activates the muscle. Thus, this is an excellent manual for many types of therapists, including physicians, physical therapists, chiropractors, naturopaths, and massage therapists.

- Stillerman, Elaine. 2009. *Modalities for Massage and Bodywork*. St. Louis, MO: Mosby. 460 pp. ISBN: 032305255X; 9780323052559.
  For those with an interest in massage therapy and bodywork, this resource explores 21 of the top modalities often used in massage practice today. Directions provided by leading experts and practitioners in each modality permit the massage therapist to incorporate these techniques into their practices. Over 265 color illustrations help clarify the concepts presented and demonstrate the techniques.

- Upledger, John E. 2001. *CranioSacral Therapy: Touchstone for Natural Healing*. Berkeley, CA: North Atlantic Books. 113 pp. ISBN: 1556433689; 9781556433689.
  In this short book, the father of craniosacral therapy discusses the background and the discovery of the healing method as well as some of his earliest work with patients as he developed his ideas more completely. Other chapters cover the guiding principles of craniosacral therapy, the flow of fluids, conditions for which craniosacral therapy is useful, and a summary of the applications of craniosacral therapy. For anyone interested in learning more about the theories and principles of craniosacral therapy, this is an excellent and important work.

- Upledger, John E., with Grossinger, Richard, Ash, Don, and Cohen, Don. 2008. *CranioSacral Therapy: What It Is, How It Works*. Berkeley, CA: North Atlantic Books. 118 pp. ISBN: 1556436955; 9781556436956.

Written by several leading practitioners of craniosacral therapy, this book builds on the writings of Upledger. The authors provide a good introduction to craniosacral therapy and its history, the philosophy that underlies it, and stories of treatments. Several chapters examine more deeply its practice by focusing on the nature of palpation as used in therapy, the healing crisis, and self-discovery and self-healing.

- Upledger, John E., and Vredevoogd, Jon D. 1983. *Craniosacral Therapy*. Chicago: Eastland Press. 367 pp. ISBN: 0939616017; 9780939616015.
  This book covers all aspects of this form of bodywork. Beginning with the craniosacral concept, the authors work through all aspects of craniosacral therapy, from terminology and palpatory skills to techniques that modify the craniosacral rhythm and the release of transverse restrictions that impair fascial mobility. Dysfunctions of the craniosacral dural membrane system and of the cranial base are covered, as are diagnosis and treatment of dysfunctions of other related structures within the craniosacral system. Thus, for anyone interested in learning more about craniosacral therapy, this is one of the best books since it helped set the field on a firm theoretical foundation.

Internet Resources

- American Massage Therapy Association, www.amtamassage.org.
  The major association for massage therapists in the United States, the AMTA has a membership of over 58,000 massage therapists. With a goal of making massage therapy an integral part of maintaining good health and of stressing is use as a complementary therapy, the ATMA sets standards and ethics for the profession, provides continuing education, publishes professional resources, educates the public, and fosters the continuing development of its members.
- Associated Bodywork & Massage Professionals, www.abmp.com/home.
  The ABMP is a national membership of both massage and bodywork practitioners and students. The association provides comprehensive liability insurance for its members and a variety of resources for massage schools and their instructors. The website includes access to *Massage & Bodywork Magazine* and a marketplace of products.
- The Biodynamic Craniosacral Therapy Association of North America, www.craniosacraltherapy.org.
  The Biodynamic Craniosacral Therapy Association of North America (BCTA/NA) promotes the biodynamic model of craniosacral therapy as developed by Franklyn Sills, which follows the work of William Garner Sutherland, DO. BCTA/NA has established a curriculum for the teaching of craniosacral therapy and provides a directory of Registered Craniosacral Therapists (RCST). The site includes a wealth of information on Biodynamic Craniosacral Therapy.
- Commission on Massage Therapy Accreditation, www.comta.org.
  The commission accredits both education institutions teaching massage therapy and bodywork and the programs themselves. The site includes a directory of schools and programs that have been accredited by COMTA.
- Federation of State Massage Therapy Boards, www.fsmtb.org.
  Composed of 30 state and territorial boards for massage therapy, the FSMTB seeks to ensure that massage therapy is practiced in a safe and effective manner. The

federation administers the MBLEx exam for licensure that is accepted in 18 states as part of the licensure requirements to practice massage therapy.

- Hellerwork International, www.hellerwork.com.
Produced by Hellerwork International, this website provides detailed information on Hellerwork Structural Integration. Pages cover topics such as a description of Hellerwork and how to become a practitioner. It also includes a directory of Hellerwork practitioners.
- Massage Network, www.massagenetwork.com.
Massage Network is a worldwide directory of massage therapists. The site also includes information about massage therapy, massage schools, and massage-related products and services.
- Massage Therapy Foundation, www.massagetherapyfoundation.org.
Composed of massage therapists, educators, clients, and vendors who sell massage supplies, the Massage Therapy Foundation seeks to advance the profession through a combination of community service projects, research, and education. The foundation provides research grants and hosts conferences in addition to maintaining a database of massage therapy research.
- Massage Therapy 101, www.massagetherapy101.com.
This is a wonderful site that provides a good introduction to massage. It covers massage therapy schools and education, massage techniques, other complementary therapies, massage equipment, and massage oils.
- MassageResource.com, www.massageresource.com.
Providing information on the Web since 1996, MassageResource.com is an excellent resource for anyone interested in therapeutic massage and bodywork. Links are provided to massage schools in the United States and Canada, a library of articles on massage, a forum related to massage, and a directory of massage therapists.
- Massagetherapy.com, www.massagetherapy.com.
Produced by the ABMP, this is a public education site for those interested in massage therapy. The site includes an e-newsletter, information about massage, a glossary of bodywork terms, a booklet on becoming a massage therapist, and a directory of massage therapists who are members of the ABMP.
- Myofascial Release Treatment Centers, www.myofascialrelease.com/home.asp.
Founded by John Barnes, the Myofascial Release Treatment Centers provide clients with the latest in myofascial release therapy. This website discusses myofascial release, the treatment programs available, and articles on the technique. In addition, the site provides information on the four treatment centers and on the seminars and courses as well as a directory of myofascial release therapists.
- Myofascial Release.com, www.myofascial-release.com.
This site presents the theory and benefits of myofascial release. The site consists of two parts, one for patients and one for practitioners. Each provides basic information on myofascial release, its benefits, and what happens during a treatment session, although the practitioners' site provides greater depth.
- National Certification Board for Therapeutic Massage and Bodywork, www.ncbtmb.com.

The NCBTMB certifies massage therapists and bodyworkers through ensuring that each certified therapist has completed appropriate instruction and passing a national certification exam. For consumers, the site offers information on massage, a glossary of terms and techniques, and a directory of certified practitioners.

- The Nurse Healers–Professional Associates International, www.therapeutic-touch.org.
  This is the official organization related to therapeutic touch as taught by Dolores Krieger and Dora Kunz. The site includes a listing of qualified teachers and qualified practitioners.
- The Rosen Institute, www.rosenmethod.org.
  This website is provided by the Rosen Institute, the major organization for those interested in the Rosen Method of bodywork and movement. The site provides an excellent introduction to the Rosen Method and discusses the history of the method and its benefits, while also listing Rosen Method training centers, practitioners, and articles.
- Rosen Method, www.rosenmethod.com.
  Produced by the Berkeley Center, this site provides basic information on the Rosen Method of bodywork. Topics such as bodywork, movement, the benefits of the method, and training are covered. The site also includes a brief biography of Marion Rosen.
- Therapeutic Touch, www.therapeutictouch.org.
  Maintained by the Pumpkin Hollow Foundation, this site includes pages on the history and reliability of therapeutic touch. It also has links to workshops, information on becoming a therapeutic touch practitioner, and ways to participate in therapeutic touch as a patient.
- Trager.com, www.trager.com.
  This site offers the reader extensive information on the Trager Approach, including its history and benefits. In addition, it provides articles, testimonials, links to national associations, and a list of training programs. The site also includes a directory of practitioners.
- United States Trager Association, www.tragerus.org.
  The United States Trager Association is the home of Trager practitioners in the United States. The site includes information on the Trager Approach and Trager Mentastics. It also has a list of practitioners and training opportunities.
- The Upledger Institute, www.upledger.com.
  The Upledger Institute promotes the work of John Upledger, the founder of craniosacral therapy. The institute sponsors training programs for those wishing to learn the light-touch therapies developed by Upledger and other therapists associated with the institute.

Periodicals/Magazines/Journals

- *International Journal of Therapeutic Massage & Bodywork: Research, Education & Practice*, published by Massage Therapy Foundation, 2008– . Quarterly. ISSN: 1916-257X. www.ijtmb.org/index.php/ijtmb.

An open access, peer-reviewed publication, the IJTMB serves the expanding needs of the therapeutic massage and bodywork profession It covers all aspects of massage and bodywork including research, education, and clinical practice.

- *Journal of Bodywork and Movement Therapies*, published by Churchill Livingstone, 1997– . Quarterly. ISSN: 1360-8592. www.elsevier.com/locate/jbmt.
  Providing articles on the latest therapeutic techniques, this journal covers all types of bodywork and movement therapies including massage therapy, physical therapy, chiropractic, structural integration, Feldenkrais Pilates, Alexander Technique, shiatsu and tui na, cranial therapy, and myofascial therapy. The articles are highly illustrated and written in a manner that makes the content immediately relevant to clinical and private practice.

- *Massage*, published by Massage Magazine, 1935– . Bimonthly. ISSN: 1057-378X. www.massagemag.com.
  Massage covers all aspects of both massage therapy and other related healing arts, especially the benefits of healing touch therapies. In addition to articles on massage and bodywork, it includes interviews with leaders in the profession, articles on techniques and the business of massage, and news on the latest trends and developments in the field.

- *Massage and Bodywork: Nurturing Body, Mind & Spirit*, published by Associated Bodywork and Massage Professionals Inc., 1988– . Bimonthly. ISSN: 1544-8827. www.massageandbodywork.com.
  Designed for both massage, bodywork, and skin care therapists, this journal presents articles on current research, massage techniques, business management, developing trends, and maintaining a healthy lifestyle.

- *Massage Today*, published by Massage Today, 200[illegible]– . Monthly. ISSN: 1531-8079. www.massagetoday.com/mpacms/mt/home.php.
  A monthly trade journal for licensed and practicing massage therapists and bodyworkers, *Massage Today* provides current reports on industry news, trends, products, services, and techniques. In addition, it gives information on trade shows, conventions, and seminars.

- *Massage World: The Massage and Body Therapists Magazine*, published by Massage Today, 2001– . Bimonthly. ISSN: 1474-4171. www.massageworld.co.uk.
  Published for anyone with an interest in massage therapy, this British magazine contains articles on massage techniques, on managing your own business, and on trends within the profession.

- *MTJ: Massage Therapy Journal*, published by American Massage Therapy Association, 1946– . Quarterly. ISSN: 0895-0814. www.amtamassage.org.
  Published by the major American association for massage therapists, *MTJ* features articles on massage techniques, research on the efficacy of massage, business advice, and news from the field.

Chapter 23

Traditional Chinese Medicine, Acupuncture, and Acupressure

Background and History

According to Chinese tradition, traditional Chinese medicine (TCM) can trace its roots back to the mythological Yellow Emperor who ruled from 2697 BC to 2598 BC. During the height of his reign, the Yellow Emperor wrote the *Huang-di Nei-jing* or *Neijing Suwen*, which laid out the principles of TCM. Others claim that the *Nei-jing* was compiled by scholars approximately 2,000 years ago. All other texts of TCM derive from *Nei-jing* since they are commentaries, interpretations, and clarifications of this basic work.

Within TCM, the human body is thought to be its own universe, and no one part of it can be understood except through its relationship to the whole. Thus, symptoms are not treated in separation from the rest of the life of the individual; the symptom must be examined to see where it fits into the entire life, being, and behavior of each person. The body itself is even understood differently in TCM based on function rather than on anatomy. TCM's concept of the spleen, for example, raises it from a single organ as it is in Western medicine to an organ whose functions are related to transformation and transportation within the body, especially turning food into qi and blood. The spleen also assists in thinking, studying, motivation, and decision making.

Such differences between TCM and Western medicine arise from the theoretical underpinnings of Chinese medicine. The basic theory is that of yin and yang, often represented by a circle with interlocking black and white sections with a small circle of the opposite color contained within each section. Yin and yang represent balance, the ultimate goal of TCM. Yin and yang are polar opposites and complements, which help explain the relationships between everything in the universe. Yin characteristics include shade, cold, rest, responsiveness, interior, inward, decrease, and tranquility. Yang, in contrast, represents sun, heat, movement, activity, light, exterior, outward, and potential. Yin and yang underlie the Chinese concept that the universe is undergoing continual change. This is reflected also in the approach to medicine that views the body as undergoing such change, with the goal of treatment being the re-establishment of balance.

A second fundamental element of TCM is the concept of qi or chi, which is usually translated as *life force* or *vital energy*, although its meaning is much broader and lies at the basis of the universe. Everything has qi, whether a mountain, a plant, or a human. The herbs used in remedies include qi, which is then transferred to the body when ingested. The goal of many treatments such as acupuncture (the use of thin needles) or tui na (a type of massage that often includes acupressure) is to increase the flow of qi in the body so that balance, and thereby health, can be restored.

The concept of an organ of the body also differs in TCM. The organ network sustains the body, and when the organs are in balance, the person is healthy. The organs are also classified as either yin or yang. The yin organs are the heart, lungs, spleen, liver, and kidneys, and sometimes the pericardium. The yang organs are the gall bladder, stomach, small intestine, large intestine, bladder, and triple burner. The triple burner is the organ most unfamiliar to Western medicine. It is not a physical organ but a pathway that makes the organs a complete system through the control of water. In addition to properties related to the physical body, the organs also have psychological components, in keeping with the idea that the body is a cosmos infused with qi.

Another concept that is essential for a basic understanding of TCM is the meridians. The meridians are the channels or pathways through which qi moves through the body. The meridians are not physical vessels that can be shown anatomically but are unseen channels that bind the body together into a whole unit. There are 12 regular meridians, each of which corresponds to one of the major organs and to the pericardium. Manipulation of the meridians through acupuncture, acupressure, or the use of herbs balances the flow of qi in the body and thereby creates or restores health.

Primary Uses and Actions

Since traditional Chinese medicine is a complete medical system, it can be used to treat any illness or disease. The concept of treatment, however, varies in many ways from allopathic or Western medicine. Since the whole cosmos of the individual is examined, treatment is tailored to each person. Diagnosis in TCM is performed through a careful observation of the patient rather than through laboratory tests. This diagnosis is performed through a process called the four examinations and consists of looking, listening and smelling (considered to be the same since they are represented by the same Chinese word), asking, and touching. Looking involves observing the patient to determine the overall appearance and state of health and may involve an examination of the face, tongue, the skin and hair, and the way the patient moves. During the listening and smelling examination, the practitioner will listen to the sound of the voice and breath and use smell to discern distinctive body odors. Asking uses questions to probe symptoms, habits, sleep, bowel and bladder functions, appetite, thirst, personal background, and medical history. Touching is considered to be the most important examination and involves feeling the pulse. Within TCM, pulse examination is a much more developed diagnostic skill than in allopathic medicine. Although there are many places in the body where a pulse can be examined, the radial artery is used primarily. The practitioner will place three fingers on the radial artery. By moving his or her fingers to different depths of the pulse, the practitioner can determine 18 different types of pulse that help determine the illness and the appropriate treatment.

Once a complete diagnosis has been made, the practitioner may use a variety of healing techniques, including herbal medicines, acupuncture, moxibustion, tui na massage, exercises such as qigong or tai chi, meditation, and food therapy, since the treatment is aimed at the whole individual, not just his or her symptoms. Chinese herbal medicines are made primarily from plants, but other ingredients from animals and minerals may also be used. In addition to using premade pills, the practitioner will often prescribe a variety of herbs that must be made into a tea for drinking since the combination of herbs will be specific to the individual being treated.

In China, there is little conflict between traditional Chinese medicine and Western medicine, and both are used by patients. In many parts of the world, however, there is little cooperation or understanding between practitioners of both modalities. This situation is changing as the practice of TCM continues to spread.

In the West, acupuncture is the most well known facet of traditional Chinese medicine. Acupuncture was introduced into the United States in the 1970s primarily as a way to provide pain relief. Since then, its use has spread and many schools of acupuncture and Oriental medicine have been established. Although still used primarily for pain control, acupuncture is now a recognized alternative medical treatment. Acupuncture uses small needles inserted into the skin at specific meridian points to help the flow of qi in the body. At times electrical stimulation may be added to the needles. Sometimes, moxibustion will accompany the insertion of needles. During moxibustion, herbs are burned over the meridian points to create heat that can also affect the flow of qi. Acupressure is based on the same meridian points as acupuncture, but the fingers, and sometimes blunt instruments, instead of needles are used to place pressure on the points.

Training

In China, training to become a practitioner of traditional Chinese medicine historically took the form of a master–apprentice relationship and this style of training can still be found today. Most TCM practitioners in China, however, now follow the standards of training for the formal Chinese Medicine Doctor (CMD) degree that is offered in a variety of colleges and universities recognized by the Ministry of Education and Ministry of Health of the People's Republic of China. Training usually takes six years.

In the United States, education in TCM is provided by a variety of schools, most of which offer the Master of Acupuncture or the Master of Oriental Medicine degree. Only three offer the accredited degree of Doctor of Acupuncture and Oriental Medicine. The Accreditation Commission for Acupuncture and Oriental Medicine (ACAOM) is recognized by the U.S. Department of Education as the national accrediting agency that accredits master's level programs in acupuncture and Oriental medicine. Currently, there are over 60 schools and colleges with accredited or candidacy status with the commission.

To practice acupuncture legally in most states, an acupuncturist must be licensed, as indicated by the designation LAc, or certified. Acupuncturists can receive certification by passing the national certification examination administered by the National Certification Commission for Acupuncture and Oriental Medicine. Most states require passing the national certification examination as a prerequisite to licensure. It is estimated that there are approximately 18,000 licensed acupuncturists in the United States, with about 12,000 maintaining an active practice. About half of American acupuncturists are located in California and New York. In some states, physicians, chiropractors, dentists, podiatrists, and naturopaths can legally practice acupuncture.

Sources

Bauer, Matthew D. 2005. *The Healing Power of Acupressure and Acupuncture: A Complete Guide to Timeless Traditions and Modern Practice*. New York: Avery.

Birch, Stephen J., and Felt, Robert L. 1999. *Understanding Acupuncture.* New York: Churchill Livingstone.

Holland, Alex. 1999. *Voices of Qi: An Introductory Guide to Traditional Chinese Medicine.* Berkeley, CA: North Atlantic Books.

Kaptchuk, Ted. 2000. *The Web That Has No Weaver: Understanding Chinese Medicine.* Chicago: Contemporary Books.

See also Herbs, Vitamins, Minerals, and Nutritional Supplements; Reflexology

Annotated Bibliography

Print Resources

- Aung, Steven K. H., and Chen, William P. D. 2007. *Clinical Introduction to Medical Acupuncture.* New York: Thieme. 324 pp. ISBN: 1588902218; 9781588902214.
  Designed for use by medical professionals and students, this is a comprehensive guide to acupuncture. The anatomy of each of the meridians or acupuncture channels is excellently presented through good diagrams and photographs with acupuncture points labeled. Brief, yet good, discussions of the various diagnostic techniques are given. Of special note are the chapters on treating selected syndromes and diseases, which list the specific acupuncture points to use during treatment.
- Baldry, Peter. 2005. *Acupuncture, Trigger Points and Musculoskeletal Pain: A Scientific Approach to Acupuncture for Use by Doctors and Physiotherapists in the Diagnosis and Management of Myofascial Trigger Point Pain.* 3rd ed. New York: Elsevier/Churchill Livingstone. 367 pp. ISBN: 0443066442; 9780443066443.
  After an introduction to traditional Chinese acupuncture and its spread from China to the rest of the world, the author introduces the principles of trigger point acupuncture. He addresses the neurophysiology of pain, myofascial trigger point pain and fibromyalgia, and the scientific evaluation of the ability of acupuncture to relieve pain. In the final section of the book, the clinical application of trigger point acupuncture is discussed in detail, with separate chapters of the chest, shoulder, neck, arm, head and face, lower back, lower limb, joints, and abdomen and pelvic regions. Designed for use by health care professionals, is it especially useful for those who treat pain, especially rheumatologists, orthopedic specialists, and physical therapists.
- Bauer, Matthew D. 2005. *The Healing Power of Acupressure and Acupuncture: A Complete Guide to Timeless Traditions and Modern Practice.* New York: Avery. 203 pp. ISBN: 1583332162; 9781583332160.
  This book is designed for those wanting a basic introduction to acupuncture and acupressure and to the theories that underlie them. The author deftly discusses the major tenets of Chinese medicine while also providing a balanced discussion of the strengths and weaknesses of both Chinese and Western medicines. He provides directions on how to find a qualified practitioner and lists conditions and diseases that have been shown through controlled clinical trials to be effectively treated by acupuncture. The final section of the book focuses on using acupressure to treat common health problems.
- Beinfield, Harriet, and Korngold, Efrem. 1992, ©1991. *Between Heaven and Earth: A Guide to Chinese Medicine.* New York: Ballantine Books. 431 pp. ISBN: 0345379748; 9780345379740.

This is an accessible, general introduction to Chinese medicine. Divided into three sections, the authors present the theory of Chinese medicine, the psychology of Chinese medicine as illustrated by five-phase theory (also known as the five elements), and the therapies used in treatment, including acupuncture, herbs, and food. Many illustrations and examples culled from the authors' own practice are used to enhance the text.

- Bensky, Dan, Clavey, Steven, and Stöger, Erich, with Gamble, Andrew. 2004. *Chinese Herbal Medicine Materia Medica*. 3rd ed. Seattle Eastland Press. 1311 pp. ISBN: 0939616424; 9780939616428.
Written as a general reference for practitioners of Chinese herbal medicine, this work is encyclopedic in scope and covers 532 herbal remedies, of which 478 are discussed at length. The 19 chapters are arranged by the action of the herbs; for example, herbs that clear heat and herbs that regulate the blood. Each entry gives the names of the herbs including the Chinese, English, pharmaceutical, Japanese, and Korean names; the standard species to be used; the text in which the herb first appeared; properties, channels entered, and key characteristics; dosage, safety issues including toxicity and herb–drug interactions; clinical use; cautions and contraindications; and actions and indications. For most herbs, a line drawing of the plant is also given.

- Birch, Stephen J., and Felt, Robert L. 1999. *Understanding Acupuncture*. New York: Churchill Livingstone. 335 pp. ISBN: 0443061793; 9780443061790.
The authors have produced a readable, up-to-date scholarly treatise on acupuncture as it is practiced around the world. The book focuses on topics such as the history of acupuncture, its theoretical basis and fundamental concepts, and its efficacy. Although it is not a textbook on how to perform acupuncture, the book does examine the practice of acupuncture, including topics such as the illnesses that acupuncture treats, the diagnosis and assessment of patients, and the treatment session.

- Cargill, Marie. 1994. *Acupuncture: A Viable Medical Alternative*. Westport, CT: Praeger. 176 pp. ISBN: 0275948811; 9780275948818.
Written for the general reader, this book introduces acupuncture, including how it works and what to expect in a visit to an acupuncturist. Chapters are also devoted to specific topics such as acupuncture and pain acupuncture anesthesia, internal medicine, cancer, and gynecology and obstetrics.

- Cassidy, Claire Monod, ed. 2002. *Contemporary Chinese Medicine and Acupuncture*. New York: Churchill Livingstone. 436 pp. ISBN: 0443065896; 9780443065897.
The goal of this book is to provide current, accurate information on Chinese medicine and acupuncture for health care professional and students. Divided into four sections, the contributors provide chapters covering the theory and modalities of Chinese medicine, the methods of delivering care, research on the effectiveness of Chinese medicine and especially acupuncture, and the profession of Oriental medicine in the United States. Although written for health care professionals, the educated reader can easily comprehend the text.

- Cerney, J. V. 1999. *Acupuncture without Needles* Rev. ed. Paramus, NJ: Prentice Hall. 320 pp. ISBN: 0735200351; 9780735200357.
Although the illustrations seem dated, the concepts covered in this book are still valid. The author does a good job presenting the use of specific types of pressure

applied to Chinese acupuncture points for the purpose of healing common ailments. After an initial chapter that discusses proper technique, the chapters present techniques to help with ailments or pain of the head, neck, chest, back and spine, gastrointestinal and abdominal system, and legs and feet. A separate chapter is devoted to the care of the sex organs.

- Deadman, Peter, and Al-Khafaji, Mazin. 2007. *A Manual of Acupuncture*. 2nd ed. Hove, East Sussex, England: Journal of Chinese Medicine Publications. 675 pp. ISBN: 0951054651; 9780951054659.
  This is a comprehensive textbook for learning acupuncture. It provides excellent instruction in selecting points for treatment and in needling. The true strength of the book, however, is its highly detailed discussions of each of the meridians and each of their associated points. Under each point, the entry provides the name of the point, its Chinese character, its location, special location notes, a diagram of its anatomical location, methods of needling, its actions, its indications, a commentary on its use, and possible combinations with other points.

- Elias, Jason, and Ketcham, Katherine. 1998. *The Five Elements of Self-Healing: Using Chinese Medicine for Maximum Immunity, Wellness, and Health*. New York: Harmony Books. 422 pp. ISBN: 0517704870; 9780517704875.
  Based primarily on the theory of the five elements (earth, metal, water, wood, and fire), this book explicates the concept of health as defined by Chinese medicine. The author presents a variety of diseases with both their Western perspective and their Chinese interpretation. He then provides various remedies to treat them, with those remedies coming from the Chinese pharmacopoeia and from Western nutritional sources and supplements.

- Ernst, Edzard, and White, Adrian, eds. 1999. *Acupuncture: A Scientific Appraisal*. Boston: Butterworth Heinemann. 162 pp. ISBN: 0750641630; 9780750641630.
  Containing chapters written by international medical specialists, this book examines the scientific evidence for the efficacy of Chinese and Western acupuncture. The evidence presented yields mixed results with some evidence indicating that acupuncture is effective for some health problems, while other evidence shows little or no efficacy.

- Fan, Warner J-W. 2003. *A Manual of Chinese Herbal Medicine*. Boston: Shambhala. 352 pp. ISBN: 1570629374; 9781570629372.
  Aimed at a general readership, this book provides an excellent introduction to traditional Chinese herbal medicine. The author presents the basic concepts such as yin-yang, qi, and the five elements in an understandable manner. Chapters also include bodily functions, cases of disease, diagnosis, herbal pharmacology, and approaches to treatment. Part 2 consists of compendia of common diseases by cause, common diseases by organ, common symptoms of disease, therapeutics, common herbs, and formulas for common compound remedies.

- Fleischman, Gary F. 1998. *Acupuncture: Everything You Ever Wanted to Know*. Barrytown, NY: Barrytown. 166 pp. ISBN: 1886449090; 9781886449091.
  This book strives to answer questions about Chinese medicine and acupuncture that many people ask. It is arranged by thematic chapters and then by questions related to

that topic. For example, in the acupuncture overview, questions about the needles are answered, and in the chapter on diet, questions related to food and meals are answered. Thus, the book is easy to read and can be consulted to find answers to specific questions that the reader may have and doesn't need to be read cover to cover.

- Focks, Claudia, März, Ulrich, and Hosbach, Ingolf. 2008. *Atlas of Acupuncture*. New York: Churchill Livingstone/Elsevier. 732 pp. ISBN: 0443100284; 9780443100284.
This is an excellent atlas to the location of acupuncture points and the main energy channels of the body. Thus, it is helpful for both beginners and for experienced practitioners who wish to learn more about seldom used points. Each point is given using anatomical drawings and photographs of the surface anatomy.
- Gach, Michael Reed. 1990. *Acupressure's Potent Points: A Guide to Self-Care for Common Ailments*. New York: Bantam Books. 251 pp. ISBN: 0553349708; 9780553349702.
After a very short introduction to acupressure and its use, this work dives straight into providing acupressure points and techniques for specific ailments. Forty-one different ailments are highlighted, from allergies to constipation, from earaches to hot flashes, and from nosebleeds to wrist pain. For each ailment, other complementary therapies and diet changes are often suggested. Diagrams show the location of the acupressure points and the entry for each point gives the point's name, cautions for its use, if any, a textual description of its location, and benefits imparted by the point. Photographs are also frequently used to demonstrate the location of the points.
- Gach, Michael Reed, and Henning, Beth Ann. 2004. *Acupressure for Emotional Healing: A Self-Care Guide for Trauma, Stress & Common Emotional Imbalances*. New York: Bantam Books. 307 pp. ISBN: 0553382438; 9780553382433.
By focusing on emotional healing, this book differs from most other books on acupressure that deal with physical ailments. The first part discusses acupressure and how to treat oneself using acupressure points the spirit of the emotions, guidelines for emotional balancing, and emotional support. The second part is a reference guide to healing common emotional complaints such as addiction, anger, depression, sexual abuse, and worry. For each complaint, detailed directions are given describing the specific points that should be used for treatment. The third section provides similar information for chronic fatigue and fibromyalgia, insomnia, menstruation and menopause, and nightmares. The final section provides a diet that will support emotional healing.
- Han, Henry, Miller, Glenn E., and Deville, Nancy. 2003. *Ancient Herbs, Modern Medicine: Improving Your Health by Combining Chinese Herbal Medicine and Western Medicine*. New York: Bantam Books. 468 pp. ISBN: 0553381180; 9780553381184.
The main goal of this work is to increase the reader's knowledge of using Chinese herbs for medical purposes. In the first part, the authors provide a good, yet brief, introduction to traditional Chinese medicine, including acupuncture and herbs. Part 2 discusses the treatment of common illnesses, including chronic and mental illnesses. Treating modern illnesses such as adrenal burnout, environmentally related illness, and HIV are the focus of Part 3, while Part 4 examines mind-body-spirit medicine, women's health, sports medicine, and anti-aging methods. The last part gives recipes for foods that match the reader's individual constitution and for medicinal herbs.

- Hartmann, David. 2009. *Acupoint Dictionary*. 2nd ed. New York: Churchill Livingstone/ Elsevier. 193 pp. ISBN: 0729538834; 9780729538831.
  This quick reference guide is helpful for administering acupuncture treatments. In addition, it discusses the 1,000 traditional Chinese medicine actions and Western signs, symptoms and disease states. Thus, it will be especially useful for students of acupuncture and TCM and for qualified health care practitioners. The treatments are listed alphabetically for the most common conditions that are encountered in routine medical practices. The author also provides a section on contraindication/ cautions and diagrams of the 14 principal channels.
- Hecker, Hans-Ulrich, Steveling, Angelika, Peuker, Elmar, Kaster, Jörg, and Liebchen, Kay. 2008. *Color Atlas of Acupuncture: Body Points, Ear Points, Trigger Points*. New York: Thieme. 328 pp. ISBN: 3131252227; 9783131252227.
  This is a handy pocket sized atlas that covers the major body and ear acupuncture points and the most frequently used trigger points. In addition to the name and location of the acupuncture points, the depth of needling, the indication, and the action according to traditional Chinese medicine are given. For trigger points, only the location is given.
- Hempen, Carl-Hermann, and Fischer, Toni. 2009. *A Materia Medica for Chinese Medicine: Plants, Minerals and Animal Products*. New York: Churchill Livingstone. 1007 pp. ISBN: 0443100942; 9780443100949.
  The chapters in this materia medica are arranged by the action of the herbs, for example herbs that release the exterior (warming and cooling acrid herbs), herbs that purge and drain, herbs that cool heat, aromatic herbs that open the orifices, herbs that dispel wind-dampness, substances that calm the spirit, and herbs that regulate the qi. Thus, this is a required resource for those who use herbs in their medical practices.
- Hicks, Angela. 2005. *The Acupuncture Handbook: How Acupuncture Works and How It Can Help You*. London: Platkus. 282 pp. ISBN: 0749924721; 9780749924720.
  This is a guide for those interested in acupuncture or receiving acupuncture treatments. In addition to discussing acupuncture and acupuncture treatments, the author gives a basic background to the theory and practice of traditional Chinese medicine. Written in an easy to understand manner, this is a good book for anyone who is curious about acupuncture.
- Hicks, Angela, Hicks, John, and Mole, Peter. 2004. *Five Element Constitutional Acupuncture*. New York: Churchill Livingstone. 404 pp. ISBN: 0443071705; 9780443071706.
  Beginning with the philosophical foundations of five element constitutional acupuncture, the authors take the reader through five element theory as applied, primarily in the West, to traditional acupuncture. After discussions of the five elements and their interactions with the organs, the book presents diagnostic and treatment techniques built on the theory of the five elements. The use of acupuncture points and the development of a treatment plan are also included.
- Holland, Alex. 1999. *Voices of Qi: An Introductory Guide to Traditional Chinese Medicine*. Berkeley, CA: North Atlantic Books. 96 pp. ISBN: 1556433263; 9781556433269.
  This short book is aimed at those interested in finding out more about traditional Chinese medicine and the treatments it offers. The author has produced an easy to read work that discusses the foundations of TCM, its theoretical framework, and the

various modalities for treatment. Chapter 4 may be of special interest since it describes a visit to a TCM practitioner, the cost, and finding a qualified practitioner.

- Hou, Joseph P., and Jin, Youyu. 2005. *The Healing Power of Chinese Herbs and Medicinal Recipes*. Binghamton, NY: The Haworth Press. 812 pp. ISBN: 0789022028; 9780789022028.

  Designed as a self-help manual, this book provides a good introduction to traditional Chinese medicine but focuses primarily on the herbs and recipes used to treat a wide variety of ailments. Eleven chapters introduce 300 herbs used to strengthen the immune system, to maintain homeostasis and harmony in the body, to invigorate the circulation system, to calm the liver and nourish the heart, to relieve colds and allergies, to relieve arthritic pain and rheumatism, to regulate digestion, to treat urinary tract disorders, and to fight infections and tumors. The last part of the book provides 245 herbal recipes that can serve as tonics and healing agents. Herbal names and recipes are given in both transliterated Chinese and in English.

- Jarmey, Chris, and Bouratinos, Ilaira. 2008. *A Practical Guide to Acu-points*. Berkeley, CA: North Atlantic Books. 354 pp. ISBN: 1556436963; 9781556436963.

  Designed not only for acupuncturists but also for bodyworkers, this guide gives comprehensive information on the acu-points of the body. Colorful detailed anatomical illustrations show the locations of the points while the text offers more specific information. In addition, the authors delineate the larger area where the point can be activated at active pressure. Thus, this will be a handy resource for those who use acupressure and certain massage techniques in their practices.

- Kaptchuk, Ted. 2000. *The Web That Has No Weaver: Understanding Chinese Medicine*. Chicago: Contemporary Books. 500 pp. ISBN: 0809228408; 9780809228409.

  This is one of the best general books on traditional Chinese medicine. The first chapter is of extreme importance since it discusses the differences between Eastern and Western medicines and their approaches to the human body. The following chapters present the basics of Chinese medicine and provide excellent discussions on the concepts of qi, blood and other bodily fluids, spirit, the organs of the body, the meridians, the origins of disease, the four examinations used in diagnosis, the eight principal patterns of disharmony that can be discerned through a patient's symptoms, and the principle patterns within the human landscape as seen and treated by Chinese medicine. Although many Chinese terms are used by necessity, the explanations are clear.

- Kenyon, Julian. 1988. *Acupressure Techniques: A Self-Help Guide*. Rochester, VT: Healing Arts Press. 222 pp. ISBN: 0892816414; 9780892816415.

  This book is intended for home use to help treat a variety of physical ailments. The author provides a basic introduction to acupuncture theory and its application in acupressure. The bulk of the book is devoted to the disorders themselves. Under each disorder, the points that should be manipulated are listed and diagrams of their locations are provided.

- Kidson, Ruth. 2008. *Is Acupuncture Right for You? What It Is, Why It Works, and How It Can Help You*. Rochester, VT: Healing Arts Press. 192 pp. ISBN: 1594772673; 9781594772672.

  Aimed at the individual who is considering acupuncture treatment or who is interested in learning more about acupuncture, this book provides information on the history of acupuncture, its fundamental principles including the meridians and the five elements, causes of disease, methods of diagnosis, and methods of treatment. The author also includes chapters on how acupuncture works by presenting case histories and on the relationship between acupuncture and modern science, although no research studies are cited. This is an easy-to-read and understandable work that may reduce apprehension for those seeking acupuncture treatment.

➤ Kohn, Livia. 2005. *Health and Long Life: The Chinese Way*. Cambridge, MA: Three Pines Press. 234 pp. ISBN: 1931483035; 9781931483032.
The purpose of this book is to present an overview of East Asian medical techniques and spirituality. Specifically, it discusses how Chinese medicine works and how the worldview embodied within it can be understood in relation to Daoism. Chapters cover topics such as qi, yin and yang, the meridian system, methods of diagnosis, acupuncture, feng shui, the Chinese pharmacopoeia, breathing, and qigong. The book is a very readable and understandable introduction to traditional Chinese medicine.

➤ Kolster, Bernard C., and Waskowiak, Astrid. 2007. *The Acupressure Atlas*. Translated by N. W. Myint. Rochester, VT: Healing Arts Press. 240 pp. ISBN: 1594771758; 9781594771750.
This is a wonderfully illustrated introduction to acupressure. After a brief survey of traditional Chinese medicine and the meridians, the energy pathways of the body, the authors provide a step-by-step explanation of how to perform acupressure using clear color images. The final section covers specific ailments that can be treated with acupressure, including sleep problems, headaches, fatigue, breathing problems, urogenital problems, digestive problems, and musculoskeletal problems.

➤ Kuhn, Aihan. 2009. *Simple Chinese Medicine: A Beginner's Guide to Natural Healing & Well-Being*. Wolfeboro, NH: YMAA Publication Center. 248 pp. ISBN: 1594391246; 9781594391248.
For the layperson who is seeking better health, this is a good introduction to traditional Chinese medicine. The contents discuss the differences between Chinese medicine and Western medicine, diagnostic methods of TCM, the use of food for healing, a healthy balanced diet and its relation to weight reduction, exercises for maintaining good health and for preventing disease, cancer prevention and healing, and TCM secrets for longevity.

➤ Lambrou, Peter T., and Pratt, George J. 2006. *Instant Emotional Healing: Acupressure for the Emotions*. New York: Broadway Books. 292 pp. ISBN: 0767903935; 9780767903936.
Using an approach they call emotional self-management, the authors present a treatment technique that combines cognitive psychology and acupressure. The purpose of the therapy is both to release negative emotions that affect functioning and to help manage life's stressors so that individual performance and effectiveness are maximized. The book discusses the background of the emotional self-management technique, the role of our emotions in our lives, the protocols for applying acupressure, and ways to maintain and optimize the effects of the treatment.

➤ Leung, Ping-Chung, Xue, Charlie Changli, and Cheng, Yung-Chi, eds. 2003. *A Comprehensive Guide to Chinese Medicine*. River Edge, NJ: World Scientific. 356 pp. ISBN: 9812386041; 9789812386045.

Aimed at both medical clinicians and patients, this book provides a wide variety of information on traditional Chinese medicine. Chapters address issues such as the intelligent use of TCM in conjunction with Western medicine, the modalities and theoretical framework of TCM, biochemistry and herbs, how acupuncture works, the state of TCM in China and around the world, clinical trials using TCM, and the future of TCM.

➤ Lin, Henry B. 2000. *Chinese Health Care Secrets: A Natural Lifestyle Approach*. St. Paul, MN: Llewellyn Publications. 512 pp. ISBN: 1567184340; 9781567184341.
After a succinct introduction to the history and philosophy of Chinese medicine, the author provides chapters that give insight into diet, sleep and rest, physical hygiene, mental hygiene, exercise, sex, and environmental hygiene. He then discusses the use of natural products, especially herbs and foods, to promote healing and methods to enhance sexual vitality, rejuvenation, and longevity. The final chapter lists specific problems and their solutions. Appendixes provide instruction in qigong and other exercises. This is an easy to read book that is full of remedies that can be immediately applied.

➤ Liu, Chongyun, Tseng, Angela, and Yang, Sue. 2005. *Chinese Herbal Medicine: Modern Applications of Traditional Formulas*. Boca Raton, FL: CRC Press. 886 pp. ISBN: 0849315689; 9780849315688.
Designed for the TCM practitioner, this resource supplies information on over 860 formulas that can be customized to meet the individual needs of patients and over 640 individual herbs that can be used either alone or in combinations to treat illness. For each formula the entry gives the components, the main indication, the preparation, the treatment principle, and comparison to other formulas. For each herb, the Chinese herb name, the common name, temperature and tastes, channels, functions, indications, and dosages are given. Of special note is the section on formulas organized by their use in allopathic medicine; for example, cardiovascular disorders or respiratory disorders.

➤ Lu, Henry C. 2005. *Traditional Chinese Medicine: How to Maintain Your Health and Treat Illness*. Laguna Beach, CA: Basic Health Publications. 207 pp. ISBN: 1591201322; 9781591201322.
Although the author provides an introduction to the theories and methods of traditional Chinese medicine, he does so in a way that differs from most other introductory books. Throughout the book he uses diseases and syndromes to provide the background in which to discuss the various modalities for treatment that are used in TCM. For example, when he presents the food and herbal cures, he lists the symptom or disease and the food or herbs that can treat it. Similarly, in his chapters on the treatment of common diseases, he lists the signs and symptoms along with the syndrome and treatment. Other chapters discuss the healing effects of exercise, the meridians and acupuncture, and the causes of diseases and treatment strategies. Overall, this is a good introduction to TCM that also has many healing techniques that an individual can try on his or her own.

➤ Maciocia, Giovanni. 2004. *Diagnosis in Chinese Medicine: A Comprehensive Guide*. New York: Churchill Livingstone. 1127 pp. ISBN: 0443064482; 9780443064487.
Containing 111 chapters, this is a comprehensive textbook for applying the wide variety of diagnostic techniques used in traditional Chinese medicine. The four

major sections of the book correspond to diagnosis through observation, questioning or interrogation, palpation, and hearing and smelling. The fifth part examines symptoms and signs, while the sixth part guides the reader in the identification of patterns. This book provides a wealth of information but is suitable only for those who are studying or practicing Chinese medicine.

- Maciocia, Giovanni. 2008. *The Practice of Chinese Medicine: The Treatment of Diseases with Acupuncture and Chinese Herbs*. 2nd ed. New York: Churchill Livingstone/Elsevier. 1501 pp. ISBN: 0443074909; 9780443074905.
  Primarily suitable for students and practitioners of traditional Chinese medicine, this work will also be a good reference for other health care providers, pharmacists, and those with an interest in TCM. In addition to general information on TCM, its main focus is the integration of acupuncture and the use of herbs in the treatment of illnesses.
- Ni, Maoshing. 2008. *Secrets of Self-Healing: Harness Nature's Power to Heal Common Ailments, Boost Your Vitality, and Achieve Optimum Wellness*. New York: Avery. 562 pp. ISBN: 1583332960; 9781583332962.
  Based primarily on the theories and remedies of traditional Chinese medicine, this book's goal is to provide information that can help heal common ailments based on five principles: diet and nutrition, herbs and supplements, exercise and acupressure, lifestyle and environment, and mind and spirit. In Part 1, the author discusses "the path to self-healing" such as taking a health inventory by examining the face, tongue, hands, and feet, employing the healing properties of herbs and supplements, and living in harmony. In the second part, he details 65 common ailments, from acne to yeast infections, and suggests remedies for self-healing. The remedies include diet, home remedies, daily supplements, herbal therapy, exercise, and acupressure as well as foods, drugs, and situations to avoid.
- Pitchford, Paul. 2002. *Healing with Whole Foods: Asian Traditions and Modern Nutrition*. 3rd rev., updated, and expanded ed. Berkeley, CA: North Atlantic Books. 753 pp. ISBN: 1556434715; 9781556434716.
  The purpose of this book is to facilitate healing through diet, especially a diet based on vegetables. Using the concepts of yin-yang, qi, and five-element theory drawn from traditional Chinese medicine, the author provides a wealth of information on specific foods and on using those foods to treat a variety of ailments. Part 1 delves into diagnosis and treatment from the Chinese perspective, while Part 2 presents the essentials of nutrition, including such topics as water, protein, oils and fats, sweeteners, salt, vitamins and supplements, and calcium. Part 3 focuses on the five elements and their relationship to the body and to nutrition. Part 4 lists major diseases and suggests dietary treatment. The final part of the book gives recipes and discusses the properties of vegetal food that are useful for treating disease.
- Reichstein, Gail. 1998. *Wood Becomes Water: Chinese Medicine in Everyday Life*. New York: Kodansha International. 215 pp. ISBN: 1568362099; 9781568362090.
  Grounded in the theory of the five elements, this book focuses on acupuncture, qigong, dietary therapy and feng shui, while also providing an introduction to the basic concepts and theories of traditional Chinese medicine. The goal is to provide information that can be used in everyday life. Thus, throughout the book, recipes,

exercises, and lifestyle suggestions are given to help relieve common ailments and to increase health.

- Schreck, Joel Harvey. 2008. *Dr. Shen's Handbook of Herbs and Acupuncture.* Point Richmond, CA: Bay Tree. 256 pp. ISBN: 0980175801; 9780980175806.
  Arranged by ailment in an A–Z format, this book lists common Chinese herbal medicines used to treat ailments from acne and allergies to weight gain and yeast infections.

- Sollars, David. 2000. *The Complete Idiot's Guide to Acupuncture and Acupressure.* Indianapolis, IN: Alpha Books. 293 pp. ISBN: 0028639421; 9780028639420.
  Written in a lighthearted style, this book still provides a wealth of good information and a clear introduction to both acupuncture and acupressure. For those interested in trying acupuncture, it will relieve any anxiety that may be present before going for a treatment. For those who wish to experiment with using acupressure to treat common ailments, the directions are clear and the illustrations helpful. Although not as detailed as some other works, this is still a good choice for those just beginning the journey into Chinese medicine.

- Stux, Gabriel, Berman, Brian, and Pomeranz, Bruce. 2003. *Basics of Acupuncture.* 5th rev. ed. New York: Springer. 352 pp. ISBN: 3540442731; 9783540442738.
  After introductory chapters on the scientific basis of acupuncture and the theories of traditional Chinese medicine, the authors provide an in-depth discussion of the meridians and each of the acupuncture points. The technique of acupuncture is then presented followed by principles of treatment and rules of point selection for a wide variety of disorders. Under each disorder, the specific points to be needled are listed. This is a work designed for the acupuncturist or the medical professional who wishes to include acupuncture in the treatment options offered to patients.

- Stux, Gabriel, and Hammerschlag, Richard, eds. 2001. *Clinical Acupuncture: Scientific Basis.* New York: Springer. 227 pp. ISBN: 3540640541; 9783540640547.
  Due to the increased interest in the use of acupuncture in the West, there has been a call for evaluating its effectiveness scientifically. This work provides a summary of research that has examined the use of acupuncture as an analgesic, the clinical efficacy of acupuncture, the use of acupuncture in the treatment of stroke patients, and clinical trials. Thus, the book may be of interest to medical researchers, practicing physicians, acupuncturists, and interested medical consumers.

- Thie, John, and Thie, Matthew. 2005. *Touch for Health: A Practical Guide to Natural Health with Acupressure Touch and Massage.* Camarillo, CA: DeVorss Publications. 370 pp. ISBN: 0875168124; 9780875168128.
  Combining applied kinesiology, the meridians as discussed in Chinese medicine, acupressure, proper posture, pain control techniques, and balancing techniques, this book seeks to provide both health care professionals and laypeople a system that can help create better functioning and overall health in their patients or themselves. The system uses kinesiology to determine the need for muscle balancing and uses acupressure touch and massage to create such balance. This book provides a complete introduction to the Touch for Health system using clear text and prolific illustrations.

- Tierra, Michael. 1998. *The Way of Chinese Herbs.* New York: Pocket Books. 474 pp. ISBN: 0671898698; 9780671898694.
  After a brief review of the theories of Chinese medicine and diagnosis, the author presents chapters on food therapy and the use of herbs to treat diseases. This is followed by a materia medica of the major Chinese medicinal herbs. For each herb, the entry provides the English name as well as the Chinese name in Western characters, common name, family, part used, energy and flavor, organ meridians affected, properties, effects and indications, contraindications, dose, recipe, and any relevant notes.
- Tsang, Patricia. 2008. *Optimal Healing: A Guide to Traditional Chinese Medicine.* San Francisco: Balance for Health Publishing. 255 pp. ISBN: 0979948495; 9780979948497.
  This is another good book that introduces the lay reader to traditional Chinese medicine, its teachings, and its approach to disease and wellness. It also seeks to help the reader integrate TCM with conventional Western medicine. The author uses a survey to help the reader understand concepts such as liver fire, hot qi, and wet heat, and then discusses common complaints and how to help heal them using the methods of TCM.
- White, Adrian, Cummings, T. M., Filshie, Jacqueline. 2008. *An Introduction to Western Medical Acupuncture.* Edinburgh: Churchill Livingstone/Elsevier. 240 pp. ISBN: 0443071772; 9780443071775.
  In most states, medical doctors can use acupuncture in their treatment of patients. This text is a practical guide to both the principles and the clinical use of medical acupuncture. The authors also cover safety issues, clinical issues, and acupuncture in clinical conditions.
- Wu, Jing-Nuan. 2005. *An Illustrated Chinese Materia Medica.* New York: Oxford University Press. 706 pp. ISBN: 0195140176; 9780195140170.
  This work focuses specifically on the herbs that are used in traditional Chinese medicine. In his introduction, the author provides a good, brief summary of the Chinese herbal theory and the use of these herbs. The entry for each herb includes its pharmaceutical name, English name, the part used, flavor, property, and channel tropism (which of the meridians it affects), functions, clinical use and major combinations, dosage and administration, and precautions. An illustration of the herb with its Chinese name accompanies each entry. There are indexes to the pharmaceutical and English names, but none for the Chinese names.
- Xinrong, Yang, ed. 2003. *Encyclopedic Reference of Traditional Chinese Medicine.* New York: Springer. 660 pp. ISBN: 3540428461; 9783540428466.
  Including more than 5,000 entries, this reference work provides short entries for herbs, drugs, and therapeutic agents used in TCM and for illnesses as defined by TCM. For each herb, drug, or agent, the origin of the item, its effect, and its indication are given. For the illnesses, which have names such as "abdominal distention due to cold deficiency," the symptoms, pathogenesis, and therapeutic principle are given. Thus, this is a work that will mainly appeal to the TCM practitioner.
- Yang, Yifan. 2010. *Chinese Herbal Medicines: Comparisons and Characteristics.* 2nd ed. New York: Churchill Livingstone/Elsevier. 254 pp. ISBN: 070203133X; 9780702031335.
  The author presents detailed information on the most commonly used Chinese herbs and medicines. Appendixes give additional information on safe dosages, common combinations of herbs, and the meanings of the Chinese words used in the

herbal names. Much of the text is in the format of question and answer that helps with practical use in a clinical setting.

Internet Resources

- The Accreditation Commission for Acupuncture and Oriental Medicine, www.acaom.org.
  The Accreditation Commission for Acupuncture and Oriental Medicine is recognized by the U.S. Department of Education as the national accrediting agency that accredits master's level programs in acupuncture and Oriental medicine. It maintains a listing of those schools that have gained or are seeking accredited status.
- Acufinder.com Acupuncture Referral Service, www.acufinder.com.
  Listing over 30,000 licensed professionals, this site helps locate acupuncturists around the world. It also provides information on a wide array of topics related to health and acupuncture, including acupuncture schools and other Web resources.
- Acupuncture.com—Gateway to Chinese Medicine, Health and Wellness, acupuncture.com.
  This is an excellent source of information on all aspects of acupuncture, whether one is a patient or a practitioner. For patients, it includes an acupuncturist locator, a listing of conditions that can be treated using acupuncture, and the basics of Chinese medicine. For practitioners, there are links to information on specific syndromes, herbology, laws and regulations, and research on the effectiveness of acupuncture and Chinese medicine.
- The American Association of Acupuncture and Oriental Medicine, www.aaaomonline.org.
  An excellent site primarily about acupuncture, the American Association of Acupuncture Oriental Medicine provides a wealth of information on the history of acupuncture and Oriental medicine, a referral service to acupuncturists in the United States, information on the use of acupuncture to treat a variety of maladies, and links to other resources related to acupuncture and Oriental medicine.
- Council of Colleges of Acupuncture and Oriental Medicine, www.ccaom.org.
  Providing information for acupuncture students, practitioners, and patients, this site is a clearinghouse to schools of acupuncture and oriental medicine as well as training, continuing education, and information for those interested in pursuing a career in acupuncture and oriental medicine.
- National Acupuncture Foundation, www.nationalacupuncturefoundation.org.
  The National Acupuncture Foundation was founded in 1991 to promote the use of acupuncture and Oriental medicine in the United States. The foundation publishes materials on the regulation of acupuncture and Oriental medicine. The site provides a wealth of links to other resources on acupuncture and Oriental medicine as well as links to state regulatory agencies.
- National Certification Commission for Acupuncture and Oriental Medicine, www.nccaom.org.
  Established in 1982, the National Certification Commission for Acupuncture and Oriental Medicine establishes, assesses, and promotes standards of competence and

safety in acupuncture and Oriental medicine. The site also provides a registry of those acupuncturists who have received NCCAOM certification in acupuncture, Oriental medicine, Chinese herbology, and Asian bodywork therapy.

Periodicals/Magazines/Journals

- *Acupuncture and Electro-Therapeutics Research: The International Journal*, published by Cognizant Communication Corp., 1976– . Quarterly. ISSN: 0360-1293. www.cognizantcommunication.com/filecabinet/Acupuncture/acu.htm.
  Covering developments in both basic and clinical research in acupuncture, electro-therapeutics and related fields, this journal seeks to improve diagnosis and treatment using modalities drawn from acupuncture and Oriental medicine.
- *Acupuncture in Medicine*, published by British Medical Acupuncture Society, 1981– . Quarterly. ISSN: 0964-5284. www.medical-acupuncture.co.uk.
  Written for medical practitioners, *Acupuncture in Medicine* is a peer-reviewed journal that publishes reports of controlled clinical trials, reviews, and case histories on acupuncture and related techniques.
- *Acupuncture Today*, published by MPA Media, 2000– . Monthly. ISSN: 1526-7784. www.acupuncturetoday.com/mpacms/at/home.php.
  Available both online and in print, *Acupuncture Today* publishes news, general articles, and research reports on a wide variety of topics such as nutrition, herbalism, Oriental medicine, and practice management.
- *The American Acupuncturist*, published by the American Association of Acupuncture and Oriental Medicine, 1978– . Quarterly. ISSN: 1520-7714. www.aaaomonline.org/default.asp?pagenumber=43.
  The American Acupuncturist covers a broad array of topics of interest to acupuncturists and Oriental medicine practitioners. The journal also covers related legislation, reports from committees of the American Association of Acupuncture and Oriental Medicine, and relevant seminars and conferences.
- *The American Journal of Chinese Medicine*, publishing by World Scientific Publishing, 1973– . Six times a year. ISSN: 0192-415X. www.worldscinet.com/ajcm/ajcm.shtml.
  As a scholarly journal, this publication covers basic science and clinical research related to Chinese medicine, including therapeutic procedures and medicinal plants.
- *Annals of Traditional Chinese Medicine*, published by World Scientific Publishing Co., 2005– . Irregular. ISSN: 1793-0138. www.worldscibooks.com/series/atcm_series.shtml.
  Generally published annually, the *Annals of Traditional Chinese Medicine* includes articles on research in traditional Chinese medicine, research methodology, clinical trials, and studies of the quality, efficacy, and safety of TCM.
- *Australian Journal of Acupuncture and Chinese Medicine*, published by Australian Acupuncture and Chinese Medicine Association, 2006– . Semi-annual. ISSN: 1833-9735. www.acupuncture.org.au/ajacm.cfm.
  This journal publishes both research and clinical practice articles on acupuncture and Chinese medicine. In addition, other articles may include reviews and reports of case histories.

- *California Journal of Oriental Medicine*, published by California State Oriental Medical Association, 1980– . Semi-annual. ISSN: 1090-1965. www.csomaonline.org/i4a/pages/index.cfm?pageid=3289.
  Dedicated to the advancement of the art, science and practice of Oriental medicine, this journal is intended for licensed acupuncturists and practitioners of Oriental medicine. It publishes peer-reviewed articles that emphasize research, clinical therapies, and the historical perspective of Oriental medicine.
- *Chinese Medicine*, published by BioMed Central Ltd., 2006– . Irregular. ISSN: 1749-8546. www.cmjournal.org/home.
  This online journal covers all aspects of research on Chinese medicine, including herbal medicine, clinical nutrition, acupuncture, tuina, qiqong, tai chi quan, and education.
- *European Journal of Oriental Medicine*, published by British Acupuncture Council, 1977– , New Series 1993– . Semi-annual. ISSN: 1351-6647. www.ejom.co.uk.
  An academic journal, the *European Journal of Oriental Medicine* seeks to provide an outlet for articles and research on Chinese medicine and other traditions of Oriental medicine.
- *International Journal of Clinical Acupuncture*, published by Allerton Press Inc., 1990– . Quarterly. ISSN: 1047-1979. www.allertonpress.com/journals/acup.htm.
  Dedicated to improving the clinical skills of acupuncture practitioners, this journal publishes articles on clinical research, the experiences of clinicians, acupuncture analgesia and therapy, case reports, news, and notices of meetings, symposia, and conferences related to acupuncture and traditional Chinese medicine.
- *Journal of Acupuncture and Tuina Science*, published by Springer, 2003– . Bimonthly. ISSN: 1672-3597. www.springer.com/medicine/complementary+%26+alternative+medicine/journal/11726.
  International in scope, this journal seeks to promote the development of acupuncture, moxibustion, and tuina therapies. The journal publishes articles that focus primarily on clinical practice and the treatment of common diseases.
- *The Journal of Chinese Medicine*, published by Journal of Chinese Medicine, 1979– . Three times a year. ISSN: 0143-8042. www.jcm.co.uk.
  Covering the entire field of traditional Chinese medicine, *The Journal of Chinese Medicine* provides practitioners, students, and researches theoretical and clinical articles on acupuncture and traditional Chinese medicine as well as on herbology, qigong, and dietary medicine.
- *Medical Acupuncture*, published by Mary Ann Liebert Inc., 1989– . Quarterly. ISSN: 1933-6586. www.liebertpub.com/publication.aspx?pub_id=233.
  Written for physicians, *Medical Acupuncture* provides information related to the use of acupuncture by those with Western medical training. Articles include evidence-based clinical studies, case reports, and research findings.
- *Thieme Almanac: Acupuncture and Chinese Medicine*, published by Thieme Medical Publishers, 2007– . Annual. No ISSN. www.thieme.com.
  Addressing both acupuncture and Chinese medicine, the *Thieme Almanac* publishes articles of interest to practitioners, teachers, researchers, and students of acupuncture

and Chinese medicine. The goal of the almanac is to increase cooperation and communication among those interested in acupuncture and traditional Chinese medicine and to present information related to legislation, training, research, and clinical practice.

Chapter 24

Yoga

Background and History

The practice of yoga began in India between 2,000 and 3,000 years ago, although its roots may go back much farther. Derived from the Sanskrit word "yuj," which means "to yoke" or "to join together," the basic concept is the integration of the human body, both internally and externally. Yoga seeks to integrate not only the physical and the spiritual but also the individual spirit with the universal. Thus, yoga is seen by many as a religious practice since its roots lie within the Hindu culture of India. Yoga, however, can be practiced by anyone and has no specific religious teachings.

The earliest treatise on yoga is the *Yoga-Sutras* written by the sage Patanjali about 2,000 years ago. Patanjali discusses all aspects of living, especially how we think and how we act. From his writings others developed the practice of yoga, because he does not specifically address the postures and breathing exercises that are usually associated with the modern concept of yoga. In Sanskrit, the term *yoga* actually encompasses a variety of other concepts, including ethical practices, self-restraint, detachment from the external world, concentration, meditation, and enlightenment (samadhi). In the Western world, yoga generally means the use of postures and breathing as a form of exercise or a way to increase one's health.

The main style of yoga that developed from the teachings of Patanjali is hatha yoga, the practice of which was not encoded into written works until the fourteenth or fifteen century, although the teachings were passed down the generations orally. Most modern forms of yogic practice can trace their origins to hatha yoga and to the sutras of Patanjali, although there are a wide variety of forms of yoga. Among other major forms are kundalini yoga, Bikram yoga, anusara yoga, integral yoga, Iyengar yoga, Jivamuku yoga, kriya yoga, Vinyasa yoga, and Kripalu yoga.

Primary Uses and Actions

Traditionally, yoga consists of two parts: asanas and pranayama. The asanas refer to the various postures that are used in the practice of yoga, while pranayama means the control of breath. The goal of the asanas is to help cure physical ailments by creating balance in the body. The asanas can tone the body, improve posture, strengthen the muscles and bones, and increase energy. Pranayama, or the control of breath, includes breathing exercises that can be used in conjunction with the asanas. As a result of the asanas and pranayama, the health of the body increases and the mind is calmed. Such healing can be physical, psychological, or spiritual.

Assuming a posture is not simply a mechanical procedure but one that should be done in a thoughtful manner so that balance is achieved and stress is removed. In performing the postures in such a way, the body and its organs are replenished with blood, they are massaged and toned, and optimum health can be achieved. Thus, yoga can be used to treat a variety of health complaints. Care must be taken, however, to ensure that the asanas are performed correctly. In addition, many pranayama exercises should be attempted only when a qualified instructor is present.

Individual postures can be used to treat specific conditions. For example, the various "mountain" postures are helpful for treating depression, strengthening the knees, reducing sciatic pain, and preventing hemorrhoids. The "full boat" posture can be used to stimulate the thyroid gland, to improve blood circulation in the abdomen, to strengthen the abdominal muscles, to relieve indigestion, and to reduce lower backache.

Training

There are a multitude of books, DVDs, and online programs that can teach basic and even advanced yogic postures. It is imperative to remember that doing the exercises incorrectly can result in injury. Thus, it is preferable to learn the postures, and especially the pranayama exercises, from a qualified instructor. The main problem, however, is that it is difficult to determine the qualifications of many yoga instructors since there are no national requirements or certification processes to become a yoga instructor.

The Yoga Alliance has been formed as one way to recognize yoga teacher training programs that offer courses that last 200 or 500 hours, depending on the level of the course. The Yoga Alliance has also developed guidelines for both the 200 and the 500 hour programs. Individuals who complete either a 200 or 500 hour yoga training program may apply to become a registered yoga teacher, which permits them to use the initials "RYT" as an indication of their status. Those who complete their training at a Yoga Alliance recognized school are automatically eligible for the RYT designation.

Other organizations also offer recognition for their yoga programs. For example, the Aerobics and Fitness Association of America offers certification as a yoga instructor to individuals who already possess their Primary Group Exercise Certification. Similarly, the American Council on Exercise offers special courses on yoga aimed for those who hold a current ACE certification, although the courses are available for others to take.

Sources

Budilovsky, Joany, Adamson, Eve, and revised with Flynn, Carolyn. 2006. *Complete Idiot's Guide to Yoga Illustrated*. 4th ed. New York: Penguin Group.

Carrico, Mara. 1997. *Yoga Journal's Yoga Basics: The Essential Beginner's Guide to Yoga for a Lifetime of Health and Fitness*. New York: Henry Holt.

Iyengar, B. K. S. 2005. *Light on Life: The Yoga Journey to Wholeness, Inner Peace, and Ultimate Freedom*. Emmaus, PA: Rodale.

See also AYURVEDA; MEDITATION

Annotated Bibliography

Print Resources

- Brown, Christina. 2003. *The Yoga Bible: The Definitive Guide to Yoga Postures*. Cincinnati: Walking Stick Press. 400 pp. ISBN: 1582972427; 9781582972428.

Featuring over 170 poses taken from a variety of yoga styles, this small book is a comprehensive guide to yoga. Color photographs and good descriptions of how to assume the poses permit almost anyone to begin a yoga practice. This work is especially handy for those who wish to add new poses to their practice. The author also includes chapters on relaxation, pranayama (breathing exercises), and yogic cleansing practices.

- Budilovsky, Joany, Adamson, Eve, and revised with Flynn, Carolyn. 2006. *Complete Idiot's Guide to Yoga Illustrated*. 4th ed. New York: Penguin Group. 282 pp. ISBN: 1592574882; 9781592574889.
  The authors provide a step-by-step guide to yoga, complete with line illustrations that help readers achieve the various postures. The text and illustrations also give good directions on how to get into and out of the postures safely and painlessly. Other sections discuss the different yoga traditions, with an emphasis on hatha yoga. The final chapter examines yoga and healing.

- Cappy, Peggy. 2006. *Yoga for All of Us: A Modified Series of Traditional Poses for Any Age and Ability*. New York: St. Martin's Griffin. 194 pp. ISBN: 0312340877; 9780312340872.
  This is a book designed for those who think that they cannot do yoga. To assist those who have physical limitations, such as problems of balance, flexibility, or strength, the author presents modifications to the traditional poses so that just about anyone can perform them. She also gives tips on breathing properly, on stretching, on relaxation methods, and on meditation.

- Carrico, Mara. 1997. *Yoga Journal's Yoga Basics: The Essential Beginner's Guide to Yoga for a Lifetime of Health and Fitness*. New York: Henry Holt. 191 pp. ISBN: 0805045716; 9780805045710.
  For the individual who is seeking an introduction to yoga, this book is highly recommended. The author discusses yoga, its history, and a variety of yoga styles. The bulk of the book is devoted to the actual practice of yoga and includes instruction on proper breathing and on a variety of postures. The postures are grouped into the basic positions: supine, prone, standing, balancing, seated, abdominals, and inversions. Separate chapters present the sun salutation, relaxation, and sample yoga practices. The final section of the book is devoted to meditation and starting a meditation practice.

- Cope, Stephen. 2006. *The Wisdom of Yoga: A Seeker's Guide to Extraordinary Living*. New York: Bantam Books. 316 pp. ISBN: 0553801112; 9780553801118.
  This book focuses on the concept of yoga, not the exercises commonly associated with it. Specifically, the author presents his interpretation of yoga as outlined in the *Yoga-Sutras* of Patanjali. He uses stories derived from his friends, students, and teachers to illustrate the principles. Thus, it is a book about living of the spirit while also confronting a life that is full of struggles and pain. The author's focus is on the eight limbs of yoga (ethical behaviors, disciplines, postures, breathing practices, sense withdrawal, concentration, meditation, and enlightenment) and how they can be applied to modern life.

- DiGirolamo, Joel. 2009. *Yoga in No Time at All: How to Practice Yoga in Your Daily Life for Improved Flexibility of Your Mind and Body*. Lexington, KY: PranaPower. 168 pp. ISBN: 0977088464; 9780977088461.

This guide is dedicated to those who think they are too busy to practice yoga. The author presents 39 poses that can be done in a very short time or in conjunction with other activities. He also provides a section on workstation ergonomics and a series of exercises that can be done during work breaks.

- Grime, Louise. 2008. *15 Minute Gentle Yoga*. New York: DK Publishing. 128 pp. ISBN: 0756629268; 9780756629267.
  This little book is helpful for those who wish to learn yoga but do not have a lot of time to devote to the exercises. The author has provided four complete mini-workouts for each day that target specific part of the body. Thus, this is an easy way to strengthen, stretch, and build your way to a healthier body.
- Iyengar, B. K. S. 2005. *Light on Life: The Yoga Journey to Wholeness, Inner Peace, and Ultimate Freedom*. Emmaus, PA: Rodale. 282 pp. ISBN: 1594862486; 9781594862489.
  Written by one of the masters of the practice of yoga, this book represents both an intimate story of Iyengar's spiritual quest and an excellent discussion of the philosophical and spiritual bases of yoga as an approach to life. It is the story of a journey inward, but in that journey all experiences are discussed. Thus, the chapters focus on the five bodies of each individual: the physical body, the energy body, the mental body, the intellectual body, and the divine body. For those who seek the spiritual teachings that lie behind the practice of asanas and pranayama, this is a book that will be worth the effort of reading.
- Iyengar, B. K. S. 2008. *Yoga: The Path to Holistic Health*. Rev. ed. New York: DK Publishing. 432 pp. ISBN: 0756633621; 9780756633622.
  This is a complete introduction to the practice of yoga, not only as exercise but also as a lifestyle. The author summarizes the philosophy of yoga and then presents the classic postures with their original Sanskrit names. He then discusses the use of yoga to relieve stress and provides a wide variety of poses that counteract stress. Next, yoga therapy and the use of specific poses to help treat ailments of the body's systems is detailed. The final chapter presents a 20 week yoga course using the asanas given in the earlier chapters. Color photographs, detailed instructions, and benefits are given for all the poses.
- Kirk, Martin, and Boon, Brooke. 2006. *Hatha Yoga Illustrated*. Champaign, IL: Human Kinetics. 233 pp. ISBN: 0736062033; 9780736062039.
  Focusing on hatha yoga, the authors present 77 different poses organized by their basic posture; for example, standing, inverted, twisting, sitting, and reclining. Color photographs accompany the directions for performing each pose. In addition, the physical benefits, the mental benefits, and any contraindications are also given. The last chapter directs the reader through 11 different routines that can be incorporated into a regular yoga practice.
- Kraftsow, Gary. 1999. *Yoga for Wellness: Healing with the Timeless Teachings of Viniyoga*. New York: Penguin/Arkana. 334 pp. ISBN: 0140195696; 9780140195699.
  The goal of this book is to present the therapeutic applications of yoga and the asanas. Part 1 provides a developmental approach to yoga and discusses the principles of yoga practice and the biomechanics of movement, including bending forward, bending backward, twisting, and extension. Part 2 focuses on yoga as a therapeutic

approach. Chapters in this part include using yoga for common aches and pains, for chronic disease, and for emotional health. With its focus on the therapeutic value of yoga and its use of clear directions and illustrations, this book will be a handy resource for those interested in pursuing the practice of yoga.

➤ Lasater, Judith. 2003. *30 Essential Yoga Poses for Beginning Students and Their Teachers.* Berkeley, CA: Rodmell Press. 248 pp. ISBN: 1930485042; 9781930485044.
For the beginning yoga student, this will be a welcome book. After an introduction to the tradition of yoga and a discussion of the student–teacher relationship, the author presents the 30 yoga poses that form the basis of many yoga exercise sequences. For each pose, good color photographs accompany the text that describes how to perform the pose. The author then describes the practice of yoga and gives a variety of pose combinations that can be used. These vary from the simple "busy days practice" to a practice that varies by the day of the week. She also provides pose combinations that can be used for specific purposes such as increasing shoulder and upper back flexibility and relieving lower back pain.

➤ McCall, Timothy B. 2007. *Yoga as Medicine.* New York: Bantam Books. 568 pp. ISBN: 0553384066; 9780553384062.
The central theme of this book is that yoga can be used as a healing technique not just for those who have a disease but for those who are healthy. The three parts of the book present yoga as medicine, the practice of yoga, and yoga therapy in action. Twenty conditions are addressed in the yoga therapy in action part including such problems as anxiety and panic attacks, asthma, depression, heart disease, insomnia, and multiple sclerosis. The chapters for each condition give an overview of the condition, how yoga can help, available scientific evidence, and specific exercises and yoga poses that can be used to help alleviate the condition.

➤ McGonigal, Kelly. 2009. *Yoga for Pain Relief: Simple Practices to Calm Your Mind & Heal Your Chronic Pain.* Oakland, CA: New Harbinger Publications. 182 pp. ISBN: 1572246898; 9781572246898.
In addition to being useful for increasing flexibility and strength, yoga can help treat pain such as back pain, knee pain, and carpal tunnel syndrome. Chapters cover topics such as understanding your pain, using the breath, moving the body, relaxation, and meditation. The final chapter helps you establish a personal yoga program that can help you make peace with your body and control your pain.

➤ Mehta, Mira. 1998. *How to Use Yoga: A Step-by-Step Guide to the Iyengar Method of Yoga, for Relaxation, Health and Well-Being.* Berkeley, CA: Rodmell Press. 96 pp. ISBN: 0962713864; 9780962713866.
This is a highly illustrated book that features the Iyengar method of yoga. In addition to providing good descriptions of 41 different poses the author outlines a 10 week course that gives daily and weekly regimens. The final section lists asanas for common problems such as headaches and backaches.

➤ Mehta, Silva, Mehta, Mira, and Mehta, Shyam. 2001. ©1990. *Yoga: The Iyengar Way.* New York: Alfred A. Knopf. 192 pp. ISBN: 0679722874; 9780679722878.
Focusing on the Iyengar method of yoga, this is a good introduction to yoga in general and to the therapeutic yoga postures as devised by B. K. S. Iyengar. The book is

divided into three parts. Part 1 focuses on the body and gives step-by-step instructions and photographs for 108 different postures. Part 2 discusses the mind, breathing techniques, control of the senses, and the philosophy of yoga. The final part examines the soul and the ultimate goals of a yogic practice.

- Miller, Olivia H. 2003. *Essential Yoga: An Illustrated Guide to Over 100 Yoga Poses and Meditations*. San Francisco: Chronicle Books. 239 pp. ISBN: 0811841154; 9780811841153.
  Focusing solely on hatha yoga, this book presents over 100 different poses that can be integrated into a yoga practice. Seven chapters provide instruction on how to create a complete yoga workout beginning with breathing exercises and progressing through warm-ups and a variety of poses. The author also presents chapters on meditation and flowing routines such as the sun and moon salutations. Chapter 6 focuses on the yoga session itself and gives examples of sessions with their suggested poses. The final chapter provides recommended sequences of poses for specific conditions such as back pain relief and cold prevention and for specific activities such as dancing and office work.
- Mohan, A. G. 2002. *Yoga for Body, Breath, and Mind: A Guide to Personal Reintegration*. Boston: Shambhala. 221 pp. ISBN: 1570629773; 9781570629778.
  In addition to providing instruction on a wide variety of poses, the author integrates breathing practices (pranayama) and meditation to create a balanced and complete yoga practice. The goal is personal integration in which the individual becomes centered, contented, and able to see life as it truly is. Instead of photographs, simple line drawings are used to represent the poses and the breathing sequence to accompany the move.
- Moyer, Donald. 2006. *Yoga: Awakening the Inner Body*. Berkeley, CA: Rodmell Press. 243 pp. ISBN: 1930485123; 9781930485129.
  The yoga exercises presented in this work are intended for home use. The first two chapters are devoted to inverted poses since these can be the most challenging for beginners. The rest of the book provides poses that focus on different parts of the body. For each pose, the author presents the props needed, the benefits of the pose as well as cautions, how to move into the pose, how to check your alignment, how to adjust while in the pose, and how to come out of the pose.
- Norberg, Ulrica. 2008. *Hatha Yoga: The Body's Path to Balance, Focus, and Strength*. New York: Skyhorse. 125 pp. ISBN: 1602392188; 9781602392182.
  This is a good introduction to one of the most popular forms of yoga. The author gives good directions on proper breathing and assuming the asanas. She also provides some of the philosophy behind the practice of yoga. Color photographs assist the novice in performing the asanas.
- Powers, Sarah. 2008. *Insight Yoga*. Boston: Shambhala. 196 pp. ISBN: 1590305981; 9781590305980.
  This is a guide to the practice of Insight Yoga as developed by the author. This style of yoga combines traditional yoga movements with the meridians of Chinese medicine and Buddhist meditation. She demonstrates a series of different yoga sequences that benefit organs, muscles, joints, tendons, and especially the mind. The result is greater physical well-being and mental and emotional clarity.

- Rosen, Richard. 2002. *The Yoga of Breath: A Step-by-Step Guide to Pranayama.* Boston: Shambhala. 304 pp. ISBN: 1570628890; 9781570628894.
  In this book, the author focuses solely on the practice of pranayama or the control of breath, which is one aspect of the practice of yoga. The purpose of pranayama is to increase prana, usually translated as life energy, in the body, thereby rejuvenating the body and permitting a transformation of the self. Although it sounds simple, the control of the breath can be difficult and the author provides both an introduction and a program that will guide the reader through the first year of the practice. Throughout the work, clear directions for each of the exercises are given as well as the philosophical background of the exercises.
- Sivananda Yoga Vedanta Centre. 2008. *Yoga Mind and Body.* New York: DK Publishing. 168 pp. ISBN: 0756636744; 9780756636746.
  Produced by the London Sivananda Yoga Centre, this guide covers all parts of starting a yoga practice. Detailed instructions help the novice perform the sun salutation and 12 basic *asanas*. The author also discusses the use of yoga for relaxation and positive thinking, proper breathing, and meditation techniques. Beautifully illustrated, the book guides helps readers understand yoga philosophy while introducing the yoga lifestyle. A final section includes a section on vegetarianism, which gives dozens of recipes.
- Turlington, Christy. 2002. *Living Yoga: Creating a Life Practice.* New York: Hyperion. 276 pp. ISBN: 0786868066; 9780786868063.
  This is a personal story of the author's spiritual journey and her discovery and practice of yoga. Contained within are good introductions to yoga in its wider context, including discussions of asanas (postures), pranayama (breathing), meditation, ayurveda, and Vastu (the art of arranging living and work spaces correctly). Although not as helpful for those seeking instruction simply on yoga postures and exercise programs, this is an engaging book about the search for the spirit in today's world.

Internet Resources

- ABC of Yoga, www.abc-of-yoga.com.
  This is a portal to a world of information on yoga. Pages discuss the different styles of yoga, the exercises and postures used in yoga practice, pranayama, meditation, yoga equipment and tools, and the effect of yoga on health. For those who are just beginning their exploration of yoga, there is a beginner's guide.
- Yoga Alliance, www.yogaalliance.org.
  With a goal of setting standards for the teaching of yoga, the website of the Yoga Alliance includes directories of registered teachers and registered schools who have complied with the minimum educational standards promulgated by the Alliance.
- Yoga Basics, www.yogabasics.com.
  As its title suggests, this site is designed for those who wish to learn the basic ideas of yoga. The site allows the user to examine the different types of yoga and their history as well as trying the basic postures used in hatha yoga. Other pages discuss the control of breath and the use of meditation.

- Yoga Site, www.yogasite.com.
  The subtitle of this site is "The Online Yoga Resource Center." As such it provides access to a wide array of yoga resources such as articles on yoga, a yoga teacher directory, a listing of workshops and retreat centers, and information on postures, meditation, pranayama, yoga therapy, and yoga styles. The site also serves as a store for yoga-related items such as mats, straps, clothing, and jewelry.
- YogaFit, www.yogafit.com.
  YogaFit, known as "Yoga for the Fitness Industry," was developed in 1994 with the purpose of teaching proper yoga techniques to fitness instructors who work in health and fitness clubs. The goal of YogaFit is to improve the health, performance, and mental acuity of both athletes and others interested in increasing their level of fitness.

Periodicals/Magazines/Journals

- *Fit Yoga*, published by Goodman Media Group, Inc., 1982– . Bimonthly. ISSN: 1932-8842. www.fityoga.com.
  Covering all aspects of yoga, *Fit Yoga* seeks to make the practice of yoga accessible to everyone. The magazine publishes interviews with yoga instructors and gurus, provides tours of yoga studios, evaluates yoga products, and supports those seeking to maximize their yoga and meditation practices.
- *Integral Yoga Magazine*, published by Integral Yoga Magazine, 1969– . Quarterly. ISSN: 0161-1380. iymagazine.org.
  The official journal of the teachings of H. H. Sri Swami Satchidananda (Sri Gurudev), *Integral Yoga Magazine* provides a forum for the practice and understanding of Integral Yoga. Drawing on many faith and wisdom traditions, the magazine strives to develop a common sense of community among those who explore the philosophy and practice of yoga.
- *International Journal of Yoga*, published by Medknow Publications, 2007– . Semi-annual. ISSN: 0973-6131. www.ijoy.org.in.
  As a multidisciplinary quarterly scientific journal whose most recent issues are available online, the *International Journal of Yoga* is dedicated to publishing research on yoga and its applications to spirituality, life sciences, physical sciences, health professions, education, and management. Published in India, the journal is the official journal of the Swami Vivekananda Yoga Anusandhana Samsthana.
- *International Journal of Yoga Therapy*, published by International Association of Yoga Therapists, 1990– . Annual. ISSN: 1531-2054. www.iayt.org.
  Published as an annual peer-reviewed journal, *IJYT* serves yoga practitioners, teachers, therapists, researchers, and other health professionals by providing scholarly and research-based reports on all aspects of yoga therapy. Each issue also contains editorials on issues related to the research and practice of yoga therapy, case studies, the practice of yoga therapy, continuing education articles, interviews, and reviews of books and DVDs.
- *International Yoga Guide*, published by Yoga Research Foundation, 1962– . Monthly. ISSN: 0277-092X. www.yrf.org.

This monthly magazine includes articles on yoga exercises, extracts from Hindu scripture with explication of its meaning, and news of activities of the International Yoga Society.

➤ *Iyengar Yoga Centre Newsletter*, published by the Iyengar Yoga Centre Society, 1984– . Bimonthly. ISSN: 1719-430X. www.iyengaryogacentre.ca/newsletter.html.
The *Iyengar Yoga Centre Newsletter* focuses on the practice and philosophy of Iyengar yoga. In addition, it examines the ancient teachings of yoga while providing a medium for the exchange of ideas and experiences in the practice of yoga.

➤ *JOY: The Journal of Yoga*, published by JOY, the Journal of Yoga, 2002– . Semi-annual. ISSN: 1541-5910. www.journalofyoga.org.
As an international and transdisciplinary journal, *JOY* publishes articles on Asian philosophy, consciousness studies, and yogic spirituality. Of special note is its examination of the philosophy of yoga, the neuroscience of yoga, the history of yoga disciplines, ayurveda, and meditation.

➤ *Self-Knowledge: A Quarterly Journal Devoted to Spiritual Thought and Practice*, published by Shanti Sadan Centre of Adhyatma Yoga and Advaita Vedanta, 1948– . Quarterly. ISSN: 0037-1556. www.self-knowledge.org.
This journal covers all aspects of the philosophy and practice of yoga while also publishing articles on spiritual development, art, science, history, and culture.

➤ *Yoga and Health*, published by Yoga Today Ltd., 1975– . Monthly. ISSN: 0953-2161. www.yogaandhealthmag.co.uk.
With some of its content available online, this is a major European yoga magazine. In addition to yoga and physical fitness, it contains articles on health issues, complementary therapies, mind, spirit, and nutrition.

➤ *Yoga Journal*, published by Yoga Journal, 1975– . Nine times a year. ISSN: 0191-0965. www.yogajournal.com.
Aimed at all those with an interest in yoga whether at the beginning or expert level, *Yoga Journal* covers all aspects of the practice of yoga as well as exploring topics on health, psychology, meditation, and spirituality.

➤ *Yoga Magazine*, published by Yoga Magazine, 2003– . Monthly. ISSN: 1478-9671. www.yogamagazine.co.uk.
Published in the United Kingdom, *Yoga Magazine* contains informative articles on a wide variety of yoga topics including yoga positions, yoga philosophy and spirituality, food and nutrition, and travel.

➤ *Yoga + Joyful Living*, published by Himalayan International Institute, 1991– . Bimonthly. ISSN: 1935-2158. www.himalayaninstitute.org/yogaplus.
Integrating both the practice of yoga and the science of ayurveda, this magazine delves into all aspects of conscious living. It also includes articles on topics such as the environment, social issues, and leadership. Each issue includes information on meditation, spiritual practice, and companies and individuals who are helping usher positive change into the world.

➤ *Yoga Therapy Today*, published by International Association of Yoga Therapists, 2005– . Three times a year. ISSN: 1945-7235. www.iayt.org.

This journal publishes articles of interest to yoga professionals and yoga therapists, primarily on the professional and practical aspects of yoga therapy. It also includes personal accounts related to the practice of yoga and yoga therapy, interviews with leaders in the field of yoga therapy, summaries of yoga research, cases studies, reviews of DVDs and books, and excerpts from recently published books on yoga therapy.

Appendix

Talking with Your Physician about Complementary and Alternative Medicine

It is very important to keep your primary care physician as well as any medical specialists you may see informed about your use of any complementary and alternative therapies. Similarly, it is important to let your complementary and alternative medicine (CAM) practitioner know about any physical ailments that you may have, any medications that you are currently taking, any surgeries you have had, and any therapies that you are undergoing. Here are some suggestions for talking to your physician about CAM:

1. Giving your physician the total picture of your approach to health care and the therapies you are using helps you stay in control of your own health while also making your physician a partner in maintaining your health.
2. Tell your physician about all of the therapies you are using, including such therapies as acupuncture, massage, chiropractic, essential oils, and special diets. Always be honest on any patient history forms that you complete. Never hide the use of any therapy, even if you think your physician will be upset with you for venturing into the world of CAM.
3. It is extremely important to let your physician know about any supplements that you may be taking, especially herbs, vitamins, and minerals. Such supplements may interact with prescription medicines. Some supplements can heighten the effects of medicines while others can cancel their benefits. Sometimes the interaction between supplements and medicines can be toxic and life threatening.
4. Your physician can often help you decide on the proper CAM therapies to use as an adjunct to traditional medicines and therapies. Physicians may be able to help you determine the safety and effectiveness of a therapy you wish to use as well as potential interactions with any current therapy, such as medications or physical therapy, you may be undergoing.
5. Your physician may also be able to help you with establishing an appropriate dosing level for herbs, vitamins, and minerals. Some supplements can have negative effects if they are taken in too high a dose and may be ineffective if taken at too low a dose.
6. Let your physician know of any recommendations made by your CAM practitioner, especially if the recommendations conflict with any made by your physician.
7. Sometimes your physician may be unfamiliar with a therapy you are using, so this is an opportunity for you to help educate him or her on other therapies and their effectiveness.

8. Some physicians are very knowledgeable about alternative therapies, so ask for their opinions. You may be surprised when one suggests using acupuncture, chiropractic, or energy healing techniques.
9. Explain why you wish to use CAM, either in place of or as an adjunct to traditional medical therapies. For example, let your doctor know that you wish to try alternative therapies so that you can avoid surgery to treat a problem or if you wish to avoid the side effects of a medicine being prescribed to treat an illness.
10. If your physician refuses to listen to you about your desire to incorporate CAM into your health care regime, consider changing physicians. Many physicians are very open to working with CAM providers to enhance the health of their patients.

Author/Title Index

Titles of books, journals, and periodicals are in italics; websites are in roman. Punctuation is ignored, and symbols and numbers treated as if spelled out, in the word-by-word alphabetization of titles.

A

B

C

D

E

F

K

L

N

O

P

T

U

V

W

About the Author

Gregory A. Crawford is director of the Penn State Harrisburg Library. He received his AB in Latin from Davidson College, his MS in library science from the University of North Carolina at Chapel Hill, and his PhD in communication, information, and library studies at Rutgers, the State University of New Jersey. In addition, he is a Reiki master/teacher, a graduate of the Surya Program for Transgradient Touch and Transgradient Counseling, and holds the Doctor of Naturopathy degree from the Trinity College of Natural Health. Thus, this book combines his interest in alternative health with his work as a librarian.